Infection Control in the Dental Office in the Era of COVID-19

Louis G. DePaola • Robert Windsor
Nisha Ganesh
Editors

Infection Control in the Dental Office in the Era of COVID-19

Springer

Editors
Louis G. DePaola
University of Maryland, Baltimore
Baltimore, MD, USA

Robert Windsor
University of Maryland, Baltimore
Baltimore, MD, USA

Nisha Ganesh
General Dentistry
Univ. of MD School of Dentistry
Baltimore, MD, USA

ISBN 978-3-031-64610-2 ISBN 978-3-031-64611-9 (eBook)
https://doi.org/10.1007/978-3-031-64611-9

This Springer imprint is published by the registered company Springer Nature Switzerland AG
The registered company address is: Gewerbestrasse 11, 6330 Cham, Switzerland

Contents

Overview of Infection Control Since the Emergence of COVID-19 and Other Emerging/Re-emerging Diseases

1

Fotini Anagnostopoulos and Monica Schneider

1.1 Impact of COVID-19 and Other Emerging Diseases on Infection Control Measures in Dentistry

Severe acute respiratory syndrome coronavirus 2 (SARS-CoV-2) is highly infectious and has been constantly detected in saliva [1]. Research has shown that virus transmission occurs through coughing, sneezing, talking, and direct contact with an infected individual; furthermore, SARS-CoV-2 can survive in aerosols and contaminate surfaces for a long time [2]. The aerosols created during dental treatment when using high-speed handpieces, ultrasonic scalers, and air and water syringes can be a source of transmission; therefore dental offices had to modify infection control procedures to prevent the transmission of infections and make dental offices safe [3]. These adjustments involve getting the patient's medical history before the dental appointment and incorporating a COVID-19 screening questionnaire that includes possible symptoms and the travel history of the patient. Only necessary items are opened in the dental operatory to minimize exposure to the patients; also patient appointments should be scheduled for longer periods to reduce the number of patients in the waiting rooms and allow for proper disinfection of the operatory [3].

In the dental office, the use of high-speed handpieces and water and air syringes produces aerosol and splatter that contains saliva and blood from the patient [4]. The dentist and dental assistant's head, arms, and facemask can become contaminated as the aerosol can reach an area of 8 feet from the patient's oral cavity. Therefore, the use of proper PPE is essential, comprising of gloves, masks, eyewear,

F. Anagnostopoulos
Department of Comprehensive Dentistry, The University of Maryland School of Dentistry, Baltimore, MD, USA
e-mail: FKing@umaryland.edu

M. Schneider (✉)
The University of Maryland School of Dentistry, Baltimore, MD, USA
e-mail: MSchneider@umaryland.edu

L. DePaola et al. (eds.), *Infection Control in the Dental Office in the Era of COVID-19*, https://doi.org/10.1007/978-3-031-64611-9_1

protective high-collared gowns, and hair covers [3]. Mask fit is key to avoid bacterial infiltration, and face shields in addition to the masks are recommended to protect forehead and eyes. Before putting and after removing personal protective equipment (PPE), it is essential to perform proper hand hygiene, and since aerosols settle and contaminate surfaces, shoe covers should be used [3].

Additional recommendations in the operatories include only opening and exposing essential instruments to be used and thoroughly disinfecting the dental chair after every patient and proper care of dental unit water lines. According to Centers for Disease Control and Prevention (CDC) recommendations, critical patient care items (penetrate soft tissue or bone) should be always heat-sterilized, and semi-critical patient care items (in contact with mucous membranes) should be heat-sterilized; however, they can also be processed using a high-level disinfectant. Noncritical patient care items can be cleaned or low-level disinfected [5]. Chlorine disinfectants used for nonmetal surfaces are effective against coronavirus; however, their use can be costly because chlorinated solutions must be prepared daily since they are not stable. High-efficiency particulate air (HEPA) filters and ultraviolet (UV) chambers are recommended in the ventilation system to reduce aerosol contamination [3].

1.2 Ethical Principles of Infection Control

The COVID-19 pandemic underscored vital lessons in ethics for individual, community, and global health decision-making. Crucial ethical choices include making the right decisions regarding masks, vaccines, and fair resource allocation. Past outbreaks of infectious diseases offer valuable insights for guiding policies and implementing ethical principles in future health crises.

More specifically, the 2003 SARS outbreak in Toronto revealed the intricate ethical considerations and the delicate balancing act required when addressing public health emergencies [6]. Decision-makers had to carefully weigh individual freedoms against the greater good of public safety and reconcile personal fears for safety with the duty to provide care. Additionally, they grappled with economic losses in light of the imperative to contain a highly contagious and deadly disease. An ethical framework was developed, which revolved around ten key ethical values and addressed five major ethical issues:

- *Balancing Individual Liberty*: The need to safeguard individual freedom had to be carefully considered against the necessity of protecting the public from harm caused by the uncontrolled movements of potentially infectious individuals.
- *Transparency:* Stakeholders needed to be fully informed about the risks and benefits that could impact their health, well-being, and personal liberty.
- *Reciprocity:* Society had a duty to ensure that those in quarantine did not suffer unfair economic penalties.
- *Privacy vs. Public Health:* While individuals have a right to privacy, the state could override this right if it significantly aided in protecting public health.

- *Avoiding Stigmatization*: Ethical considerations emphasized the importance of avoiding the linking of ethnicity with illness to prevent unwarranted stigma in communities.

In addition to these ethical values and issues, several other significant challenges emerged during the outbreak:

- *Healthcare Workers' Dilemma:* Balancing duty of care with the need to protect oneself, an intensely personal decision with vital implications for managing the pandemic.
- *Access to Care:* Individuals with serious illnesses such as cancer and heart disease were denied medical and dental care. Anxious patients also suffered from the loss of contact and emotional support from their families.
- *Fair Decision-Making:* Weighing the risks, benefits, and opportunity costs was essential, especially in preserving equity between the interests of SARS patients and those in need of urgent treatment for other diseases. *Procedural fairness* was crucial in decision-making.
- *Global Solidarity*: Reinforcing cooperation, transparency, honesty, and effective communication became imperative, given the interdependence of nations and the shared responsibility in managing public health crises.

Practicing ethics, what is right, fair, and good, goes beyond laws, encompassing principles safeguarding individual integrity, the profession, and our social contract with the public. The American Dental Association (ADA) has established comprehensive guidelines to uphold ethical standards in dentistry, including five key principles [7]. Additional recommendations were set during the pandemic to navigate these uncertain times while maintaining the Standard of Care [8]:

Autonomy The principle of self-determination and self-governance based on the ethical theory of deontology.

- Our primary duty is to enable patients to participate in treatment decisions, considering their needs, desires, and skills, while protecting their privacy (protection of person) and confidentiality (protection of data).
- Patients should also be accurately educated about the risks of viral infections, including the potential need to share identifiable information for contact tracing and public health purposes (public health exception to HIPAA) in order to contain the viral spread and obtaining informed consent by discussing treatment risks, benefits, and alternatives [7–9].
- Available alternate treatments, e.g., root canal therapy vs. extraction, may present conflicts between patient preferences and performing a high-risk treatment.

Nonmaleficence Cardinal principle to "first and foremost do no harm" certainly remains consistent while adhering to government declarations and guidelines [8, 9].

- Dentists must inform patients if they or any staff members have COVID-19.
- Screening of patients for symptoms, travel history, and fever is essential.
- Quality of care should not be compromised, despite increased sterilization measure costs. Strict protocols should be followed, including waste management and proper donning/doffing steps. Social distancing and staggered appointments with substantial time lag and minimum number of accompanying attendants while avoiding handshakes help limit office occupancy and transmission of virus.
- Use new recommended equipment such as high-volume evacuators, high-efficiency (particularly) air filters and ultraviolet sterilization units.
- Adherence to universal precautions, sanitization, and sterilization guidelines is mandatory. Office protocols should be regularly reviewed with patients, following current guidance from sources like the CDC, ADA, and United States Occupational Safety and Health Administration (OSHA).
- Patients must receive adequate notice if the dental office needs to close due to COVID-19.
- Collaboration with other dentists in the community is encouraged; when unsure about what to do or feel unqualified, we are ethically obligated to seek consultation or refer to specialists or other professionals who may have more updated skills, expertise, or equipment [9].
- Keeping knowledge and skills current and designating appropriate tasks to auxiliary members while protecting their well-being are essential [9].
- Deferring treatment for the larger good of the community to ensure no wastage of PPE when precious resources are already in short supply may be acceptable, but indefinitely postponing care raises nonmaleficence concerns [10].
- Prescribing antibiotics against stewardship policies [10].

Beneficence
Do and promote good—based on the ethical theory of utilitarianism.

- Dentists should prioritize promoting good by providing *timely and competent care* when serving the patient and the public at large.
- In cases of *limited resources* like personal protective equipment (PPE), allocation should prioritize emergencies or be shared with facilities facing shortages.
- Dental workplaces should foster respect and collaboration in the *workplace environment.* Employees should not feel undue pressure or judgment if they believe they are unable to perform their duties [8].

Justice
Dentists must uphold principles of fairness.

- Avoid any discrimination based on race, color, creed, national origin, sexual orientation, gender identity, age, or disability [8, 9].
- Justice is violated with dental practice suspensions, impacting fairness regardless of age or disease status. Infection control costs hinder economically disadvantaged populations, breaching equality, equity, and justice principles [10].

Veracity
Accurate, consistent, and truthful individual as well as community-centered communication is essential, particularly during public health emergencies like COVID-19 [11].

- Any advertisement to the public, such as posting on social media negative COVID test results without explaining the scientific significance/test limitations would contain misleading information and suggest daily testing, thereby compromising veracity [9].
- Dentists should not waive co-payments, overbill, or provide unnecessary services [7].

While principles may overlap, they form the basis of professional ethical conduct. For examples in the case of charging an additional fee for PPE, costs should be uniform *(justice)*, accurately represented *(veracity)*, and explained to patients, with a notice that the patient will sign to acknowledge that they have read and understand the fee and its purpose respecting their *autonomy* [9].

1.2.1 Challenges

It is perhaps not hyperbole to describe pandemic-related circumstances as creating *a perfect storm* in oral health care in the United States. Risk factors are elevated, access for the most vulnerable is limited, safety concerns are heightened, and the economy presents substantial challenges for patients and providers alike [12, 13].

The nature of dental work raises concerns about COVID-19 transmission, challenging ethical guidelines. Initially, dentists had to treat emergency cases (pain/bleeding/infection), despite infection risks. This was necessary due to limited scientific evidence [14]. The SARS-CoV-2 virus, found in patients' nasopharyngeal and salivary secretions, spreads primarily through respiratory droplets, aerosols, and fomites. The risk for dental practitioners and staff is exacerbated by asymptomatic transmission as well as close physical proximity between practitioners and patients [12]. Adhering to guidelines presented challenges as well: uncomfortable PPE; extended hours to treat urgent needs as well as catch up with patients not seen at the beginning of the pandemic; pressure to shorten procedures; compromised adherence to infection control, diagnosis, and treatment quality; and violating *beneficence and nonmaleficence principles*.

Neglected minor preventable issues escalated into costly treatments. Practitioner fatigue and burnout was observed across the globe. Additionally, the pandemic severely impacted dental staff, academic personnel, students, and researchers' training, reducing care quality [15].

Preventive dental care plays a crucial role in shaping oral health disparities [12, 16]. The substantial unemployment rate among oral health professionals during the pandemic exacerbated restrictions on oral healthcare access, overlooking the integral role of oral health in overall well-being [12]. The implementation of heightened safety and infection control measures raised expenses, leading to rationing and denial of care. This further complicated access for marginalized communities grappling with elevated infection rates following the *inverse care law*: people who mostly need care are least likely to receive it [17].

1.2.2 Solutions

Amid the urgent need for solutions, ethical considerations seemed to take a backseat to developing and delivering solutions. Robotic systems were swiftly deployed for tasks like disinfection and elderly care, reducing human contact. The Montreal Declaration outlines 10 AI ethical principles, including *well-being, autonomy, data protection, solidarity, equity, caution, responsibility, and sustainability* [18]. *Prioritizing the common good, safety, responsible technology use, legal questions regarding liability, and vandalism prevention* is emphasized in roboethics [18]. Tele-dentistry, tele-triage, and telemonitoring played vital roles in minimizing virus risks [15].

Dentists, leveraging their head and neck expertise, swiftly acquired skills for swabbing procedures and can aid in early disease detection by reporting unusual oral symptoms to public health authorities, extending their role beyond dentistry [19]. Surgical masks offered around 80% filtration for micrometer-sized particles, while respirators achieved 99% for particles up to 6 nanometers. Based on the principle of universal precautions, understanding that we may not know whether a patient has the potential for disease transmission or not, this heightened level of protection could be used [20]. In cases where dental offices cannot perform emergency procedures, hospital consultation is the advisable alternative.

Upholding high care standards and maintaining trust and honesty during the pandemic are crucial. Balancing personal risk and professional duty as well as using models like Ozar's when faced with ethical dilemmas is essential (overall health trumping over oral health, patient autonomy, and aesthetic concerns) [21].

1.3 Recent Outbreaks in the Dental Office

According to the Occupational Safety and Health Administration, dentists performing aerosol-generating procedures are classified as having a very high exposure risk. Very high exposure risk is defined as "those with high potential for exposure to known or suspected sources of COVID-19 during specific medical, postmortem, or laboratory procedures" [5]. Bitencourt et al. published a systematic review on the prevalence of SARS-CoV-2 among oral healthcare workers worldwide; they reported that between February 2020 and April 2021, 9.3% of oral healthcare workers were infected by SARS-CoV-2 virus [22]. However, it is challenging to establish if the infections are caused by an occupational risk or exposure in the community because household exposures are a significant factor for infection transmission [22]. It has been reported that the incidence of COVID-19 among Canadian dentists is low infection compared to the general population. In addition, results from studies in the United States and France performed in the early phases of the pandemic also show low prevalence compared to the general population [23].

Lately, the outbreak of monkeypox (Mpox) has been concerning with over 85,000 cases reported by January 2023 [24]. The CDC has reported the virus can be transmitted from one person to another by airborne contact, direct body fluids from an infected person, or during pregnancy from the mother to the fetus. Present research has shown that Mpox does not spread until the patient shows symptoms. Dentists play a key role in preventing the spread of the virus by recognizing the symptoms at the initial stages [24, 25]. In addition, measles could also be transmitted in the dental office; it infected approximately 870,000 people globally in 2019. The virus transmits by coughing and sneezing and by direct contact with secretions; it infects the respiratory tract and spreads affecting various tissues, for example, lymphoid tissues, gastrointestinal tract, and skin. The recent outbreaks of SARS-CoV-2, Mpox, and measles present common symptoms that include fever, fatigue, and severe headaches. These common symptoms can potentially result in misdiagnosis and lead to disease progression. Oral healthcare workers are essential in supporting prevention by first completing a detailed assessment of the patient's medical history and differing dental treatment if the patient is presenting signs and symptoms of infection, and the dentist should also refer the patient to the primary physician for diagnosis and treatment [26].

1.4 Summary and Conclusion

This chapter presented an overview of infection control in the context of COVID-19 and other emerging or re-emerging diseases in dental settings, emphasizing its importance in maintaining safe oral healthcare, especially due to the highly contagious nature of COVID-19. The impact of COVID-19 on infection control measures in dentistry, including the need for comprehensive infection control systems, proper use of personal protective equipment (PPE), ventilation systems, instrument sterilization, and surface disinfection procedures is discussed. Special attention is given to the generation of aerosols during dental procedures, which can contribute to disease transmission.

The ADA, CDC, and OSHA's guidelines emphasize ethical principles, patient autonomy, confidentiality, beneficence, justice, and truthfulness, ensuring that dental care is provided ethically and responsibly during the pandemic. Infection control is a fundamental aspect of ethical and evidence-based oral health care, ensuring safety for patients and providers while respecting cultural competence. Consistency across all communities is vital, with routine, meticulous daily, weekly, monthly, and annual maintenance checklists serving as ethical standards for care delivery. Dental practitioners and auxiliary personnel have an ethical duty to stay updated on infection control guidelines to minimize disease spread [11]. Patient awareness and appreciation of dentistry's infection control and its purpose were heightened during the pandemic; protocols made patient and employee screening common and training on infection control became valued.

The pandemic restricted oral health promotion and prevention programs and services. Following the *common risk approach* by integrating oral health into primary health care is essential due to shared risk factors with chronic systemic diseases [27]. Leveraging information technology to educate vulnerable groups, who struggle to access oral health services due to mobility constraints and social determinants, is a priority. Additionally, balancing personal risk and professional duty became paramount, requiring re-imagination and reconfiguration in dental practice.

References

1. Induri SNR, et al. Protective measures against COVID-19: dental practice and infection control. Healthcare (Basel). 2021;9(6):679.
2. van Doremalen N, et al. Aerosol and surface stability of SARS-CoV-2 as compared with SARS-CoV-1. N Engl J Med. 2020;382(16):1564–7.
3. Patel M. Infection control in dentistry during COVID—19 pandemic: what has changed? Heliyon. 2020;6(10):e05402.
4. Sabino-Silva R, Jardim ACG, Siqueira WL. Coronavirus COVID-19 impacts to dentistry and potential salivary diagnosis. Clin Oral Investig. 2020;24(4):1619–21.
5. Centers for Disease Control and Prevention (CDC); Infection prevention and control in dental settings—sterilization. 2019 [cited 2023 Oct 1].
6. Singer PA, et al. Ethics and SARS: lessons from Toronto. BMJ. 2003;327(7427):1342–4.
7. American Dental Association; The ADA principles of ethics and code of conduct. 2023 [cited 2023 Oct 2].
8. American Dental Association. Guidance on continuing to practice ethically during COVID-19. ADA [Internet]. 2020:1–4.
9. American Dental Association; Dental practice reopening. following the American Dental Association principles of ethics and code of professional conduct. J Am Dent Assoc. 2020;151(10):798–800.
10. Ramanarayanan V, Sanjeevan V, Janakiram C. The Covid-19 uncertainty and ethical dilemmas in dental practice. Indian J Med Ethics. 2021;Vi(2):1–3.
11. Scarlett MI, Grant LE. Ethical oral health care and infection control. J Dent Educ. 2015;79(5 suppl):S45–7.
12. Elster N, Parsi K. Oral health matters: the ethics of providing oral health during COVID-19. HEC Forum. 2021;33(1–2):157–64.
13. Weintraub JA. Oral health and COVID-19: increasing the need for prevention and access. Prev Chronic Dis. 2020;17:E93.
14. Kathree BA, et al. COVID-19 and its impact in the dental setting: a scoping review. PLoS One. 2020;15(12):e0244352.
15. Goriuc A, et al. The impact of the COVID-19 pandemic on dentistry and dental education: a narrative review. Int J Environ Res Public Health. 2022;19(5)

16. Ahluwalia R, Aggarwal R, Sharma K. Bioethical dilemmas in dentistry in the cOVID-19 Era. Global Bioethics Enquiry. 2020;8:66.
17. Watt G. The inverse care law revisited: a continuing blot on the record of the National Health Service. Br J Gen Pract. 2018;68:562–3.
18. Maddahi Y, et al. RoboEthics in COVID-19: a case study in dentistry. Front Robot AI. 2021;8:612740.
19. Seneviratne CJ, Lau MWJ, Goh BT. The role of dentists in COVID-19 Is beyond dentistry: voluntary medical engagements and future preparedness. Front Med (Lausanne). 2020;7:566.
20. Coulthard P. Dentistry and coronavirus (COVID-19)—moral decision-making. Br Dent J. 2020;228(7):503–5.
21. Ozar DT, Sokol DJ. Dental ethics at chairside: professional principles and practical applications. Washington, DC: Georgetown University Press; 2002.
22. Bitencourt FV, et al. Prevalence of SARS-CoV-2 infection among oral health care workers worldwide: a meta-analysis. Community Dent Oral Epidemiol. 2023;51(5):718–28.
23. Madathil S, et al. The incidence of COVID-19 among dentists practicing in the community in Canada: a prospective cohort study over a 6-month period. J Am Dent Assoc. 2022;153(5):450–459.e1.
24. Srivastava S, et al. The global monkeypox (Mpox) outbreak: a comprehensive review. Vaccines (Basel). 2023;11(6):1093.
25. Mahdi SS, et al. Monkeypox resurgence and its implications for dentistry—a scoping review. Ig Sanita Pubbl. 2023;80(2):49–59.
26. Hamdana AH, et al. Monkeypox virus and other emerging outbreaks: an overview and future perspective. Inquiry. 2023;60:469580231175437.
27. Kadriye P, et al. The impacts of the Covid-19 pandemic on dental public health and ethical issues. J Adv Res Health Sci. 2021;4(1):83–95.

Overview of Infectious Diseases of Concern to Dental Practitioners: Airborne Pathogens

2

Martina Majstorovic and Glenn Canares

2.1 Introduction

Infectious diseases that can be transmitted by the airborne route are particularly concerning to healthcare workers, inclusive of dental healthcare workers (DHCWs). Daily exposure to oral/nasal secretins generated during the performance of dental treatment puts DHCWs are high-risk for exposure to these infections, While many organisms do not survive in this aerosol; some microorganisms can withstand drying and evaporation and still remain infectious. These are known as droplet nuclei and are very small (<5 u) and very light. Consequently, these organisms can remain suspended in the air (airborne) for long periods of time, and the infectious particles can be widely dispersed by air currents. This is known as airborne transmission. Furthermore, medical and dental procedures can generate infectious aerosols which may be inhaled by a susceptible person. This airborne route of transmission allows organisms to efficiently enter the upper and lower respiratory tracts. The most transmissible diseases are spread by the airborne route. This chapter will review the most commonly circulating airborne pathogens of concern to DHCWs.

2.2 COVID-19

COVID-19 is a disease caused by severe acute respiratory syndrome coronavirus-2 (SARS-CoV-2). The disease first emerged in Wuhan, China, in December 2019 and by March 2020 and spread across the globe, causing the world pandemic [1, 2]. Within the first 2 years of the COVID-19 pandemic, more than 450 million cases

M. Majstorovic · G. Canares (✉)
Department of Pediatric Dentistry, The University of Maryland School of Dentistry, Baltimore, MD, USA
e-mail: mmajstorovic@umaryland.edu; GCanares1@umaryland.edu

L. DePaola et al. (eds.), *Infection Control in the Dental Office in the Era of COVID-19*, https://doi.org/10.1007/978-3-031-64611-9_2

were reported worldwide and over 100 million in EU/EEA alone [3]. SARS-CoV-2 is primarily spread via respiratory droplets/aerosols, and the most common mode of acquiring infection is from an infected person who sneezes, coughs, speaks, sings, or breathes in close proximity to other people [4–10]. Droplets can be inhaled or deposited in the nose, mouth, and eyes, so special measures of precaution have been implemented (including wearing masks) and were required as mandatory during the pandemic [11].

As to pathogenesis, clinical conditions can vary in severity. Individuals may present without symptoms (asymptomatic) but also with a wide range of mild or severe symptoms, which can be life-threatening. The most common/typical symptoms are fever, cough, general weakness, fatigue and muscle pain, and loss of smell and taste [12–16]. In certain cases, an individual can experience other, less common symptoms, such as sore throat, headache, general ache and pain, diarrhea, skin rash/discoloration of fingers and toes, and red/irritated eyes (conjunctivitis). More severe symptoms, leading to potential serious complications include difficulties with breathing, shortness of breath (dyspnea/apnea), loss of speech and confusion, and chest pain [17–25]. Due to virus mutations and a variety of symptoms, clinical picture may be rather diverse, however, most of the time mimics flu [16, 25, 26].

In the United States, variants of SARS-CoV-2 can be tracked in the following link: https://www.who.int/en/activities/tracking-SARS-CoV-2-variants/

Variants can be tracked globally in the following link: https://www.who.int/activities/tracking-SARS-CoV-2-variants

Recently reported cases include symptoms that mimic Kawasaki disease (KD) shock syndrome. Younger population/children with hyperinflammation disorder have been reported from several countries. Severe acute respiratory syndrome coronavirus-2 (SARS-CoV-2) was confirmed as the main cause of this severe acute respiratory syndrome known as *multisystem inflammatory syndrome (MIS-C)*. This is a new disease entity, and scientific evidence is still insufficient to distinguish it clearly from Kawasaki disease. MIS-C develops 4–6 weeks following SARS-CoV-2 infection with high titers of anti-SARS-CoV-2 antibodies, which confirms the diagnosis. It mainly represents with cardiovascular pathology, although overall, it implies a multisystem disorder. Current treatment guidelines recommend the use of intravenous immunoglobulin and high-dose corticosteroids as the first-line treatment. In general, mortality rates of MIS-C are lower compared to adult forms of severe COVID-19 disease [24, 27–29]. Research shows that due to evolution and fast adaptation of the SARS-CoV-2, some variants with mutations in the spike protein show an increased transmissibility [30–36].

Currently, vaccines are the only safe tools to prevent infection, although they do not provide long-term immunity. Booster doses are required to maintain the level of antibodies which may be considered protective. So far, all COVID-19 vaccines have rather high efficacy against the original strain and the variants of concern and are well tolerated. However, as to quality of protection, it greatly varies depending on the type of vaccine and additional booster doses. Questions remain regarding a booster dose and vaccine combinations/heterologous vaccination as well as waning immunity and the duration of immunity. Overall, the benefits of COVID-19 vaccination outweigh the risks, despite rare but potentially serious adverse effects [37]. Levels of antibodies after vaccines could last for at least 6 months but are expected to decrease over time [38–41]. Some observational studies report decreasing effectiveness (42–57%) at 4–6 months for mRNA vaccines [42–45].

Useful COVID-19 links

1. *Transmission of SARS-CoV-2 and implications for infection prevention precautions is available in the link:*
   (a) https://www.who.int/news-room/commentaries/detail/transmission-of-sars-cov-2-implications-for-infection-prevention-precautions
2. *Interim recommendations for the use of inactivated COVID-19 vaccine are available in the links:*
   (a) https://www.who.int/publications/i/item/WHO-2019-nCoV-vaccines-SAGE_recommendation-inactivated-2023.1
   (b) https://iris.who.int/bitstream/handle/10665/372713/WHO-2019-nCoV-vaccines-SAGE_recommendation-inactivated-2023.1-eng.pdf?sequence=1

2.3 Respiratory Syncytial Virus (RSV)

In general, due to mode of transmission of respiratory viruses and other respiratory pathogens, including the most recent RSV, but also influenza virus and SARS-CoV-2, an increasing number of hospitalization and disease-related complications emerged, thus creating pressure on healthcare systems. Respiratory syncytial virus (RSV) infection causes mild disease but can also present with severe clinical manifestations. Populations most prone to infection are individuals with comorbidities, children <5 years (particularly infants under 6 months), and adults ≥65 years.

Current data reveal an increased circulation of RSV infection. National data representing breakdown by EU/EEA countries are available in the following link: https://www.ecdc.europa.eu/sites/default/files/documents/RRA-20221128-473.pdf

RSV transmission occurs via respiratory tract or eyes but also by skin contact and contact with the surface contaminated with the virus (where RSV can survive for up to several hours). Incubation is usually 3–8 days. Infections progress from the upper to the lower respiratory system, resulting in mucus hypersecretion, which could lead to thick plug formation and fatal outcome. Due to the severity of the disease, infants with severe RSV should be hospitalized. Symptoms of infection are presented as bronchiolitis (inflammation of bronchioles) and pneumonia (inflammation of the alveolar spaces in the lungs) [46–48].

In children, pneumonia manifests with fever, nausea, wheezing, chills, and chest pain. In addition, symptoms indicating bronchiolitis include dyspnea and tachypnea, with overall general fatigue and malaise [49–51]. RSV is highly contagious, and due to its pathogenesis in children, it is considered one of the most likely single pathogens to cause death in infants <1 years [52]. RSV pathogenesis in adults and elderly population presents with symptoms like influenza virus, including typical mild fever, runny nose and nasal congestion, cough, dyspnea, and wheezing [53, 54].

Several vaccines have been in developing stages, particularly for infants, pregnant women, and older adults. However, neither licensed vaccines nor specific treatments (other than palliative/supportive) are available to prevent RSV infection [55]. Currently, passive immune prophylaxis with the RSV preventive antibodies (generic name nirsevimab/trade name Beyfortus) is recommended for high-risk infants. As opposed to traditional vaccines which represent immunization that stimulates the recipient's immune system to produce antibodies, nirsevimab is an immunization that provides antibodies directly to the recipient.

2.4 Measles

Measles virus (MV) is the prototype member of the genus *Morbillivirus*, the subfamily *Paramyxovirinae* and the family *Paramyxoviridae* [56]. MV is highly contagious and is transmitted via the respiratory tract. Systemic infection with clinical signs appears after 9–19 days, with typical prodromal symptoms including fever and malaise, associated with cough, coryza, and conjunctivitis (the three "C's"). Pathognomonic signs in this prodromal stage are the so-called Koplik's spots, which are most likely observed on the buccal mucosa. Patients further develop a maculopapular skin rash, which typically starts behind the ears and spreads around the face, trunk, and extremities [57, 58] (Figs. 2.1, 2.2 and 2.3).

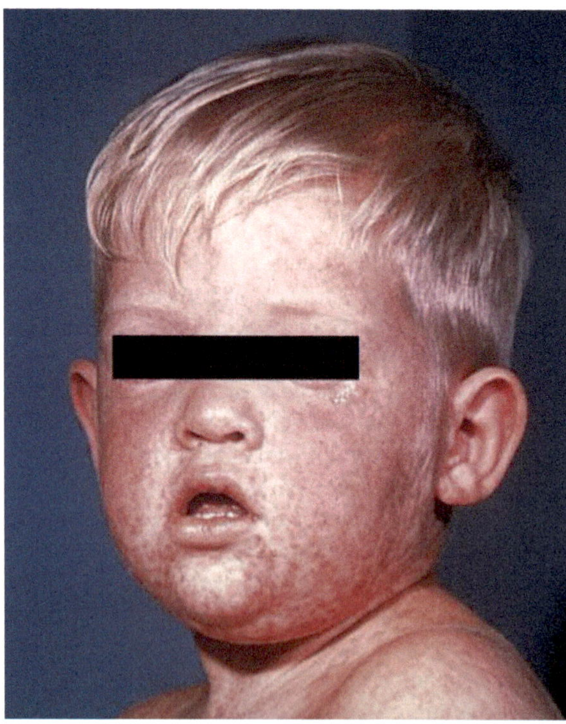

Fig. 2.1 Face of boy after 3 days with measles rash. (Courtesy of the CDC Image Library: https://www.cdc.gov/measles/symptoms/photos.html)

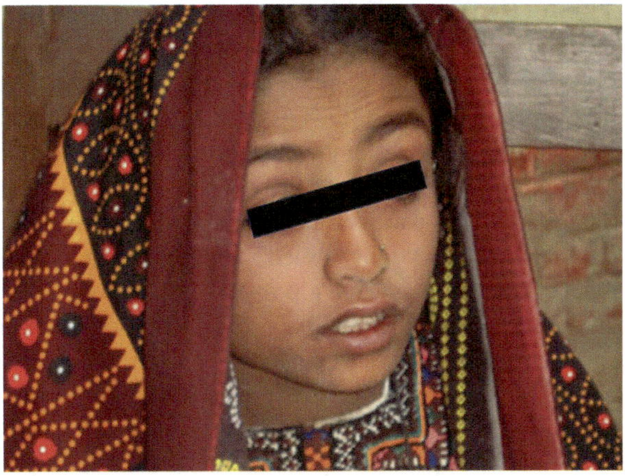

Fig. 2.2 The girl pictured presented with all the classical signs and symptoms of measles, including a blotchy rash, fever, cough, and runny nose. (Courtesy of the CDC Image Library: https://phil.cdc.gov/Details.aspx?pid=19728)

The girl pictured presented with all the classical signs and symptoms of measles, including a blotchy rash, fever, cough, and runny nose.

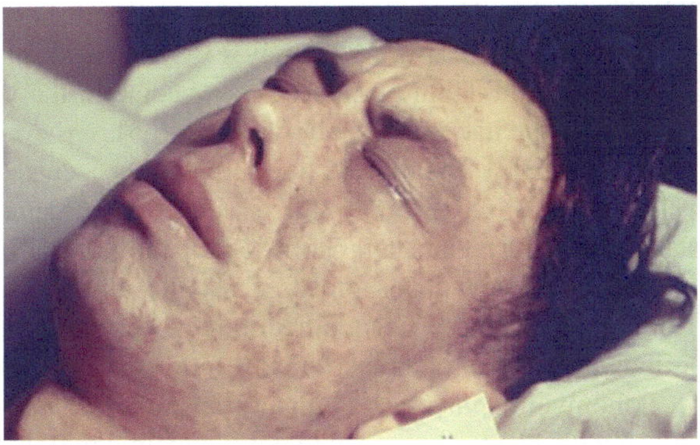

Fig. 2.3 This image depicted a close, left lateral view of a patient's face, revealing the onset of a macular rash due to measles. (Courtesy of the CDC Image Library: https://phil.cdc.gov/Details.aspx?pid=22149)

This image depicted a close, left lateral view of a patient's face, revealing the onset of a macular rash due to measles.

Measles infection is usually self-limiting. Symptoms resolve in 2–3 weeks due to the clearance of the virus by the immune system, following recovery and lifelong immunity. However, severe measles-associated central nervous system (CNS) complications may develop in the form of acute disseminated encephalomyelitis (ADEM), measles inclusion body encephalitis (MIBE), or subacute sclerosing panencephalitis (SSPE) [59]. A transient immune suppression may last over 2 years after infection leading to opportunistic infections and increased mortality risk [60].

2.5 Poliomyelitis

Poliomyelitis is a highly infectious disease which is caused by a virus belonging to the *Picornaviridae* family. It has been even mentioned in ancient Egyptian paintings and carvings. In the year 1840, polio was known as Heine-Medin disease due to the contributions of physicians Jakob Heine and Karl Oskar Medin [61]. In the United States, localized paralytic polio epidemics appeared in the 1900s. In 1916, the US public health authorities issued a directive regarding an epidemic of polio as more than 27,000 patients were reported, and fatality was more than 6000 in the country and over 2000 deaths in New York City alone [62]. Epidemic began to appear each summer. With the highest peak in 1940s to 1950s, leading to mandatory quarantine [62, 63]. The last reported case in the United Kingdom was in the year 1984, whereas between 1985 and 2002, 40 cases of paralytic polio were reported [64].

Clinical symptoms range from mild cases of respiratory illness, gastroenteritis, and malaise to severe forms of paralysis. Based on clinical features, it can be categorized as infection without symptoms (asymptomatic), mild illness (abortive poliomyelitis), aseptic meningitis (nonparalytic poliomyelitis), and paralytic poliomyelitis. In its severe form, the disease may cause crippling deformities and may be life-threatening. No cure has been implemented; however, it can be prevented by vaccination and is given routinely to children as inactivated poliovirus vaccine (IPV). Salk and Sabin introduced the vaccine in the year 1950 (oral polio vaccine (OPV) and the inactivated polio vaccine) [65].

In 2000–2001, an outbreak of poliomyelitis occurred in Dominican Republic and Haiti [66]. In 2013, only three countries remained polio-endemic—Nigeria, Pakistan, and Afghanistan. Global eradication of polio is imperative else the threat of an outbreak will hover forever. Currently, all the governments worldwide, in collaboration with the WHO, unified in the effort to maintain a polio-free population, as the threat for an outbreak remains forever [65].

Poliomyelitis undergoes human transmission but is also suspected in any individual with a history of travel to polio-endemic regions. Acute poliomyelitis is diagnosed in any individual older than 15 years of age with acute flaccid paralysis or specifically suspected by a physician. Laboratory tests include one of the following criteria: isolation of polio virus and intratypic differentiation (wild polio virus), vaccine-derived polio virus, and Sabin-like poliovirus (which is intratypic differentiation performed by a WHO-accredited polio laboratory) [67].

2.6 Monkeypox

Monkeypox (MPX) spreads through close contact with infectious material from skin lesions of an infected person, respiratory droplets, and through fomites. The overall risk is considered as moderate for persons having multiple sexual partners and low for the broader population.

Monkeypox cases as reported by countries within EU/EEA are available in the following link: https://www.ecdc.europa.eu/en/publications-data/data-mpox-monkeypox-cases-eueea

As to pathogenesis, it has been recommended to diagnose for orthopoxviruses and review available smallpox vaccines, antivirals, and personal protective equipment (PPE).

The likelihood of MPX spreading in persons having multiple sexual partners is considered high. Although most cases present with mild disease symptoms, monkeypox virus (MPXV) may cause severe disease in young children, pregnant women, and immunosuppressed individuals. However, the likelihood of cases with severe morbidity cannot be accurately estimated yet [68]. Symptoms usually develop 21 days from the last exposure to a case. Cases should remain isolated until their rash heals completely and by avoiding contact with immunosuppressed persons and abstaining from sexual activity and close physical contact. Most cases can remain at home with supportive/palliative care.

Clinical features typically include rash, but other symptoms include fever, chills, swollen lymph nodes, exhaustion, muscle aches, headache, and respiratory symptoms (Figs. 2.4 and 2.5).

Recent concerns regarding the possible emergence of monkeypox virus have been raised due to some reports of the clinical signs which resemble to monkey pox/smallpox [69, 70].

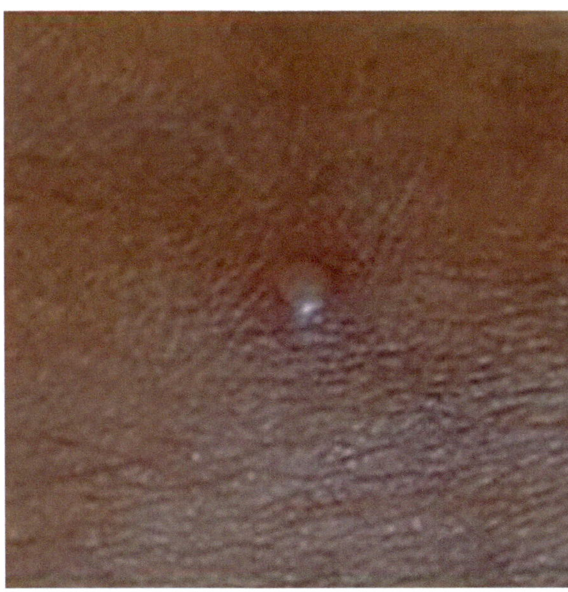

Fig. 2.4 Examples of Monkeypox rash. Source: Courtesy of CDC: https://www.cdc.gov/poxvirus/mpox/clinicians/clinical-recognition.html

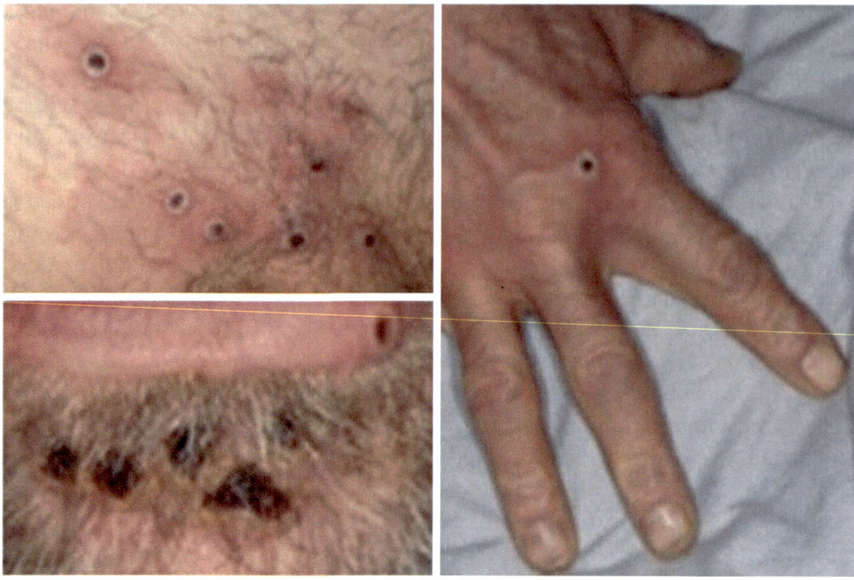

Fig. 2.5 Examples of Monkeypox rashes. Source: Courtesy of GOV.UK: https://www.gov.uk/government/news/ukhsa-latest-findings-into-monkeypox-outbreak

2.7 The WHO and the Immunization Agenda 2030

The World Human Organization entered a new decade by implementing a global immunization plan, to make vaccines available to every individual. Regional and state levels are expected to raise and support global awareness about vaccine-preventable diseases, which has been recently presented by the Immunization Agenda 2030.

Global efforts were made in incorporating new strategies and creating a safer environment worldwide. The Immunization Agenda 2030 plan focuses on access to high-quality and affordable primary healthcare with universal health coverage, which includes the initiative of preventing diseases through global immunization. To maintain high standards and accurate planning in providing immunization, global and regional indicators are selected by countries and tailored in the context of specific regional needs.

Details are available in the following link: https://www.who.int/teams/immunization-vaccines-and-biologicals/strategies/ia2030

2.8 Vaccine-Preventable Diseases

Certain diseases still represent a huge health concern worldwide, as activity and mutations of most viruses seem to be driven by climate and environmental factors. Research documented that environmental factor resulting from climate change may significantly impact the dynamics of infections, survival of the viruses outside the host, and dampening of immunity. In addition, environmental disasters, such as flooding, water contamination, and malnutrition but also, most importantly, the structure of the health systems account for activation/reactivation of some viral strains [71–74].

Potential association between environmental factors and emergence of certain diseases, as well as transmission of pathogens, have been related primarily to enteric diseases, vector-borne diseases (such as mosquito-borne diseases), and airborne diseases (influenza, COVID-19, and RSV). Most common enteric diseases include cholera [75, 76], enteritis caused by rotavirus [77–79], and enteric fever caused by *Salmonella enterica* [80, 81].

2.9 The United States

Most recent data for the US population estimate that flu infections, pneumococcal pneumonia, and chronic hepatitis B have raised in the last decade or so, resulting in the increased number of hospitalization due to serious complications possibly leading to deaths. In addition, a significant number of adults suffer from shingles, with severe consequences of experiencing rash and long-term pain/postherpetic neuralgia.

Therefore, a continuous effort toward preventing complications related to vaccine-preventable diseases was prioritized. Due to currently available vaccines, certain diseases are preventable, and as such, most of them are considered for routine immunization, based on CDC recommendations and in accordance with the recent updates of the vaccine-preventable immunization schedule.

2.10 EU/UK and Recent COVID-19 Pandemic

EU population is under surveillance for vaccine-preventable diseases (listed in *Decision 2000/96/EC*), based on the unique criteria for selecting the communicable diseases and related special health issues which are covered by epidemiological surveillance within the EU population network [82, 83]. Pursuant to Decision No 2119/98/EC of the European Parliament and of the Council on serious cross-border threats to health, Commission Decision 2000/96/EC established a list of communicable diseases and special health issues to be covered by epidemiological surveillance in the Community of EU network [83]. Therefore, European Centre for Disease Prevention and Control (ECDC) supervises and continues eradicating vaccine-preventable diseases through rather rigorous campaigns, promoting benefits, effectiveness, and safety of vaccines [84].

With the most recent COVID-19 pandemic and continuous and ubiquitous presence of influenza virus, new vaccines are being developed, and adjustments to the current vaccine protocols have been made accordingly. However, some vaccines are underutilized due to major challenges regarding opposition in the population against immunization.

Vaccine-preventable diseases under EU surveillance are cholera, congenital rubella syndrome (CRS), COVID-19, cryptosporidiosis, diphtheria, hepatitis B, human papillomavirus, invasive *Haemophilus influenzae* disease, invasive pneumococcal disease, Japanese encephalitis, measles, meningococcal disease, mumps, pertussis (whooping cough), poliomyelitis, rabies, rotavirus infection, rubella (German measles), seasonal influenza, smallpox, tetanus, thyroid and parathyroid fever, varicella (chickenpox), and yellow fever [85].

Case classification for each infectious disease is based on clinical, laboratory, and epidemiological criteria. Clinical criteria include common clinical symptoms which represent an indicative, clear picture of the disease. Laboratory criteria comprise of relevant laboratory tests used for diagnosing and confirming the case. Epidemiological criteria are confirmed pending establishment of epidemiological link, i.e., confirmed transmission, exposure, and/or exposure to the virus [83].

COVID-19 is currently under surveillance in EU, and each state/member of EU is required to report a confirmed case in any individual meeting at least one of the following criteria: SARS-CoV-2 nucleic acid detection, SARS-CoV-2 r antigen in a clinical specimen detection (excluding self-tests performed outside healthcare settings), and SARS-CoV-2 isolation in a clinical specimen.

Overview of the regional indicators as specified by the country (EU/EEA) are available in the link:

https://covid19-country-overviews.ecdc.europa.eu/key_epidemiological_indicators.html

References

1. Ochani R, Asad A, Yasmin F, Shaikh S, Khalid H, Batra S, Sohail MR, Mahmood SF, Ochani R, Hussham Arshad M, Kumar A, Surani S. COVID-19 pandemic: from origins to outcomes. A comprehensive review of viral pathogenesis, clinical manifestations, diagnostic evaluation, and management. Infez Med. 2021;29(1):20–36.
2. Chen H, Guo J, Wang C, Luo F, Yu X, Zhang W, Li J, Zhao D, Xu D, Gong Q. Clinical characteristics, and intrauterine vertical transmission potential of COVID-19 infection in nine pregnant women: a retrospective review of medical records. Lancet. 2020;395:809–15. https://doi.org/10.1016/s0140-6736(20)30360-3.
3. https://www.ecdc.europa.eu/en/covid-19/questions-answers/questions-answers-basic-facts
4. Wang J, Du G. COVID-19 may transmit through aerosol. Ir J Med Sci. 2020;189:1143. https://doi.org/10.1007/s11845-020-02218-2.
5. Morawska L, Cao J. Airborne transmission of SARS-CoV-2: the world should face the reality. Environ Int. 2020;139:105730. https://doi.org/10.1016/j.envint.2020.105730.
6. Hinds WC, Zhu Y. Aerosol technology: properties, behavior, and measurement of airborne particles. Hoboken: Wiley; 2022.
7. Judson SD, Munster VJ. Nosocomial transmission of emerging viruses via aerosol-generating medical procedures. Viruses. 2019;11:940. https://doi.org/10.3390/v11100940.
8. Li Q, Guan X, Wu P, Wang X, Zhou L, Tong Y, Ren R, Leung KS, Lau EH, Wong JY, Xing X. Early transmission dynamics in Wuhan, China, of novel coronavirus–infected pneumonia. N Engl J Med. 2020;382:1199. https://doi.org/10.1056/NEJMoa2001316.
9. Burke RM, et al. Active monitoring of persons exposed to patients with confirmed COVID-19—United States, January–February 2020. MMWR Morb Mortal Wkly Rep. 2020;69:245.

10. World Health Organization (WHO) 2020. Modes of transmission of virus causing COVID-19: implications for IPC precaution recommendations: Scientific Brief, 27 Mar 2020. https://apps.who.int/iris/handle/10665/331601
11. Jayaweera M, Perera H, Gunawardana B, Manatunge J. Transmission of COVID-19 virus by droplets and aerosols: a critical review on the unresolved dichotomy. Environ Res. 2020;188:109819. https://doi.org/10.1016/j.envres.2020.109819.
12. Huang C, Wang Y, Li X, Ren L, Zhao J, Hu Y, Zhang L, Fan G, Xu J, Gu X. Clinical features of patients infected with 2019 novel coronavirus in Wuhan, China. Lancet. 2020;395:497–506. https://doi.org/10.1016/s0140-6736(20)30183-5.
13. Sharma A, Ahmad Farouk I, Lal SK. COVID-19: a review on the novel coronavirus disease evolution, transmission, detection, control and prevention. Viruses. 2021;13(2):202. https://doi.org/10.3390/v13020202.
14. Chams N, Chams S, Badran R, Shams A, Araji A, Raad M, Mukhopadhyay S, Stroberg E, Duval EJ, Barton LM, Hajj Hussein I. COVID-19: a multidisciplinary review. Front Public Health. 2020;8:383. https://doi.org/10.3389/fpubh.2020.00383.
15. Rahman S, Montero MTV, Rowe K, Kirton R, Kunik F Jr. Epidemiology, pathogenesis, clinical presentations, diagnosis and treatment of COVID-19: a review of current evidence. Expert Rev Clin Pharmacol. 2021;14(5):601–21. https://doi.org/10.1080/17512433.2021.1902303.
16. Cui X, Zhao Z, Zhang T, Guo W, Guo W, Zheng J, Zhang J, Dong C, Na R, Zheng L, Li W, Liu Z, Ma J, Wang J, He S, Xu Y, Si P, Shen Y, Cai C. A systematic review and meta-analysis of children with coronavirus disease 2019 (COVID-19). J Med Virol. 2021;93(2):1057–69. https://doi.org/10.1002/jmv.26398.
17. Vardavas CI, Mathioudakis AG, Nikitara K, Stamatelopoulos K, Georgiopoulos G, Phalkey R, Leonardi-Bee J, Fernandez E, Carnicer-Pont D, Vestbo J, Semenza JC, Deogan C, Suk JE, Kramarz P, Lamb F, Penttinen P. Prognostic factors for mortality, intensive care unit and hospital admission due to SARS-CoV-2: a systematic review and meta-analysis of cohort studies in Europe. Eur Respir Rev. 2022;31(166):220098. https://doi.org/10.1183/16000617.0098-2022.
18. Webb GJ, Marjot T, Cook JA, Aloman C, Armstrong MJ, Brenner EJ, Catana MA, Cargill T, Dhanasekaran R, García-Juárez I, Hagström H, Kennedy JM, Marshall A, Masson S, Mercer CJ, Perumalswami PV, Ruiz I, Thaker S, Ufere NN, Barnes E, Barritt AS 4th, Moon AM. Outcomes following SARS-CoV-2 infection in liver transplant recipients: an international registry study. Lancet Gastroenterol Hepatol. 2020;5(11):1008–16. https://doi.org/10.1016/S2468-1253(20)30271-5.
19. Vai B, Mazza MG, Delli Colli C, Foiselle M, Allen B, Benedetti F, Borsini A, Casanova Dias M, Tamouza R, Leboyer M, Benros ME, Branchi I, Fusar-Poli P, De Picker LJ. Mental disorders and risk of COVID-19-related mortality, hospitalisation, and intensive care unit admission: a systematic review and meta-analysis. Lancet Psychiatry. 2021;8(9):797–812. https://doi.org/10.1016/S2215-0366(21)00232-7.
20. Zuccon W, Comassi P, Adriani L, Bergamaschini G, Bertin E, Borromeo R, Corti S, De Petri F, Dolci F, Galmozzi A, Gigliotti A, Gualdoni L, Guerra C, Khosthiova A, Leati G, Lupi G, Moscato P, Perotti V, Piantelli M, Ruini A, Sportelli S, Susca M, Troiano C, Benelli G, Buscarini E, Canetta C, Merli G, Scartabellati A, Melilli BSCG, Sfogliarini R, Pellegatta G, Viganò G. Intensive care for seriously ill patients affected by novel coronavirus sars—CoV—2: experience of the Crema Hospital, Italy. Am J Emerg Med. 2021;45:156–61. https://doi.org/10.1016/j.ajem.2020.08.005.
21. Raman B, Bluemke DA, Lüscher TF, Neubauer S. Long COVID: post-acute sequelae of COVID-19 with a cardiovascular focus. Eur Heart J. 2022;43(11):1157–72. https://doi.org/10.1093/eurheartj/ehac031.
22. Akbarialiabad H, Taghrir MH, Abdollahi A, Ghahramani N, Kumar M, Paydar S, Razani B, Mwangi J, Asadi-Pooya AA, Malekmakan L, Bastani B. Long COVID, a comprehensive systematic scoping review. Infection. 2021;49(6):1163–86. https://doi.org/10.1007/s15010-021-01666-x.

23. Bisaccia G, Ricci F, Recce V, Serio A, Iannetti G, Chahal AA, Ståhlberg M, Khanji MY, Fedorowski A, Gallina S. Post-acute sequelae of COVID-19 and cardiovascular autonomic dysfunction: what do we know? J Cardiovasc Dev Dis. 2021;8(11):156. https://doi.org/10.3390/jcdd8110156.
24. Furqan M, Chawla S, Majid M, Mazumdar S, Mahalwar G, Harmon E, Klein A. COVID-19 vaccine-related myocardial and pericardial inflammation. Curr Cardiol Rep. 2022;24(12):2031–41. https://doi.org/10.1007/s11886-022-01801-6.
25. Mohamadian M, Chiti H, Shoghli A, Biglari S, Parsamanesh N, Esmaeilzadeh A. COVID-19: virology, biology and novel laboratory diagnosis. J Gene Med. 2021;23(2):e3303. https://doi.org/10.1002/jgm.3303.
26. Majumder J, Minko T. Recent developments on therapeutic and diagnostic approaches for COVID-19. AAPS J. 2021;23(1):14. https://doi.org/10.1208/s12248-020-00532-2.
27. Cattalini M, Della Paolera S, Zunica F, Bracaglia C, Giangreco M, Verdoni L, Meini A, Sottile R, Caorsi R, Zuccotti G, Fabi M, Montin D, Meneghel A, Consolaro A, Dellepiane RM, Maggio MC, La Torre F, Marchesi A, Simonini G, Villani A, Cimaz R, Ravelli A, Taddio A, Rheumatology Study Group of the Italian Pediatric Society. Defining Kawasaki disease and pediatric inflammatory multisystem syndrome-temporally associated to SARS-CoV-2 infection during SARS-CoV-2 epidemic in Italy: results from a national, multicenter survey. Pediatr Rheumatol Online J. 2021;19(1):29.
28. Whittaker E, Bamford A, Kenny J, Kaforou M, Jones CE, Shah P, Ramnarayan P, Fraisse A, Miller O, Davies P, Kucera F, Brierley J, McDougall M, Carter M, Tremoulet A, Shimizu C, Herberg J, Burns JC, Lyall H, Levin M, PIMS-TS Study Group and EUCLIDS and PERFORM Consortia. Clinical characteristics of 58 children with a pediatric inflammatory multisystem syndrome temporally associated with SARS-CoV-2. JAMA. 2020;324(3):259–69. https://doi.org/10.1001/jama.2020.10369.
29. Kabeerdoss J, Pilania RK, Karkhele R, Kumar TS, Danda D, Singh S. Severe COVID-19, multisystem inflammatory syndrome in children, and Kawasaki disease: immunological mechanisms, clinical manifestations and management. Rheumatol Int. 2021;41(1):19–32. https://doi.org/10.1007/s00296-020-04749-4.
30. Van Dorp L, Richard D, Tan CCS, Shaw LP, Acman M, Balloux F. No evidence for increased transmissibility from recurrent mutations in SARS-CoV-2. Nat Commun. 2020;11:5986.
31. Volz E, Mishra S, Chand M, Barrett JC, Johnson R, Geidelberg L, et al. Transmission of SARS-CoV-2 lineage B.1.1.7 in England: insights from linking epidemiological and genetic data. medRxiv. 2020; https://doi.org/10.1101/2020.12.30.20249034
32. Tegally H, Wilkinson E, Giovanetti M, Iranzadeh A, Fonseca V, Giandhari J, et al. Emergence and rapid spread of a new severe acute respiratory syndrome-related coronavirus 2 (SARS-CoV-2) lineage with multiple spike mutations in South Africa. medRxiv. 2020; https://doi.org/10.1101/2020.12.21.20248640
33. Davies NG, Abbott S, Barnard RC, Jarvis CI, Kucharski AJ, Munday JD, et al. Estimated transmissibility and impact of SARS-CoV-2 lineage B.1.1.7 in England. Science. 2021;372:372.
34. Public Health England. SARS-CoV-2 variants of concern and variants under investigation; 2021. p. 68.
35. Campbell F, Archer B, Laurenson-Schafer H, Jinnai Y, Konings F, Batra N, et al. Increased transmissibility and global spread of SARS-CoV-2 variants of concern as at June 2021. Eur Secur. 2021;26:2100509.
36. The Scientific Pandemic Influenza Group on Modelling, Operational sub-group (SPI-M-O) for the Scientific Advisory Group for Emergencies (SAGE). SPI-M-O: Consensus statement on COVID-19, 30 Jun 2021 (Internet) GOV.UK; 2021.
37. Agafonova E, Reshetnikova I, Rizvanova F. Mucosal immunity after novel COVID-19 infection—virus-induced immunosuppression: preliminary study. BioNanoScience. 2022;12(4):1473–81. https://doi.org/10.1007/s12668-022-01020-x.
38. Barouch DH, Stephenson KE, Sadoff J, Yu J, Chang A, Gebre M, et al. Durable humoral and cellular immune responses following Ad26.COV2.S vaccination for COVID-19. medRxiv. 2021. https://doi.org/10.1101/2021.07.05.21259918.

39. Doria-Rose N, Suthar MS, Makowski M, O'Connell S, McDermott AB, Flach B, et al. Antibody persistence through 6 months after the second dose of mRNA-1273 vaccine for Covid-19. N Engl J Med. 2021;384:2259–61.
40. Naaber P, Tserel L, Kangro K, Sepp E, Jürjenson V, Adamson A, et al. Dynamics of antibody response to BNT162b2 vaccine after six months: a longitudinal prospective study. Lancet Reg Health Eur. 2021;10:100208. https://doi.org/10.1016/j.lanepe.2021.100208.
41. Pegu A, O'Connell S, Schmidt SD, O'Dell S, Talana CA, Lai L, et al. Durability of mRNA-1273 vaccine–induced antibodies against SARS-CoV-2 variants. Science. 2021;373:1372–7.
42. Andrews N, Tessier E, Stowe J, Gower C, Kirsebom F, Simmons R, et al. Vaccine effectiveness and duration of protection of Comirnaty, Vaxzevria and Spikevax against mild and severe COVID-19 in the UK. medRxiv. 2021; https://doi.org/10.1101/2021.09.15.21263583
43. Puranik A, Lenehan PJ, Silvert E, Niesen MJM, Corchado-Garcia J, O'Horo JC, et al. Comparison of two highly-effective mRNA vaccines for COVID-19 during periods of Alpha and Delta variant prevalence. medRxiv. 2021. https://doi.org/10.1101/2021.08.06.21261707.
44. Goldberg Y, Mandel M, Bar-On YM, Bodenheimer O, Freedman L, Haas EJ, et al. Waning immunity of the BNT162b2 vaccine: a nationwide study from Israel. medRxiv. 2021. https://doi.org/10.1101/2021.8.24.21262423.
45. Tartof SY, Slezak JM, Fischer H, Hong V, Ackerson BK, Ranasinghe ON, et al. Effectiveness of mRNA BNT162b2 COVID-19 vaccine up to 6 months in a large integrated health system in the USA: a retrospective cohort study. Lancet. 2021;398:1407–16.
46. Welliver TP, Garofalo RP, Hosakote Y, Hintz KH, Avendano L, Sanchez K, et al. Severe human lower respiratory tract illness caused by respiratory syncytial virus and influenza virus is characterized by the absence of pulmonary cytotoxic lymphocyte responses. J Infect Dis. 2007;195:1126–36. https://doi.org/10.1086/512615.
47. Aherne W, Bird T, Court SD, Gardner PS, McQuillin J. Pathological changes in virus infections of the lower respiratory tract in children. J Clin Pathol. 1970;23:7–18. https://doi.org/10.1136/jcp.23.1.7.
48. Persson BD, Jaffe AB, Fearns R, Danahay H. Respiratory syncytial virus can infect basal cells and alter human airway epithelial differentiation. PLoS One. 2014;9:e102368. https://doi.org/10.1371/journal.pone.0102368.
49. Scott JA, Wonodi C, Moïsi JC, Deloria-Knoll M, DeLuca AN, Karron RA, et al. The definition of pneumonia, the assessment of severity, and clinical standardization in the Pneumonia Etiology Research for Child Health study. Clin Infect Dis. 2012;54(Suppl. 2):S109–16. https://doi.org/10.1093/cid/cir1065.
50. Nascimento-Carvalho AC, Ruuskanen O, Nascimento-Carvalho CM. Comparison of the frequency of bacterial and viral infections among children with community-acquired pneumonia hospitalized across distinct severity categories: a prospective cross-sectional study. BMC Pediatr. 2016;16:105. https://doi.org/10.1186/s12887-016-0645-3.
51. Pickles RJ, DeVincenzo JP. Respiratory syncytial virus (RSV) and its propensity for causing bronchiolitis. J Pathol. 2015;235:266–76. https://doi.org/10.1002/path.4462.
52. Lozano R, Naghavi M, Foreman K, Lim S, Shibuya K, Aboyans V, et al. Global and regional mortality from 235 causes of death for 20 age groups in 1990 and 2010: a systematic analysis for the global burden of disease study 2010. Lancet. 2012;380:2095–128. https://doi.org/10.1016/S0140-6736(12)61728-0.
53. Mochizuki H, Todokoro M, Arakawa H. RS virus-induced inflammation and the intracellular glutathione redox state in cultured human airway epithelial cells. Inflammation. 2009;32:252–64. https://doi.org/10.1007/s10753-009-9128-0.
54. Bonville CA, Rosenberg HF, Domachowske JB. Macrophage inflammatory protein-1alpha and RANTES are present in nasal secretions during ongoing upper respiratory tract infection. Pediatr Allergy Immunol. 1999;10:39–44. https://doi.org/10.1034/j.1399-3038.1999.101005.
55. Mazur NI, Higgins D, Nunes MC, Melero JA, Langedijk AC, Horsley N, Buchholz UJ, Openshaw PJ, McLellan JS, Englund JA, Mejias A, Karron RA, Simões EA, Knezevic I, Ramilo O, Piedra PA, Chu HY, Falsey AR, Nair H, Kragten-Tabatabaie L, Greenough A,

Baraldi E, Papadopoulos NG, Vekemans J, Polack FP, Powell M, Satav A, Walsh EE, Stein RT, Graham BS, Bont LJ, Respiratory Syncytial Virus Network (ReSViNET) Foundation. The respiratory syncytial virus vaccine landscape: lessons from the graveyard and promising candidates. Lancet Infect Dis. 2018;18(10):e295–311. https://doi.org/10.1016/S1473-3099(18)30292-5.
56. De Vries RD, Duprex WP, de Swart RL. Morbillivirus infections: an introduction. Viruses. 2015;7:699–706. https://doi.org/10.3390/v7020699.
57. Yanagi Y, Takeda M, Ohno S. Measles virus: cellular receptors, tropism and pathogenesis. J Gen Virol. 2006;87:2767–79. https://doi.org/10.1099/vir.0.82221-0.
58. Griffin DE. Fields virology. 6th ed. Philadelphia: Lippincott Williams & Wilkins; 2013.
59. Mina MJ, Metcalf CJ, de Swart RL, Osterhaus AD, Grenfell BT. Long-term measles-induced immunomodulation increases overall childhood infectious disease mortality. Science. 2015;348:694–9. https://doi.org/10.1126/science.aaa3662.
60. Schneider-Schaulies S, Schneider-Schaulies J. Curr Top Microbiol Immunol. 2009;330:243–69.
61. Bodian D, Horstmann DM. Polioviruses. In: Horsfall FL, Tamm I, editors. Viral and rickettsial infections of man. 4th ed. Philadelphia: JB Lippincott & Co; 1965. p. 430–73.
62. Melnick JL. Current status of poliovirus infections. Clin Microbiol Rev. 1996;9(3):293–300.
63. Trevelyan B, Smallman-Raynor M, Cliff A. The spatial dynamics of poliomyelitis in the United States: from epidemic emergence to vaccine-induced retreat, 1910–1971. Ann Assoc Am Geogr. 2005;95(2):269–93.
64. Polio: the green book, Chapter 26; 18 Jan 2013. https://www.gov.uk/government/publications/polio-the-green-book-chapter-26. Accessed 24 Oct 2023.
65. Mehndiratta MM, Mehndiratta P, Pande R. Poliomyelitis: historical facts, epidemiology, and current challenges in eradication. Neurohospitalist. 2014;4(4):223–9. https://doi.org/10.1177/1941874414533352.
66. He Y, Mueller S, Chipman PR, et al. Complexes of poliovirus serotypes with their common cellular receptor, CD155. J Virol. 2003;77(8):4827–35.
67. Commission Implementing Decision (EU) 2018/945. https://eur-lex.europa.eu/legal-content/EN/TXT/PDF/?uri=CELEX:32018D0945. Accessed 15 Nov 2023.
68. Damon IK. Status of human monkeypox: clinical disease, epidemiology and research. Vaccine. 2011;30(29 Suppl 4):D54–9. https://doi.org/10.1016/j.vaccine.2011.04.014.
69. Petersen E, Kantele A, Koopmans M, Asogun D, Yinka-Ogunleye A, Ihekweazu C, Zumla A. Human monkeypox: epidemiologic and clinical characteristics, diagnosis, and prevention. Infect Dis Clin N Am. 2019;33(4):1027–43. https://doi.org/10.1016/j.idc.2019.03.001.
70. Bunge EM, Hoet B, Chen L, Lienert F, Weidenthaler H, Baer LR, Steffen R. The changing epidemiology of human monkeypox—a potential threat? A systematic review. PLoS Negl Trop Dis. 2022;16(2):e0010141. https://doi.org/10.1371/journal.pntd.0010141.
71. Metcalf CJE, Walter KS, Wesolowski A, Buckee CO, Shevliakova E, Tatem AJ, et al. Identifying climate drivers of infectious disease dynamics: recent advances and challenges ahead. Proc Biol Sci. 2017;284:20170901.
72. Patz JA, Epstein PR, Burke TA, Balbus JM. Global climate change and emerging infectious diseases. JAMA. 1996;275:217–23.
73. Reiner RC, King AA, Emch M, Yunus M, Faruque A, Pascual M. Highly localized sensitivity to climate forcing drives endemic cholera in a megacity. Proc Natl Acad Sci USA. 2012;109:2033–6.
74. Foxman EF, Storer JA, Vanaja K, Levchenko A, Iwasaki A. Two interferon-independent double-stranded RNA-induced host defense strategies suppress the common cold virus at warm temperature. Proc Natl Acad Sci USA. 2016;113:8496–501.
75. Cash BA, Rodó X, Kinter JL. Links between tropical Pacific SST and cholera incidence in Bangladesh: role of the eastern and central tropical Pacific. J Clim. 2008:4647–63. https://doi.org/10.1175/2007JCLI2001.1.

76. Cash BA, Rodó X, Kinter JL, Yunus M. Disentangling the impact of ENSO and Indian Ocean variability on the regional climate of Bangladesh: implications for cholera risk. J Clim. 2010;23:2817–31.
77. Tate JE, Burton AH, Boschi-Pinto C, Parashar UD. Global, regional, and national estimates of rotavirus mortality in children <5 years of age, 2000–2013. Clin Infect Dis. 2016;62:S96–S105.
78. Martinez PP, King AA, Yunus M, Faruque ASG, Pascual M. Differential and enhanced response to climate forcing in diarrheal disease due to rotavirus across a megacity of the developing world. Proc Natl Acad Sci. 2016;113:4092–7.
79. Levy K, Hubbard AE, Eisenberg JNS. Seasonality of rotavirus disease in the tropics: a systematic review and meta-analysis. Int J Epidemiol. 2009;38:1487–96.
80. Thindwa D, Chipeta MG, Henrion MYR, Gordon MA. Distinct climate influences on the risk of typhoid compared to invasive non-typhoid Salmonella disease in Blantyre, Malawi. Sci Rep. 2019;9:20310.
81. Karkey A, Arjyal A, Anders KL, Boni MF, Dongol S, Koirala S, et al. The burden and characteristics of enteric fever at a healthcare facility in a densely populated area of Kathmandu. PLoS One. 2010;5:e13988.
82. International Committee on Taxonomy of Viruses (ICTV). Virus taxonomy: the classification and nomenclature of viruses. The 9th report of the ICTV. 2011. Available at: https://ictv.global/report_9th
83. European Centre for Disease Prevention and Control. EU case definitions. https://www.ecdc.europa.eu/en/all-topics/eu-case-definitions. Accessed 15 Nov 2023.
84. European Vaccination Information Portal. https://vaccination-info.europa.eu/en. Accessed 15 Nov 2023.
85. European Centre for Disease Prevention and Control. Vaccine-preventable diseases. https://www.ecdc.europa.eu/en/immunisation-vaccines/facts/vaccine-preventable-diseases. Accessed 15 Nov 2023.

Overview of Infectious Diseases of Concern to Dental Practitioners: Blood-Borne and Related Pathogens

3

Joy Void-Holmes and Deborah Cartee

3.1 Hepatitis A (HAV)

3.1.1 Definition and History

The hepatitis A virus (HAV), a positive-stranded RNA virus that is part of the Hepatovirus species within the broader Picornaviridae family, has a longstanding and extensive historical relationship with humans, spanning several millennia [1]. The symptoms, which closely mirror contemporary manifestations of hepatitis A, were chronicled in ancient Chinese documents dating back approximately 5000 years [2]. The disease was first accurately defined in the seventeenth century, often within the context of military campaigns. The inaugural outbreak on American soil transpired in Norfolk, VA, in 1812, and the disease saw a significant increase during the Civil War, culminating in over 40,000 recorded cases [2, 3]. The frequent emergence of this disease during times of warfare fostered terms such as "kriegsikterus" or "jaunisse des camps" [4]. The extent of affliction was particularly overwhelming during World War II, with an estimated 16 million cases [2].

Formerly known as "infectious hepatitis," hepatitis A was initially differentiated from hepatitis B in the 1940s due to the latter's extended incubation period [3]. The development of serologic testing led to a definitive diagnosis of hepatitis B. By the 1970s, advancements in the identification of the virus and the establishment of additional serologic tests further distinguished hepatitis A from other non-B hepatitis variants [3].

J. Void-Holmes (✉)
Dr. Joy, RDH, Jell-Ed Education Consulting, Bowie, MD, USA
e-mail: info@drjoyrdh.com

D. Cartee
Department of Advanced Oral Sciences and Therapeutics, The University of Maryland School of Dentistry, Baltimore, MD, USA
e-mail: dcartee@umaryland.edu

L. DePaola et al. (eds.), *Infection Control in the Dental Office in the Era of COVID-19*, https://doi.org/10.1007/978-3-031-64611-9_3

3.1.2 Statistics in the USA and Worldwide

Since its discovery in 1966, HAV was rife in the USA, particularly in western states and among children aged 2–18 [3]. In 1996, vaccinations were recommended for high-risk groups, eventually extending to all children by 2006 and homeless individuals by 2019 [3]. This resulted in a 95.5% decrease in acute HAV cases from 1996 to 2011. However, recent outbreaks among drug users and the homeless led to a rise in adult cases [3]. In 2018, 12,474 acute HAV cases were reported, with an incidence rate of 3.8 per 100,000 population [3]. Despite improved vaccination coverage, especially among children and adolescents, it remains low among adults. Challenges persist as seen in outbreak-associated cases reported in multiple states between 2016 and 2021 [3]. In 2021, 5728 HAV cases were documented in the USA, although under-reporting suggests the actual figure is closer to 11,500 [5]. After yearly increases since 2015, the incidence began to decline in 2020, with a 43% reduction in cases between 2020 and 2021 [5]. Nonetheless, the number of cases in 2021 is still four times higher than in 2015 [5].

An analysis of Global Burden of Disease (GBD) 2019 data revealed that despite a stable age-standardized incidence rate (ASIR) of HAV from 1990 to 2019, the number of cases increased by 13.90% [6]. The highest ASIR in 2019 was in sub-Saharan Africa, with significant increases in low and low-middle socio-demographic index (SDI) regions. High-income regions like Asia Pacific, Oceania, and Australasia also saw an upward trend, despite good sanitation [6]. The increase in HAV cases globally is attributed to population growth, especially in low-income and middle-income countries, and immigration [6]. The disease is more prevalent in low-income regions due to poor sanitation, but incidence rates have decreased in most middle-income regions [6]. Despite improved sanitation and hygiene, high-income regions are seeing more HAV cases, particularly among adults [3, 6]. The availability of a HAV vaccine has reduced the disease incidence in many countries, but it still increased in some high and low endemic countries due to poor sanitary conditions and hygienic practices [3] (Fig. 3.1).

3.1.3 How Is HAV Transmitted

The HAV virus primarily spreads through the fecal-oral route, a mechanism that involves an uninfected person ingesting food or water contaminated with the feces of an infected individual [3, 7]. This mode of transmission is especially prevalent within family settings if an infected person, without practicing proper hand hygiene, prepares food [3, 7]. Additionally, the virus can be contracted through close physical contact, such as oral–anal sex, with an infected person [3, 7]. Casual contact, however, does not lead to the spread of the virus [3]. The fecal-oral route is the main pathway for HAV infection either through the consumption of contaminated food or water or direct contact with an infected person [3, 7]. During the prodromal phase of the disease, the virus can be found in the blood, and instances of transmission

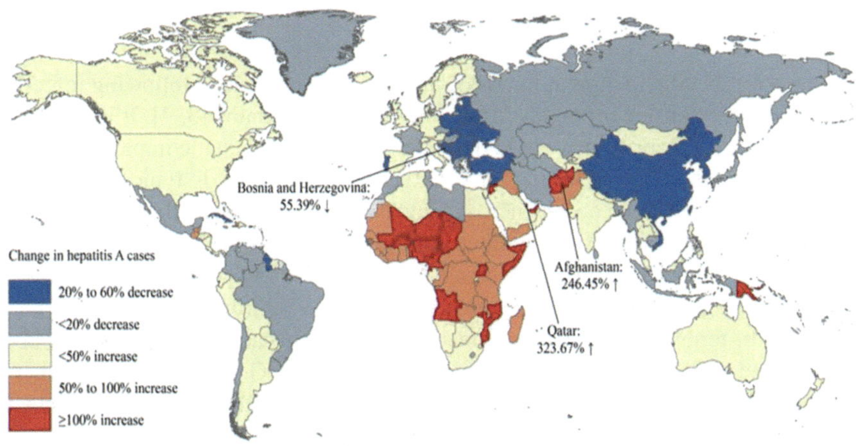

Fig. 3.1 Source: Cao et al. [6]

through blood transfusion or organ transplantation have been recorded, though these are rare [3]. Despite the detectable presence of HAV in saliva, there is no confirmed evidence of transmission through this medium [3]. Waterborne outbreaks are uncommon, particularly in the USA, but when they do occur, they are typically linked to inadequately treated water or water contaminated with sewage [3, 7].

3.1.4 Pathogenesis and Signs/Symptoms of HAV Infection

Typically, HAV incubates within a period of 14–28 days, presenting symptoms that can range from mild to severe [3, 5, 7]. These manifestations can include fever, malaise, anorexia, diarrhea, nausea, abdominal discomfort, dark urine, and jaundice, although it is important to note that not all infected persons will exhibit all these symptoms [3, 5, 7]. Adults are more likely to display significant signs and symptoms compared to children, and the severity of the disease and mortality rates tend to escalate with age [3, 5]. Notably, children under the age of 6 seldom show noticeable symptoms, with only 10% developing jaundice [3, 5]. In some instances, hepatitis A may relapse, leading to an additional acute episode following the initial recovery, which is typically followed by complete recuperation [3, 5].

The period of viral shedding lasts for 1–3 weeks, with individuals being most contagious 1–2 weeks before the onset of illness when the concentration of HAV in stool is highest [3, 5]. The risk of transmission then gradually diminishes and is minimal 1 week post-symptom onset. While symptoms usually last less than 2 months, between 10% and 15% of symptomatic persons may experience extended or recurring disease for up to 6 months [3, 5]. HAV can endure outside the body for several months, contingent on environmental conditions, with an average incubation period of 28 days (ranging from 15 to 50 days) [3, 5, 7].

3.1.5 Treatment of Hepatitis A

There is no specific treatment for HAV, and the recovery period following infection can be quite extensive, often lasting several weeks to months [3, 7]. It is crucial to circumvent medications that could potentially exacerbate hepatic impairment, such as acetaminophen and paracetamol [3]. Hospital admission is typically not warranted unless there is an occurrence of acute liver failure [7]. The focus of therapeutic strategies is primarily on patient comfort and ensuring adequate nutritional status, which may include replenishing fluids lost due to symptoms like vomiting and diarrhea [3]. Notably, HAV does not progress to a chronic or long-term infection [3]. In terms of potential re-infection with the hepatitis A virus, it has been established that the development of Immunoglobulin G antibodies early in the infection process confers enduring immunity against the disease, thereby preventing subsequent infections [3].

3.1.6 HAV Disease-Relevance to Dentistry

The significance of hepatitis A in dentistry is emphasized by recent research, which has illuminated the potential for HAV transmission within a dental environment [8]. This transmission was associated with inadequate hand hygiene protocols implemented by a dentist who, interestingly, contracted the infection despite having been administered a hepatitis A vaccine as post-exposure prophylaxis [8]. To our current understanding, this represents the first documented instance of such a scenario [3].

Research has shown that HAV can endure on surfaces and adapt to a wide range of biological and non-biological environments, thereby indicating that human hands and surfaces significantly contribute to the spread of HAV [9]. However, it is disconcerting to note that only a minority of oral healthcare providers (HCPs) consistently adhere to recommended hygiene practices [10]. Moreover, there is a scarcity of detailed data regarding the transmission of infection by HCPs contaminated due to poor hand hygiene practices. In a systematic review of outbreaks attributed to HCPs, nearly 43.2% of the reports categorized hand hygiene compliance as "insufficient" [11]. While the importance of proper hand hygiene cannot be overstated for HCPs, it may be especially advisable to reinforce adherence to pertinent infection control guidelines among those exposed to HAV [11]. Even though vaccination is not recommended across the board, HCPs working in high-risk areas might want to contemplate it as an extra preventive strategy [11].

3.2 Hepatitis B (HBV)

3.2.1 Description of the Hepatitis B Virus

Hepatitis B (HBV) is a member of the hepadnavirus family. HBV infects mainly the liver but can also infect the kidneys and pancreas in humans and chimpanzees. HBV is a small, enveloped DNA virus also known as a Dane particle. This is a particularly stable virus, making it very resistant to disinfection. This makes HBV able to live for a long time outside of the body, therefore making cross contamination and infection much more likely [12]. It can survive outside the body for at least 7 days and still be capable of causing infection [13].

The disease manifests in two forms: acute and chronic hepatitis B. Acute hepatitis B is a short-term condition that arises within 6 months of exposure to the virus, with symptoms varying from mild to severe [14]. In contrast, chronic hepatitis B is a long-term infection that may persist for a lifetime, leading to serious health complications such as liver damage, cirrhosis, liver cancer, and potentially death [14]. The probability of developing chronic hepatitis B is largely dependent on the age at which an individual contracts the virus. Infants are at the highest risk, with about 90% developing chronic infection [14]. This risk decreases with age, with nearly all children over 6 years and adults recovering completely without developing a chronic condition [14].

3.2.2 Statistics in the USA and Worldwide

Hepatitis B virus (HBV) is a significant global health concern. In the USA, it is estimated that up to 2.4 million people are chronically infected [15]. Rates of acute hepatitis B infection have notably risen by 50–450% in states affected by the opioid crisis [15]. The Centers for Disease Control and Prevention (CDC) reported 2157 acute hepatitis B cases in 2020, which equates to an incidence rate of 0.7 cases per 100,000 population [13]. However, the actual number of cases is likely much higher due to under-reporting, with estimates suggesting there were around 14,000 cases that year [13]. Despite a decade of stability, the rate of acute hepatitis B decreased by 32% after 2019, potentially due to fewer people seeking healthcare and testing during the COVID-19 pandemic [13]. Interestingly, rates among all racial/ethnic groups decreased from 2005 to 2012 but remained largely unchanged from 2013 to 2019, with rates ranging from 0.2 cases per 100,000 among Asian/Pacific Islander persons to 0.7 case per 100,000 among non-Hispanic White and non-Hispanic Black persons [13].

The prevalence of chronic HBV infection is also high, with an estimated 580,000 to 1.17 million people affected in the USA alone [13]. Two-thirds of these individuals may be unaware of their infection [13]. Chronic hepatitis B disproportionately impacts people born outside the USA; 69% of the U.S. population living with chronic HBV infection are non–U.S.-born, despite only accounting for 14% of the general population [13]. More than 50% of people living with chronic hepatitis B are of Asian, Pacific Islander, or African descent, making hepatitis B and the resulting liver cancer one of the largest health disparities for these groups [15]. The weighted average chronic hepatitis B prevalence for all foreign-born people in the USA in 2018 was about 3% [15]. Around 59% of those U.S. residents with chronic hepatitis B in the USA in 2018 emigrated from Asia, 19% from the Americas, and 15% from Africa [15].

Globally, the burden of hepatitis B infection is highest in the WHO Western Pacific Region and the WHO African Region, with 116 million and 81 million people chronically infected, respectively [16, 17]. In total, approximately 296 million people worldwide, including over 6 million children under the age of 5, are affected by hepatitis B [17]. HBV contributes to an estimated 820,000 deaths annually, and 25% of chronic hepatitis B infections progress to liver cancer [17]. Despite the high rates of infection, thousands of people die each year from hepatitis B-related causes, such as liver cancer. In 2020, there were 1752 reported hepatitis B-associated deaths in the USA, corresponding to an age-adjusted death rate of 0.45 cases per 100,000 population [13].

3.2.3 Pathogenesis and Signs/Symptoms of HBV Infection

HBV can be an acute, short-term illness in some that are infected, but for others, it can turn into a long term, chronic infection. Whether or not a person develops a chronic infection is dependent on the immune response. If hepatitis B surface antigen (HBsAg) and hepatitis B e antigen (HBeAg) components of the virion are detected in the person's blood, this indicates an ongoing infection. Specifically, HBeAg indicates that the virus is replicating, and the person infected has high levels of HBV [12]. Acute infection may or may not cause symptoms. Symptoms generally appear after an incubation period of 90 days and include fever, fatigue, loss of appetite, nausea and vomiting, abdominal pain, dark urine, joint pain, and jaundice. Symptoms can last up to 6 months [12]. It takes a long time after initial infection for liver damage to occur. Infected hepatocytes are destroyed through the body's cell mediated immune response. A weaker initial immune response will result in less symptoms, but also a lower chance of clearing the infection.

As infants and young children have a weaker immune response, they are generally less likely to clear the infection and therefore develop chronic infection more often as opposed to less than 5% of adults [12]. For this reason, immunosuppressed people are more likely to develop a chronic infection as well [18]. Coinfection of HBV infected individuals with HCV, HIV, and HDV is common. HCV is found in 10–15% of patients with HBV. These individuals are more likely to have acquired the virus through IV drug use and are more likely to develop liver cirrhosis when compared to those infected with either virus alone. HDV is a type of satellite virus that requires HBV to cause infection [19]. This occurs more commonly in the Mediterranean region as well as South America [20]. This can lead to a severe episode of acute hepatitis, even in a patient who previously had asymptomatic HBV [20]. Lastly, HIV is seen in 6–13% of patients infected with HBV in areas where both viruses are endemic, such as sub-Saharan Africa [21]. These patients are also more likely to experience liver disease, especially in those that are immunocompromised due to low CD4 T cell counts [18]. The World Health Organization estimates that 80% of all cases of Primary Hepatocellular Carcinoma are due to chronic HBV infection [16]. This type of cancer has a very high mortality rate and is one of the three most common causes of cancer death worldwide [16].

3.2.4 Treatment of Hepatitis B

Certain individuals are more at risk for contracting HBV or for being a carrier of the virus. Those that engage in high-risk IV drug behaviors are at risk through parenteral exposure. Others at risk and who should therefore be screened are those that are from countries with higher HBV prevalence, men who have intercourse with men or others that may be exposed through sexual contact, HIV/HCV infected individuals, infants born to HBV infected mothers, pregnant women, and blood/tissue donors [18].

As noted earlier, people who have acute or chronic HBV infection will have the presence of hepatitis B surface antigen (HBsAg) in their blood. The body makes this in order to fight the virus, and this is what is used to make the hepatitis B vaccine. Hepatitis B surface antibody (anti-HB's) will be present in the blood of someone who has immunity either from a previously cleared infection of from receiving the vaccination [18].

If a patient is found to be positive for HBsAg, they should be counseled on preventing the transmission of the virus to others. It is also recommended that they limit or abstain from drinking alcohol, as that could exacerbate liver damage [13]. Treatment HBV infection differs depending on whether the condition is acute or chronic. Acute HBV infection does not have a specific treatment, and care primarily revolves around ensuring the patient's comfort [16]. This includes maintaining a healthy diet and adequate hydration to counteract potential dehydration caused by vomiting and diarrhea [16]. Chronic HBV infection, on the other hand, can be managed with oral medications such as tenofovir or entecavir [16]. These treatments can slow the progression of cirrhosis, decrease incidences of liver cancer, and improve long-term survival [16]. However, it is important to note that most individuals who begin treatment for hepatitis B will likely need to continue it for life [16]. It is possible for those that have been on antiviral therapy to develop drug resistance. In this case, it is possible to test for genotype resistance and alter the drug therapy as necessary [22].

Estimations suggest that 12–25% of people with chronic HBV infection will require treatment, based on setting and eligibility criteria [16]. The ongoing 2023 update of the World Health Organization's Hepatitis B treatment guidelines aims to broaden treatment eligibility, thereby increasing the proportion of individuals receiving treatment [16]. Outcomes can vary greatly depending on the socio-economic setting. In low-income environments, most people with liver cancer are diagnosed late in the disease progression and often die within months [16]. Conversely, in high-income countries, earlier detection and access to surgery and chemotherapy can extend life expectancy by several months to a few years [16]. Liver transplantation is an option for patients with cirrhosis or liver cancer in technologically advanced countries, although success rates vary [16]. Pregnant patients testing positive for HBsAg with HBV-DNA levels exceeding 200,000 IU/ML should receive antiviral therapy as per the American Association for the Study of Liver Diseases (AASLD) to reduce the risk of perinatal HBV transmission [13]. For comprehensive guidelines on treating chronic hepatitis B, refer to the AASLD's practice guidelines [13]. Regular monitoring and care are crucial for preventing liver damage and potential hepatocellular carcinoma in patients with chronic HBV infection

[13]. A vaccine is available for providing immunity to HBV infection. It is recommended for all infants and children under 19 years of age, those at risk from sexual exposure, those at risk of parenteral exposure including health care workers, those who are traveling to high-risk countries, and those that are infected with HIV or HCV [22]. The vaccine should be given as three intramuscular injections, with the second and third being at 1 and 6 months from the first dose [22]. Even if an individual has already been exposed to HBV, the vaccine can prevent infection. Certain individuals should receive post-vaccination testing to confirm their immunity and include infants born to HBV positive mothers, health care workers, hemodialysis patients, immunocompromised patients, and sex partners of known infected persons. There are three single-antigen hepatitis B vaccines available in the USA which include Engerix-B, Recombivax HB, and Heplisav-B. Two combination vaccines available are Pediarix and Twinrix [13, 22].

3.2.5 HBV-Relevance to Dentistry

It is critical that healthcare workers who are at high risk of percutaneous exposure to HBV get vaccinated. This includes those in dental practice. Healthcare works should also receive post vaccination testing to ensure that presence of anti-HBs, therefore confirming their immunity.

If a healthcare worker is positive for HBV, they are still able to practice, however should always maintain standard precautions to prevent transmission of the virus. They should not perform exposure-prone procedures, however, if their HBV-DNA serum levels exceed 1000 IU/mL. It should be reduced through treatment and maintained below this level [23]. A careful medical history is critical in determining a patient's safety during dental procedures. All standard precautions should be followed to prevent infection of healthcare workers as well as cross contamination to other patients through infected surfaces or instruments. As liver disease is the most common outcome of chronic HBV infection, dental practitioners should be aware of common oral manifestations of liver dysfunction such as jaundice, bleeding, fetor hepaticus (distinctive breath odor), cheilitis, atrophic tongue, xerostomia, and bruxism [24]. Liver function should also be evaluated as certain clotting factors may be affected by liver dysfunction. This could cause excessive bleeding during dental procedures. Metabolism of certain medications may also be affected by liver disease. The prevention of the spread of HBV is of utmost importance to the dental profession, both for the safety of the practitioners and the patients.

3.3 Hepatitis C (HCV)

3.3.1 Description of Hepatitis C Virus

Hepatitis C (HCV) is a blood-borne virus of the family Flaviviridae that often results in chronic liver infection. HCV is a small, enveloped RNA virus that targets human hepatocytes that was first discovered in 1989 [25]. For some people, the infection is acute, and they are able to clear it on their own but in 70–85% of cases, it becomes a chronic infection.

Acute Hepatitis C is a new infection that occurs within the first 6 months after someone is exposed to the hepatitis C virus, often not showing any symptoms. Hepatitis C can be a short-term illness, but for most people, acute infection leads to chronic infection.

Chronic Hepatitis C can be a "silent" lifelong and life threatening infection. Left untreated, chronic hepatitis C can cause serious health problems, including liver damage, cirrhosis (scarring of the liver), liver cancer, and even death.

Most people who become infected are not aware because they do not show any signs of illness. Chronic infection can lead to more serious complications such as liver cirrhosis, hepatocellular carcinoma, and even death.

3.3.2 HCV Statistics in the USA and Worldwide

There were 107,300 cases of newly reported chronic HVC infections during 2020. There were 40.7 newly reported cases of chronic hepatitis C per 100,000 people. The incidence rate of acute HCV has more than doubled since 2013, and increased 15% from 2019 [26] (Figs. 3.2 and 3.3).

Globally, an estimated 58 million people have chronic HCV infection, with about 1.5 million new infections occurring per year. There are an estimated 3.2 million adolescents and children with chronic HCV infection. WHO estimated that in 2019, approximately 290,000 people died from hepatitis C, mostly from cirrhosis and hepatocellular carcinoma (primary liver cancer). Direct-acting antiviral medicines (DAAs) can cure more than 95% of persons with hepatitis C infection, but access to diagnosis and treatment is low [27] (Figs. 3.2, 3.3, and 3.4).

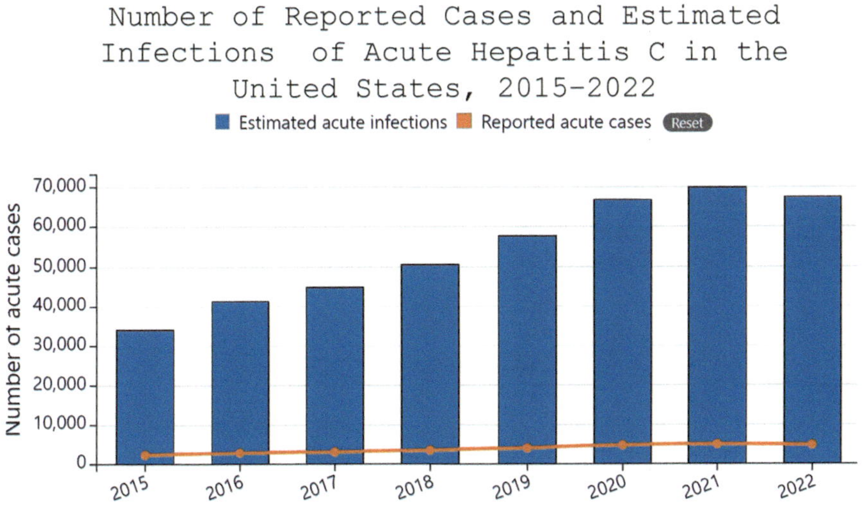

Fig. 3.2 Source: 2014–2021 Reported Hepatitis C Cases & Estimated Infections - US Centers for Disease Control and Prevention

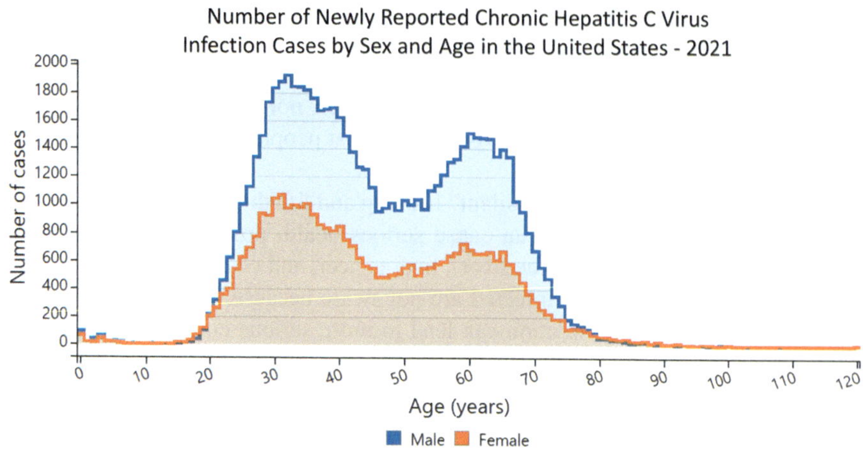

Fig. 3.3 Source: 2021 Newly Reported Chronic Hepatitis C by Sex & Age - US Centers for Disease Control and Prevention

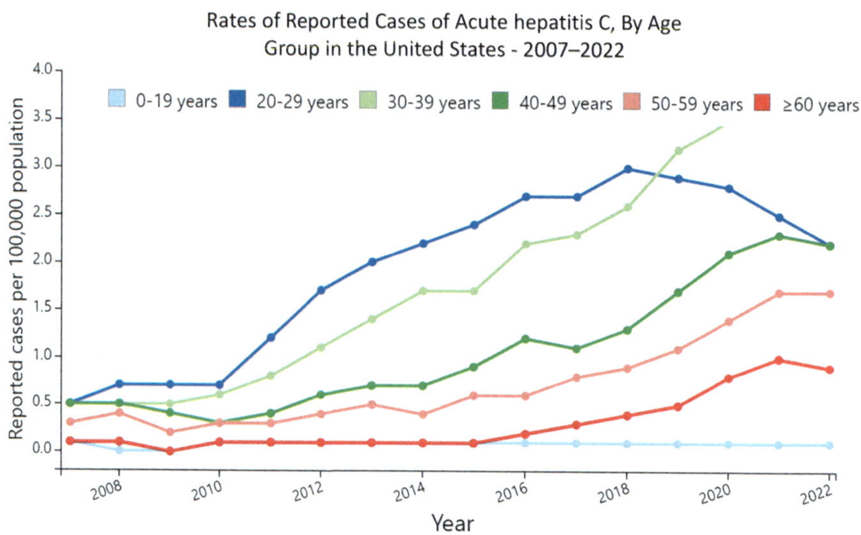

Fig. 3.4 Source: Rates* of reported cases† of acute hepatitis C, by age group — United States, 2007–2022; 2022, US Centers for Disease Control and Prevention

3.3.3 How Is HCV Transmitted?

HCV only infects humans and chimpanzees. It can be transmitted in blood, semen, and vaginal secretions. This is most commonly seen in patients receiving blood transfusions or organs, needlesticks in the healthcare setting, sharing drug needles and through sexual intercourse. Almost all those infected with HIV (greater than 90%) who are or were intravenous drug users are also infected with HCV [12].

Better detection and screening have greatly reduced the incidence of HCV transmission among those receiving blood transfusions or organs, but due to the chronic, asymptomatic nature of the virus, transmission remains rampant through the other routes [12].

3.3.4 Pathogenesis and Signs/Symptoms of HCV Infection

HCV coats itself with low-density lipoprotein or very low-density lipoprotein which binds to the appropriate receptor on hepatocytes. The virus will then replicate and release proteins that inhibit cell death via apoptosis. This allows for persistent infection in liver cells and therefore chronic infection [12]. Utilizing direct-acting antiviral medicines (DAAs) can cure more than 95% of persons with hepatitis C infection but access to diagnosis and treatment is low [27].

Acute infection of HCV has symptoms similar to hepatitis A and hepatitis B infection but usually milder. The viremia lasts about 4–6 months. Infected individuals may experience fever, fatigue, nausea, loss of appetite, and abdominal pain. Jaundice will also be noted in 70–80% of adults [12]. More than 70% of infected individuals will be asymptomatic after initial infection but will go on to have persistent, chronic infection with the virus. It is unknown why these infections become chronic, but through study of the immune response, it can be noted that there is little CD4 or CD8 T cell response in these cases. The predominant symptom in these cases is chronic fatigue [28].

After 10–15 years of persistent infection, the disease will often progress to active hepatitis. After 20 years, 20% will progress to cirrhosis followed by liver failure. After 30 years of chronic infection, 5% of those infected will develop hepatocellular carcinoma. These outcomes are more likely to occur with alcohol use as well as certain medications [12].

3.3.5 Treatment of HCV

It is critical to prevent transmission of this pathogen by avoiding high-risk behavior such as IV drug use and unprotected sexual intercourse. HCV infection can be detected via a blood test and should be considered in those who are considered high risk. If an individual is found to have the HCV virus in their blood, they then need to undergo tests to determine what liver damage has already occurred. This may include identification of certain biomarkers, liver function tests or liver biopsy. It is also important that they reduce their risk of liver damage, which would include abstaining from alcohol and avoiding certain medications.

Antiviral medications are used to treat hepatitis C. The treatment is successful if there is no virus in the body at least 12 weeks after completion of the medications. The selection of medication will depend on the genotype, presence of liver damage and other medical conditions that the patient has [29]. Antiviral medications are used to treat hepatitis C. The treatment is successful if there is no virus in the body at least 12 weeks after completion of the medications. The selection of medication will depend on the genotype, presence of liver damage and other medical conditions that the patient has [29]. Treatment is not recommended for those with acute hepatitis C infection. They should be monitored for persistent infection to see if it is still present after 6 months. In severe cases, a liver transplantation may be the only treatment option. However, it is likely that the virus will return and infect the new liver, so patients must receive antiviral medication to prevent this [29]. There are currently no vaccines available for hepatitis C.

3.3.6 HCV Relevance to Dentistry

All healthcare personnel should adhere to the appropriate standard precautions by using personal protective equipment, to avoid both exposure to the patient and to the healthcare practitioner. Transmission via blood splatter has been reported but the risk is very low. After needlestick or sharps exposure to a patient with HCV positive blood, the risk of infection is 0.1% [29].

It is critical for the dental professional to take a careful medical and social history of the patient to screen for those that may be at risk. Patients in the acute stage of hepatitis C infection should not be treated except for emergency care. In a patient with known liver disease, liver function tests must be conducted to assess a patient's clotting abilities, as these factors are affected by liver damage. Liver disease may also interfere with the metabolism of certain drugs [30]. Oral manifestations of liver dysfunction include mucosal jaundice, petechiae, bleeding, cheilitis, smooth and atrophic tongue, xerostomia, and bruxism [31].

3.4 Hepatitis D (HDV)

3.4.1 Definition and History

Hepatitis D virus (HDV) infection, a severe hepatic inflammatory condition, is transmitted parenterally and independently replicates within hepatocytes [32]. However, it necessitates the presence of hepatitis B surface antigen for propagation [32, 33]. Hepatic cell damage arises either directly due to HDV's cytotoxic effects or as a result of a host-mediated immune response [32]. Notably, perinatal transmission is a rare occurrence. Risk factors associated with HDV infection include blood transfusions and intravenous drug abuse [32, 33].

HDV, identified as a "satellite virus," induces liver disease and can only infect individuals who are simultaneously infected with the hepatitis B virus (HBV) [33]. The HDV infection can be acute or progress to a chronic, long-lasting illness. The infection can be acquired either concomitantly with HBV, termed coinfection, or as a superinfection in individuals already chronically infected with HBV [33].

An HBV/HDV coinfection refers to the simultaneous infection with both viruses, whereas an HDV superinfection refers to the acquisition of HDV by a person already chronically infected with HBV [33]. While acute HBV/HDV coinfections may resolve, HDV superinfection can expedite the progression of the pre-existing HBV infection, culminating in liver cirrhosis and liver failure [33]. These outcomes are observed within 5–10 years in 70–80% and within 1–2 years in 15% of individuals with chronic HBV/HDV infection [33].

HDV was first identified in 1977 in patients with chronic HBV infection and was initially believed to be an unrecognized HBV antigen [32]. Subsequent research revealed the HDV nuclear antigen to be part of a new pathogen, initially referred to as the delta agent [32]. HDV is considered a hybrid virus as it utilizes hepatitis B surface antigen (HBsAg) as its envelope protein, enabling it to infect only those patients concurrently harboring HBV [32]. Interestingly, HBV replication is suppressed in individuals infected with HDV, although the reasons for this phenomenon remain elusive [32].

3.4.2 Statistics in the USA and Worldwide

The prevalence of HDV infection within the USA is relatively low, with the majority of cases presenting in individuals who have migrated to the country or visited from regions exhibiting high endemicity of HDV [33, 34]. As hepatitis D is not a condition that requires national notification, the precise incidence of hepatitis D cases within the USA remains undetermined [33]. Hepatitis D exhibits a higher incidence in regions such as Eastern and Southern Europe, the Mediterranean area, the Middle East, West and Central Africa, East Asia, and the Amazon Basin of South America [33].

Hepatitis D virus (HDV) is categorized into eight distinct genotypes, each circulating in specific global regions and sharing common transmission routes and risk demographics. HDV genotype 1 is predominantly found in North America, Europe, the Middle East, and North Africa. HDV genotypes 2 and 4 are prevalent in East Asia, while genotype 3 is exclusive to the Amazon Basin in South America. Lastly, HDV genotypes 5 through 8 are observed in West and Central Africa [27].

3.4.3 How Is HDV Transmitted

The hepatitis D virus (HDV) is primarily disseminated through activities that involve percutaneous exposure or punctures through the skin. It can also be transmitted, albeit to a lesser degree, via mucosal contact with infectious bodily fluids such as blood, semen, and saliva [33, 35]. The modes of transmission include sexual intercourse with an infected individual, sharing needles, syringes, or drug-preparation equipment during injection-drug use, and contact with the blood or open sores of an infected person [32, 33, 35]. Transmission from mother to child at birth is possible but infrequent. Other potential routes of transmission include needle sticks or sharp instrument exposures and sharing personal items like razors and toothbrushes with an infected person [32, 33, 35]. The transmission pathways for HDV largely mirror those of hepatitis B virus (HBV), occurring via broken skin (through injections, tattooing, etc.) or contact with infected blood or blood products

[33, 35]. Vaccination against HBV provides protection against HDV coinfection; thus, the expansion of childhood HBV immunization programs has led to a global decline in the incidence of hepatitis D [32, 33, 35]. Chronic carriers of HBV are susceptible to HDV infection. Individuals who lack immunity to HBV, whether due to natural disease or immunization via the hepatitis B vaccine, are at risk of contracting HBV, which subsequently places them at risk for HDV infection [32, 33, 35]. Certain demographics are more likely to experience HBV and HDV coinfection, including indigenous populations, individuals who inject drugs, and those living with hepatitis C virus or HIV infection. The risk of coinfection is potentially elevated in recipients of hemodialysis, men who have sex with men, and commercial sex workers [32, 33, 35].

3.4.4 Pathogenesis and Signs/Symptoms of HDV Infection

Hepatitis D Virus (HDV) is a unique virus that replicates exclusively in hepatocytes, causing primary liver damage [36]. Its structure consists of an RNA genome, hepatitis D antigen (HDAg), and a hepatitis B virus (HBV) lipoprotein envelope [32]. HDV infection can only occur simultaneously with HBV infection, often leading to acute hepatitis B and D [32]. While most patients recover, roughly 5% develop chronic infection [32]. The pathogenesis of HDV is complex and thought to involve both immune-mediated liver damage and a direct cytopathic effect on hepatocytes [32]. In superinfected chronic HBsAg carriers, HDV can lead to severe acute hepatitis or exacerbation of existing chronic hepatitis B [32]. This superinfection often progresses into chronic hepatitis D, leading to increased morbidity and complications [32].

Variations in immune responses during acute and chronic HDV infection may explain the persistence of superinfection [36]. Insufficient and delayed immune responses can fail to clear the infection, establishing chronic infection [36]. Conversely, an exaggerated immune response can lead to fulminant hepatic failure in a small percentage of patients [36]. Woodchuck models have been instrumental in studying HDV pathogenesis and testing new treatments [36]. However, current immunization strategies have proven ineffective against superinfection, indicating the need for alternative vaccine development [36]. Lastly, HDV genotype influences disease progression. Genotype 1 can rapidly progress to cirrhosis, Genotype 2 is less associated with severe disease, while Genotype 3 often causes severe acute hepatitis progressing to liver failure [32]. Despite this knowledge, the interaction between HDV and HBV remains unclear, and triple infections with HBV, HCV, and HDV can occur, further complicating the disease course [32].

Acute hepatitis D virus (HDV) infection presents symptoms like fever, fatigue, nausea, vomiting, and jaundice, similar to other types of acute viral hepatitis [35]. Individuals coinfected with HBV/HDV may experience symptoms ranging from mild to severe, with less than 5% developing chronic infections [35]. However, acute liver failure is more common in these individuals. HDV superinfection accelerates chronic HBV progression in 70–90% of cases, often leading to cirrhosis a decade earlier than HBV alone [35]. Over 95% of adults clear both viruses when simultaneously acquired, but HDV becomes chronic in over 80% of superinfections [35]. Chronic HDV infection typically results in rapid liver disease progression, with 70–80% of chronic HDV superinfections leading to cirrhosis and liver failure within 5–10 years [35].

3.4.5 Treatment of Hepatitis D

Pegylated interferon-alpha is traditionally the preferred therapeutic strategy for managing hepatitis D virus (HDV) infection, with a treatment course extending to at least 48 weeks, irrespective of the patient's response [37]. This regimen typically elicits a low viral response rate, yet it is associated with a diminished likelihood of disease progression [38]. However, this method carries substantial adverse effects and is contraindicated in patients with decompensated cirrhosis, active psychiatric conditions, and autoimmune diseases [39].

Bulevirtide has recently been identified as an emerging potential treatment for hepatitis D [40]. Despite the lack of FDA approval for chronic hepatitis D, interferon alpha (IFN alpha) has shown promise in a multitude of clinical trials [41]. It is often the preferred form of treatment according to expert guidelines, with a weekly administration persisting for at least 1 year [42]. The key objective of this treatment is to inhibit HDV replication, indicated by the non-detection of HDV RNA in serum and HDAg in the liver [43]. Treatment goals include the normalization of alanine aminotransferase (ALT) levels and the reduction of inflammation as observed in liver biopsies [39].

In circumstances where the disease advances to cirrhosis, liver transplantation emerges as the sole viable option [44]. There is currently no specific treatment for HDV infection. New therapies are presently being evaluated [37].

Overall, there is a pressing need to lessen the global impact of chronic hepatitis B and develop safe, effective, and affordable treatments for hepatitis D [38]. Current therapeutic options for hepatitis D are limited, and the optimal treatment plan remains uncertain, particularly as there are no known treatments for acute hepatitis D [39]. This underscores the importance of ongoing research and development in this field [41].

3.4.6 HDV Disease-Relevance to Dentistry

Although HDV is recognized as the most severe form of viral hepatitis, information about this virus is notably scarce, especially when compared to other types of viral hepatitis. Within the field of dentistry, the role and implications of the hepatitis D virus (HDV) have been inadequately explored and reported, leaving a significant gap in our understanding [45]. While there are no known instances of HDV transmission within dental contexts, it is crucial to consider that an estimated 5% of individuals infected with hepatitis B virus (HBV) also harbor HDV [45]. This suggests that there may be an unrecognized rate of HDV transmission via dental procedures [45].

Historically, most documented cases of HBV transmission in dental settings date back to the period between 1975 and 1989, a time when HDV serologic testing was neither routine nor widely accessible. This lack of testing could potentially obscure the true prevalence and impact of HDV within dental settings [45].

For dental practitioners, maintaining a heightened awareness of blood-borne pathogens is essential for ensuring their safety and that of their patients. Given that HDV depends on HBV for replication and shares similar transmission routes, the prevention of HDV infection is intrinsically tied to HBV prevention, primarily through vaccination [46].

3.5 Hepatitis E (HEV)

3.5.1 Definition and History

Hepatitis E is inflammation of the liver caused by the hepatitis E virus (HEV). Hepatitis E is an RNA virus that exists in both enveloped and non-enveloped forms and was first recognized in the early 1980s [47]. The virus is a member of the Hepeviridae family. It has at least four known mammalian genotypes (named 1–4), which belong to a single serotype.

The virus is shed in the stools of infected persons and enters the human body through the intestine. It is transmitted mainly through contaminated drinking water. The infection is usually self-limiting and resolves within 2–6 weeks. Occasionally a serious disease known as fulminant hepatitis (acute liver failure) develops, which can be fatal.

Genotypes 1 and 2 have been found only in humans. Genotypes 3 and 4 circulate in several animals including pigs, wild boars and deer without causing any disease, and occasionally infect humans [48].

Genotype 1 is the most prevalent HEV genotype and is widely distributed in several countries in Asia and Africa. Genotype 1 has also been identified among indigenous cases of hepatitis E in South America. In Europe, North America and Australia cases due to genotype 1 have occurred in persons who had traveled to Asia or Africa. The distribution of HEV genotype 2 has been focal, with the majority of cases reported from Mexico, Nigeria, Namibia and a few other West African countries [48].

Despite the ubiquity of HEV genotype 3 in the swine population, clinically apparent human infections with this genotype have been reported almost entirely in developed countries and is more common in older adults. In recent years, HEV genotype 4 has been found to circulate in animals in India and China and has been found in several European countries; most human cases of hepatitis due to HEV genotype 4 have been reported in mainland China and Taiwan [49].

3.5.2 Statistics in the USA and Worldwide

Hepatitis E virus (HEV) is a leading cause of acute viral hepatitis in developing countries. A global burden of disease study estimated that HEV genotypes 1 and 2 account for approximately 20.1 million HEV infections, 3.4 million symptomatic cases, 70,000 deaths, and 3000 stillbirths annually [48].

In developing countries, where HEV genotypes 1 and 2 are the causes of hepatitis E, the disease mainly affects young adults (aged 15–39 years), with preponderance in males. In pregnant women, hepatitis caused by HEV genotype 1 has a high mortality rate [50]. The ratio of symptomatic to asymptomatic infection has been estimated to range from 1:2 to 1:10 or more in outbreak settings and may be dependent on age at infection.

3.5.3 How Is HEV Transmitted

Hepatitis E infection is found worldwide and is common in low- and middle-income countries with limited access to essential water, sanitation, hygiene, and health services. Fecal contamination of drinking water is a major route of HEV transmission [48]. In these areas, HEV genotypes 1 and 2 predominate. Sporadic disease occurs in endemic countries, with periodic large epidemics. Some of these outbreaks have occurred in areas of conflict and humanitarian emergencies such as war zones and camps for refugees or internally displaced populations, where sanitation and safe water supply pose special challenges. The overall burden of disease due to hepatitis E is greatest in parts of the world where clean drinking water is scarce,

In industrial countries, hepatitis E infection is infrequent, with only occasional sporadic cases. Most of these cases are caused by genotype 3 virus and are triggered by infection with virus originating in animals, usually through ingestion of undercooked animal meat (including animal liver, particularly pork). These cases are not related to contamination of water or other foods [51].

Certain population subgroups are at greater risk for severe disease following HEV infection. These include pregnant women, persons with pre-existing liver disease and immunosuppressed persons [52]. Due to the nature of their living conditions, including overcrowding and poor hygiene, displaced persons and refugees experience the highest attack rates whenever outbreaks occur. Travelers from industrialized countries to areas where hepatitis E is endemic are at risk of exposure to the virus if water sources are contaminated. During epidemics, fulminant hepatitis E occurs with a disproportionately high rate among pregnant women [50, 53, 54]. The disease is typically most severe during the third trimester of pregnancy [55, 56].

While in the general population mortality from hepatitis E ranges from 0.1% to 4%, among women in the third trimester of pregnancy, it can range from 10% to 50%.

3.5.4 Symptoms

The incubation period following exposure to HEV ranges from 2 to 10 weeks, with an average of 5–6 weeks. The infected persons excrete the virus beginning from a few days before to 3–4 weeks after onset of the disease [57].

In areas with high disease endemicity, symptomatic infection is most common in young adults aged 15–40 years. In these areas, although infection does occur in children, it often goes undiagnosed because they typically have no symptoms or only a mild illness without jaundice.

Typical signs and symptoms of hepatitis include:

- an initial phase of mild fever, reduced appetite (anorexia), nausea, and vomiting lasting for a few days;
- abdominal pain, itching, skin rash, or joint pain;
- jaundice (yellow color of the skin), dark urine and pale stools; and
- a slightly enlarged, tender liver (hepatomegaly).

These symptoms are often indistinguishable from those experienced during other liver illnesses and typically last 1–6 weeks.

In rare cases, acute hepatitis E can be severe and result in fulminant hepatitis (acute liver failure). These patients are at risk of death. Pregnant women with hepatitis E, particularly those in the second or third trimester, are at increased risk of acute liver failure, fetal loss and mortality. Up to 20–25% of pregnant women can die if they get hepatitis E in third trimester [50].

Cases of chronic hepatitis E infection have been reported in immunosuppressed people, particularly organ transplant recipients on immunosuppressive drugs, with genotype 3 or 4 HEV infection. These remain uncommon.

Transfusion transmission of HEV occurs and is well documented; however, its contribution to the overall disease burden is limited [51, 58, 59].

3.5.5 Diagnosis

Cases of hepatitis E are not clinically distinguishable from other types of acute viral hepatitis. However, diagnosis can often be strongly suspected in appropriate epidemiologic settings, for example, when several cases occur in localities in known disease-endemic areas, in settings with risk of water contamination when the disease is more severe in pregnant women or if hepatitis A has been excluded.

Definitive diagnosis of hepatitis E infection is usually based on the detection of specific anti-HEV immunoglobulin M (IgM) antibodies to the virus in a person's blood; this is usually adequate in areas where the disease is common. Rapid tests are available for field use.

Additional tests include reverse transcriptase polymerase chain reaction (RT-PCR) to detect the hepatitis E virus RNA in blood and stool. This assay requires specialized laboratory facilities. This test is particularly needed in areas where hepatitis E is infrequent and in uncommon cases with chronic HEV infection.

3.5.6 Treatment of Hepatitis E

There is no specific treatment capable of altering the course of acute hepatitis E. As the disease is usually self-limiting, hospitalization is generally not required. It is important to avoid unnecessary medications that can adversely affect liver function, e.g., acetaminophen, paracetamol.

Hospitalization is required for people with fulminant hepatitis and should also be considered for symptomatic pregnant women.

Immunosuppressed people with chronic hepatitis E benefit from specific treatment using ribavirin, an antiviral drug. In some specific situations, interferon has also been used successfully.

3.5.7 Prevention

The one currently licensed hepatitis E vaccine (HEV 239 vaccine, Hecolin®) is considered a promising vaccine which has shown a high degree of efficacy against hepatitis E disease in 16–65-year-old healthy subjects in China [60].

Prevention is the most effective approach against HEV infection. Transmission of HEV can be reduced by:

- maintaining quality standards for public water supplies; and
- establishing proper disposal systems for human feces.

On an individual level, infection risk can be reduced by:

- maintaining hygienic practices; and
- avoiding consumption of water and ice of unknown purity.

3.5.8 HEV Disease-Relevance to Dentistry

HEV is common in many parts of the developing world where sanitation is poor. It is not common in the USA, where people have access to clean drinking water. Most cases in the USA involve people who have recently traveled to countries where hepatitis E is common [61].

3.6 Human Immunodeficiency Virus (HIV)

3.6.1 Definition and History

Human immunodeficiency virus, commonly known as HIV, is a virus that can eventually become AIDS if left untreated. AIDS, which stands for acquired immunodeficiency syndrome, will eventually lead to death. Currently, there are no treatments that can completely cure the HIV virus, so once you are infected, you will have it for life [62]. HIV is classified as a retrovirus and works by targeting the body's immune system, specifically CD4 T cells, making it difficult for the body to fight off infections. If this is allowed to continue and progress to AIDS, the body will eventually succumb to opportunistic infections, which is what eventually leads to death [62].

HIV first appeared in the USA in the Early 1980s. The AIDS epidemic was first reported on June 5, 1981 in a report describing Pneumocystis pneumonia in previously healthy, gay men in Los Angeles [63].

On September 24, 1982, the CDC used the term "AIDS" for the first time and released the first case definition. It was also discovered at this time that transmission occurred through blood transfusion as well as perinatally. In September of 1983, the CDC identified all major routes of HIV transmission as well as the first recommendations to prevent occupational exposure in healthcare workers [63]. The original source of HIV infection in humans has been identified as simian immunodeficiency virus, (SIV) which is found in a type of chimpanzee in Central Africa. It was likely transmitted to humans through their blood when they were hunted for food consumption. The virus likely spread through Africa and then to other parts of the world [62].

3.6.2 Statistics in the USA and Worldwide

According to the CDC in 2021, the annual number of HIV diagnoses decreased 7% (36,136 people aged 13 and older) from 2017 to 2021in the USA and six dependent areas [64, 65]. However, 2021 diagnoses represent an 18% increase from the previous year, likely due to the identification and reporting of HIV diagnoses missed in 2020 due to the impact of the COVID-19 pandemic on access to HIV testing, care-related services, and case surveillance activities in state and local jurisdictions. HIV diagnosis trends varied for different groups of people.

HIV continues to have a disproportionate impact on certain populations, particularly racial and ethnic minorities and gay, bisexual, and other men who have sex with men (MSM).

The number of HIV diagnoses in the USA have steadily declined from 2010 to 2019 except for an increase from 2013 to 2014; another exception has been documented from 2020 to 2021; however, data for 2020 should be interpreted with caution due to the impact of the COVID-19 pandemic on access to HIV testing, care-related services, and case surveillance activities in state and local jurisdictions (Figs. 3.5 and 3.6).

The data continues to show a strong male prevalence when compared to females as well as a higher incidence in black or African Americans. The age groups 20–24 and 25–29 are among the highest groups affected [65] (Fig. 3.7).

Worldwide HIV Data While HIV continues to be a major global public health issue, claiming 40.4 million [32.9–51.3 million] lives so far; there is excellent progress globally in reducing the number of new HIV infections as well as deaths associated with HIV/AIDS. In 2022, 630,000 [480,000–880,000] people died from

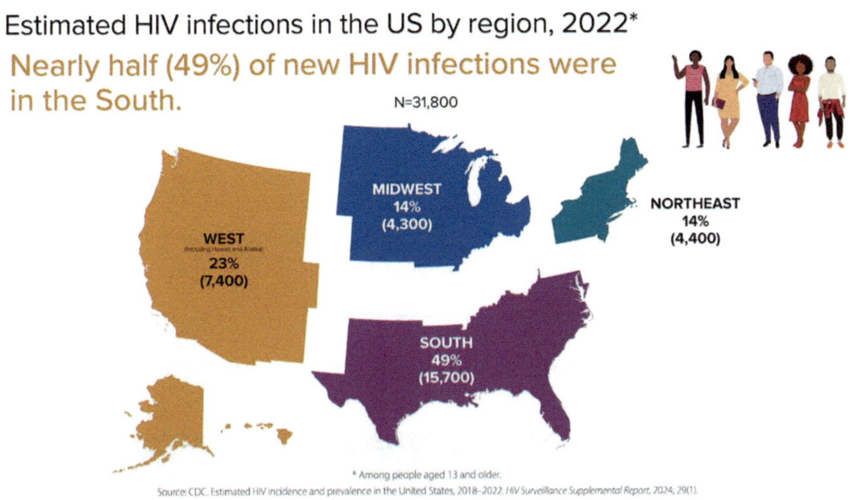

Fig. 3.5 Source: https://www.hiv.gov/hiv-basics/overview/data-and-trends/statistics. HIV.gov, 2022, US Centers for Disease Control and Prevention

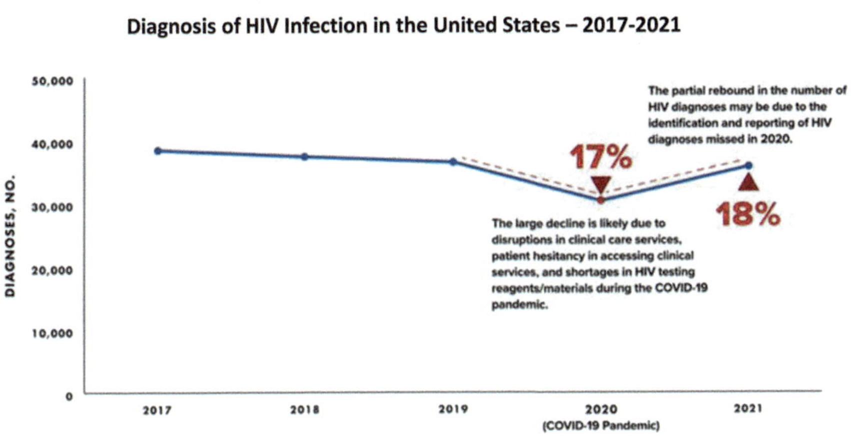

Fig. 3.6 Source: HIV Surveillance Reports; Resource Library - HIV/AIDS - US Centers for Disease Control and Prevention

HIV-related causes globally. Since 2010, HIV-related deaths have been reduced by 51%, from 1.3 million [970,000–1.8 million]. The global HIV epidemic claimed 69% fewer lives in 2022 since the peak in 2004. Approximately 84,000 [56,000–120,000] children died from HIV-related causes in 2022.

Many countries are on their way to eliminate new HIV infections in children. Antiretroviral therapy (ART) has also become more readily available worldwide which has significantly helped in reducing lives lost. At the end of 2022,

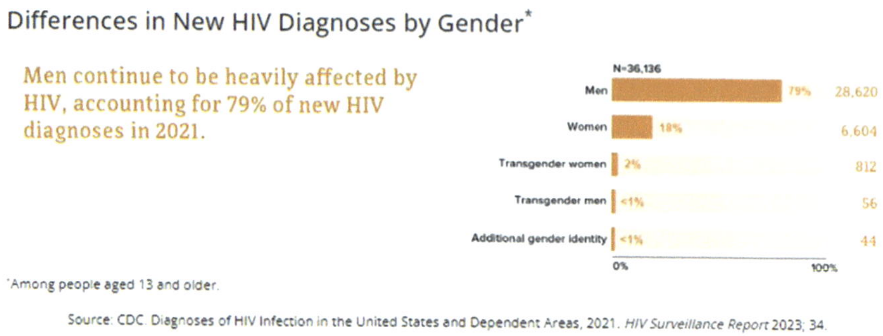

Fig. 3.7 Source: HIV Surveillance Reports; Resource Library - HIV/AIDS - US Centers for Disease Control and Prevention

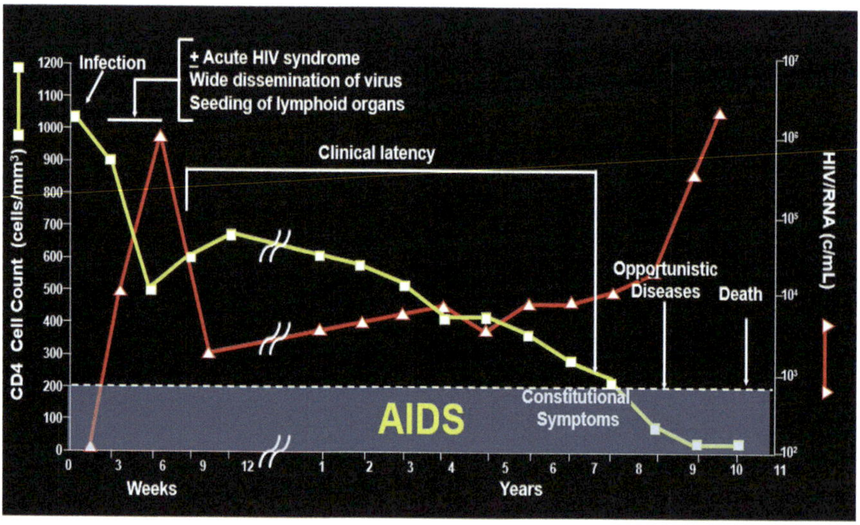

Fig. 3.8 Natural History of HIV/AIDS. Source: Naif [71]

29.8 million people were accessing antiretroviral therapy, up from 7.7 million in 2010. As of 2022, Africa still remains the highest among people living with HIV. The number of newly infected people worldwide dropped from 3 million in 2000 to 1.8 million in 2016 and the number do deaths dropped from 1.9 million in 2005 to 1.0 million in 2016 according to data from UNAIDS/WHO [66]. The number of newly infected people and the number of deaths worldwide continues to decline.

According to HIV.gov, an estimated 1.3 million individuals worldwide acquired HIV in 2022, *marking a 38% decline in new HIV infections since 2010* and 59% since the peak in 1995 [67] (Fig. 3.8).

3.6.3 Situation and Trends

At the end of 2022, 76% [65–89%] of people living with HIV were accessing antiretroviral therapy, up from 24% [21–29%] in 2010 [68].

- Globally, there were 1.2 million [940,000–1.5 million] pregnant women with HIV in 2022, of which an estimated 82% [64–98%] received antiretroviral drugs to prevent mother-to-child transmission [68].
- At the end of 2022, there were 1.5 million [1.2–2.1 million] children living with HIV globally, down from 2.5 million [2.0–3.5 million] in 2010 [68].

3.6.4 How Is HIV Transmitted?

HIV is transmitted most commonly from anal or vaginal sex and through the sharing of needles or syringes. In more rare cases, HIV has been documented as being transmitted through oral sex, blood transfusions, or organ/tissue transplants. Proper testing of donors has almost completely eliminated this issue in the USA. It is also possible, although again very rare, that it can be transmitted from eating food that has been pre-chewed by an HIV infected person, being bitten by a person with HIV, and contact with broken skin, wounds or mucous membranes. It is also possible for HIV to be transferred from an HIV-positive mother to her baby during pregnancy, birth or breastfeeding, although this is also rare. HIV is not transmitted through casual touching, sharing toilets, closed-mouth kissing, saliva, tears, sweat, or insects [69].

3.6.5 Pathogenesis and Early Signs/Symptoms of HIV Disease

Initial infection of HIV can begin without symptoms and lasts about 3 months until seroconversion. At this point, HIV-specific antibodies can be identified in the blood. However, about 40–90% of people will have flu-like symptoms during this acute phase such as fever, chills, rash, muscle aches, etc. This stage is highly contagious, even though the individual may not show a positive HIV diagnosis during this time [70].

HIV usually progresses very slowly, often taking years for a person to exhibit signs and symptoms. During this initial infection, the virus is actively replicating in the lymph nodes and blood stream. HIV mainly infects and destroys CD4 T cells, gaining entry through the CD4+ protein on the surface. HIV can also infect other cells involved in the immune response, using various coreceptors to gain entry. As mentioned earlier, if left untreated, HIV will progress to the symptomatic stage of the disease, AIDS, which is defined as a CD4 T cell count of less than 200 mm. This is when you will likely notice opportunistic infections such as *Mycobacterium tuberculosis*, Cytomegalovirus (CMV), toxoplasmosis, and candidiasis, conditions that are rare in an otherwise healthy individual [71]. The graph below shows the initial surge in viral load with the corresponding decrease in CD4 T cells. During the latent period, the CD4 T cell count will slowly decrease if left untreated, which will eventually lead to the development of AIDS. Death eventually occurs from opportunistic infections [71].

3.6.6 HIV-Late Signs and Symptoms

If HIV is left untreated, the disease will progress to AIDS. Symptoms of AIDS can include rapid weight loss, recurring fever, extreme fatigue, prolonged lymph node swelling, sores, and pneumonia. Red, brown, pink or purplish blotches may be noted under the skin or inside the mouth, nose or eyelids. Neurologic symptoms such as memory loss and depression may also be noted [69].

Opportunistic infections are less commonly seen today in patients with HIV due to advancements in treatment. However, some of the more commonly seen opportunistic infections that are likely to be found in a patient with advanced HIV or AIDS are: Candidiasis, deep fungal infections, CMV, Herpes Simplex Virus, Kaposi's Sarcoma, Tuberculosis, and pneumonia [69].

3.6.7 Treatment of HIV Disease

Although HIV cannot be cured at this time, there are treatments designed to slow the progression. These drugs can essentially let the patient lead a normal life if taken daily. These drugs are called antiretrovirals (ARV). They are given in combination with other ARV's, which is known as antiretroviral therapy (ART). The goal of ART is to significantly reduce the viral load in a patient's body, therefore reducing your chance of transmission to others. Treatment with ART should begin immediately after diagnosis and continue for life. This will reduce the risk of any secondary or opportunistic infections that would otherwise affect a person with a weakened immune system. It is possible for a person to develop resistance to drugs used to treat HIV. This can happen especially if you do not follow exact guidelines for taking the medications as prescribed. There are also tests to determine which drugs you may be resistant to if that is suspected, and the medications can then be tailored to the patient for the most effective treatment [72].

There are many different antiretrovirals available today, and the specific combination of drugs depends on the current status of the patient. Each country has a drug approval process, and new antiretroviral drugs are approved each year.

3.6.8 HIV Disease-Relevance to Dentistry

Patients that are HIV positive can be treated routinely in the dental office if standard precautions are followed by the practitioner and staff. It is important to obtain a detailed medical history from the patient as well as their most recent lab values and treatments to determine their current disease status. A high CD4 T cell count, and low viral load would indicate an effective treatment regimen. Dental treatment may be affected if a patient is severely immunocompromised as wound healing would likely be impaired. A patient with a very high viral load would also be more likely to be contagious, so elective treatment may be delayed until this is brought to more manageable levels. Other things to consider are abnormal bleeding due to low platelet counts, glucose intolerance and hyperlipidemia as a result of medications used in treatment.

Dentists can be the first to detect the presence of opportunistic infections. Oral conditions that correlate with advanced HIV and/or AIDS such as candidiasis, herpes virus, and other chronic ulcers, Kaposi's sarcoma, and lymphoma are seen on routine dental exams. A thorough head and neck exam is critical for all patients, but specifically important in patients with known HIV diagnosis to detect any potential changes in disease status [73].

References

1. Shouval D. The history of hepatitis A. Clin Liver Dis. 2020;16(Suppl 1):12–23. https://doi.org/10.1002/cld.1018.
2. Feinstone SM. History of the discovery of hepatitis A virus. Cold Spring Harb Perspect Med. 2019;9,5:a031740. https://doi.org/10.1101/cshperspect.a031740.
3. CDC—Hepatitis A—Pinkbook. Centers for Disease Control and Prevention, U.S. Department of Health & Human Services. www.cdc.gov/vaccines/pubs/pinkbook/hepa.html. Accessed 21 Oct 2023.
4. Thomas RE, et al. Mortality and morbidity among military personnel and civilians during the 1930s and World War II from transmission of hepatitis during yellow fever vaccination: systematic review. Am J Public Health. 2013;103(3):e16–29. https://doi.org/10.2105/AJPH.2012.301158.
5. Hepatitis A Q&As for Health Professionals. Centers for Disease Control and Prevention, U.S. Department of Health & Human Services. www.cdc.gov/hepatitis/hav/havfaq.htm. Accessed 21 Oct 2023.
6. Cao G, et al. The global trends and regional differences in incidence and mortality of hepatitis A from 1990 to 2019 and implications for its prevention. Hepatol Int. 2021;15(5):1068–82. https://doi.org/10.1007/s12072-021-10232-4.
7. Hepatitis A. World Health Organization. www.who.int/news-room/fact-sheets/detail/hepatitis-a. Accessed 20 Oct 2023.
8. Vinograd A, Ben-David D, Gozlan Y, Mor O, Mor Z, Sheffer R, Savion M. Hepatitis A virus transmission in a dental clinic setting. Infect Control Hosp Epidemiol. 2023;44(4):692–3. https://doi.org/10.1017/ice.2023.16.
9. Mbithi JN, Springthorpe VS, Boulet JR, Sattarl SA. Survival of hepatitis A virus on human hands and its transfer on contact with animate and inanimate surfaces. J Clin Microbiol. 1992;30:757–63.

10. Oosthuysen J, Potgieter E, Fossey A. Compliance with infection prevention and control in oral healthcare facilities: a global perspective. Int Dent J. 2014;64:297–311.
11. Danzmann L, Gastmeier P, Schwab F, Vonberg RP. Healthcare workers causing large nosocomial outbreaks: a systematic review. BMC Infect Dis. 2013;13:98.
12. Murray PR, Rosenthal KS, Pfaller MA. Medical microbiology. 7th ed. Philadelphia: Elsevier Mosby; 2005.
13. Centers for Disease Control and Prevention (CDC). Viral hepatitis, hepatitis B frequently asked questions for health professionals. Updated 30 Mar 2022. https://www.cdc.gov/hepatitis/hbv/hbvfaq.htm#treatment.
14. Centers for Disease Control and Prevention (CDC). Viral hepatitis, hepatitis B frequently asked questions for the public. Updated 9 Mar 2023. https://www.cdc.gov/hepatitis/hbv/bfaq.htm.
15. Hepatitis B Foundation. Facts and figures. 2021. https://www.hepb.org/what-is-hepatitis-b/what-is-hepb/facts-and-figures/. Accessed 13 Nov 2023.
16. World Health Organization. Hepatitis B. World Health Organization. 2024. www.who.int/news-room/fact-sheets/detail/hepatitis-b#:~:text=Care%20for%20acute%20hepatitis%20B,medicines%2C%20including%20tenofovir%20or%20entecavir.&text=improve%20long%20term%20survival.
17. Centers for Disease Control and Prevention. Fast facts on global hepatitis B. n.d. https://www.cdc.gov/globalhealth/immunization/diseases/hepatitisb/data/fast-facts.html. 2021Accessed 13 Nov 2023.
18. Lok AS, McMahon BJ. Chronic hepatitis B. Hepatology. 2007;45(2):507–39. https://aasldpubs.onlinelibrary.wiley.com/doi/10.1002/hep.21513.
19. Shahriar S, et al. Insights into the coinfections of human immunodeficiency virus-hepatitis B virus, human immunodeficiency virus-hepatitis C virus, and hepatitis B virus-hepatitis C virus: prevalence, risk factors, pathogenesis, diagnosis, and treatment. Front Microbiol. 2022;12:780887. https://doi.org/10.3389/fmicb.2021.780887.
20. Afify S, et al. Survival and outcomes for co-infection of chronic hepatitis C with and without cirrhosis and COVID-19: a multicenter retrospective study. World J Gastroenterol. 2021;27(42):7362–75. https://doi.org/10.3748/wjg.v27.i42.7362.
21. Huang C-R, Lo SJ. Hepatitis D virus infection, replication and cross-talk with the hepatitis B virus. World J Gastroenterol. 2014;20(40):14589–97. https://doi.org/10.3748/wjg.v20.i40.14589.
22. Gupta A, Fine SM, Vail RM, et al. Prevention and management of hepatitis B virus infection in adults with HIV. Baltimore (MD): Johns Hopkins University; 2022. https://www.ncbi.nlm.nih.gov/books/NBK584516/.
23. Lutwick L. Hepatitis B in the dental health care worker: a review of current recommendations for preventing occupational infection. Pediatr Dent. 2004;26(5):417–22. https://www.aapd.org/globalassets/media/publications/archives/lutwick-04-04.pdf. Accessed 13 Nov 2023.
24. Åberg F, Helenius-Hietala J. Oral health and liver disease: bidirectional associations—a narrative review. Dent J. 2022;10(2):16. https://doi.org/10.3390/dj10020016.
25. Centers for Disease Control and Prevention (CDC). Viral hepatitis, hepatitis C information. Updated 31 Oct 2023. https://www.cdc.gov/hepatitis/hcv/.
26. 2020 Hepatitis C | Viral hepatitis surveillance report. Centers for Disease Control and Prevention, U.S. Department of Health & Human Services. www.cdc.gov/hepatitis/statistics/2020surveillance/hepatitis-c.htm. Accessed 18 Oct 2023.
27. Hepatitis C. World Health Organization www.who.int/news-room/fact-sheets/detail/hepatitis-c. Accessed 23 Oct 2023.
28. Mayo Clinic. Hepatitis C, diagnosis. Updated 23 Aug 2023. https://www.mayoclinic.org/diseases-conditions/hepatitis-c/diagnosis-treatment/drc-20354284.
29. Centers for Disease Control and Prevention (CDC). Viral hepatitis, hepatitis C questions and answers for health professionals. Updated 31 Oct 31 2023. https://www.cdc.gov/hepatitis/hcv/hcvfaq.htm#section4.
30. Zeisel MB, Felmlee DJ, Baumert TF. Hepatitis C virus entry. In: Bartenschlager R, editor. Hepatitis C virus: from molecular virology to antiviral therapy. Current topics in microbiology

and immunology, vol. 369. Berlin: Springer; 2013. https://link.springer.com/chapter/10.1007%2F978-3-642-27340-7_4.
31. Oral health topics, hepatitis viruses. American Dental Association. www.ada.org/en/member-center/oral-health-topics/hepatitis-viruses. Published 26 Mar 2019. Accessed 23 Oct 2023.
32. Masood U, John S. Hepatitis D. [Updated 12 Sep 2022]. In: StatPearls. Treasure Island (FL): StatPearls Publishing; 2023. https://www.ncbi.nlm.nih.gov/books/NBK470436/.
33. Hepatitis D questions and answers for health professionals. Centers for Disease Control and Prevention, U.S. Department of Health & Human Services. www.cdc.gov/hepatitis/hdv/hdv-faq.htm#section1. Accessed 21 Oct 2023.
34. Kamili S, Drobeniuc J, Mixson-Hayden T, Kodani M. Delta hepatitis: toward improved diagnostics. Hepatology. 2017;66:1716–8.
35. Hepatitis D. World Health Organization. www.who.int/news-room/fact-sheets/detail/hepatitis-d#:~:text=The%20routes%20of%20HDV%20transmission,child%20is%20possible%20but%20rare. Accessed 18 Oct 2023.
36. Abbas Z, Afzal R. Life cycle and pathogenesis of hepatitis D virus: a review. World J Hepatol. 2013;5(12):666–75. https://doi.org/10.4254/wjh.v5.i12.666.
37. Ferenci P, et al. Treatment of chronic hepatitis D with bulevirtide—a fight against two foes—an update. Cells. 2022;11(22):3531. https://doi.org/10.3390/cells11223531.
38. Olsen K, et al. Recent treatment advances and practical management of hepatitis D virus. Clin Med. 2023;23(4):403–8. https://doi.org/10.7861/clinmed.2022-0556.
39. Xu HY, Yang JO, Chen PH, Han S-HB. Bulevirtide and emerging drugs for the treatment of hepatitis D. Expert Opin Biol Ther. 2023;23(12):1245–53. https://doi.org/10.1080/14712598.2023.2273260.
40. Abbas Z, et al. Interferon alpha for chronic hepatitis D. Cochrane Database Syst Rev. 2011;(12):CD006002. https://doi.org/10.1002/14651858.CD006002.pub2.
41. European Association for the Study of the Liver. Electronic address: easloffice@easloffice.eu and European Association for the Study of the Liver. EASL clinical practice guidelines on hepatitis delta virus. J Hepatol. 2023;79(2):433–60. https://doi.org/10.1016/j.jhep.2023.05.001.
42. Pons JA. Role of liver transplantation in viral hepatitis. J Hepatol. 1995;22(1 Suppl):146–53.
43. Farci P, Niro GA. Current and future management of chronic hepatitis D. Gastroenterol Hepatol. 2018;14(6):342–51.
44. Kushner T, et al. Liver transplantation for hepatitis D virus in the United States: a UNOS study on outcomes in the MELD era. Transplant Direct. 2021;8(1):e1253. https://doi.org/10.1097/TXD.0000000000001253.
45. Mahboobi N, Porter SR, Rizzetto M, Alavian SM. Hepatitis D virus: an overview for dentists. J Adv Med Med Res. 2019;29(4):1–8. https://doi.org/10.9734/jammr/2019/v29i430081.
46. Dahiya P, Kamal R, Sharma V, Kaur S. Hepatitis—prevention and management in dental practice. J Educ Health Promot. 2015;4:33. https://doi.org/10.4103/2277-9531.157188. PMID: 26097847; PMCID: PMC4456879.
47. Balayan MS, Zamyatina NA, Mikhailov MI, et al. Serological survey on hepatitis E virus infection in an endemic area: diagnosis potential of enzyme immunoassay for detection of IgG antibody. Clin Diagn Virol. 1994;2(4–5):297–304.
48. Kim JH, Nelson KE, Panzner U, et al. A systematic review of the epidemiology of hepatitis E virus in Africa. BMC Infect Dis. 2014;14:308.
49. Rein DB, Stevens GA, Theaker J, et al. The global burden of hepatitis E genotypes 1 and 2 in 2005. Hepatology. 2012;55(4):988–97.
50. Nelson KE, Kmush B, Labrique AB. The epidemiology of hepatitis E virus infections in developed countries and among immunocompromised patients. Expert Rev Anti-Infect Ther. 2011;9(12):1133–48.
51. Khuroo MS, Kamili S. Aetiology, clinical course and outcome of sporadic acute viral hepatitis in pregnancy. J Viral Hepat. 2003;10(1):61–9.
52. Kamar N, Bendall R, Legrand-Abravanel F, et al. Hepatitis E. Lancet. 2012;379(9835):2477–88.
53. Hepatitis E Vaccine Working Group. Hepatitis E: epidemiology and disease burden. Geneva: World Health Organization; 2014. https://terrance.who.int/mediacentre/data/sage/

SAGE_Docs_Ppt_Oct2014/8_session_hepE/Oct2014_session8_HepE_burden.pdf. Accessed Oct 2023.
54. Tsega E, Krawczynski K, Hansson BG, et al. Hepatitis E virus infection in pregnancy in Ethiopia. Ethiop Med J. 1993;31(3):173–81.
55. Ramalingaswami V, Purcell RH. Waterborne non-A, non-B hepatitis. Lancet. 1988;1(8585):571–3.
56. Kumar A, Beniwal M, Kar P, et al. Hepatitis E in pregnancy. Int J Gynaecol Obstet. 2004;85(3):240–4.
57. Khuroo MS, Kamili S. Aetiology and prognostic factors in acute liver failure in India. J Viral Hepat. 2003;10(3):224–31.
58. Hewitt PE, Ijaz S, Brailsford SR, Brett R, et al. 2. Hepatitis E virus in blood components: a prevalence and transmission study in southeast England. Lancet. 2014;384:1766–73.
59. Huzly D, Umhau M, Bettinger D, et al. Transfusion-transmitted hepatitis E in Germany, 2013. Euro Surveill. 2014;19:20812.
60. Proffitt A. First HEV vaccine approved. Nat Biotechnol. 2012;30:300. https://doi.org/10.1038/nbt0412-300a. Accessed Oct 2023.
61. World Health Organization. Hepatitis E questions and answers for the public. https://www.who.int/news-room/fact-sheets/detail/hepatitis-e. Accessed Oct 2023.
62. Centers for Disease Control (CDC). https://www.cdc.gov/hiv/basics/whatishiv.html. Centers for Disease Control and Prevention (CDC). HIV/aids; HIV basics. Updated 30 Jun 2022. https://www.cdc.gov/hiv/basics/whatishiv.html
63. Centers for Disease Control and Prevention (CDC). HIV and AIDS timeline. Updated 9 Jan 9 2023. https://npin.cdc.gov/pages/hiv-and-aids-timeline#1980.
64. Centers for Disease Control and Prevention (CDC). Health, United States, 2016, May 2017. https://www.cdc.gov/nchs/data/hus/hus16.pdf#034.
65. Centers for Disease Control and Prevention (CDC). Murphy SL, et al. Natl Vital Stat Rep. 2017;66(6). https://www.cdc.gov/nchs/data/nvsr/nvsr66/nvsr66_06.pdf.
66. World Health Organization. HIV/AIDS, prevent HIV, test and treat all—WHO support for country impact. Progress report 2016. https://www.who.int/hiv/pub/progressreports/2016-progress-report/en/.
67. HIV.gov. Global statistics | HIV.gov. 2023. https://www.hiv.gov/hiv-basics/overview/data-and-trends/global-statistics/. Accessed 14 Nov 2023.
68. World Health Organization. Data on the HIV/AIDS response. 2023. https://www.who.int/data/gho/data/themes/hiv-aids/data-on-the-hiv-aids-response. Accessed 14 Nov 2023.
69. U.S. Department of Health & Human Services. HIV.gov. Symptoms of HIV. Updated 16 Jun 2022. https://www.hiv.gov/hiv-basics/overview/about-hiv-and-aids/how-is-hiv-transmitted.
70. U.S. Department of Health & Human Services. HIV.gov. How is HIV transmitted? Updated 15 Jun 2022. https://www.hiv.gov/hiv-basics/overview/about-hiv-and-aids/symptoms-of-hiv.
71. Naif HM. Pathogenesis of HIV infection. Infect Dis Rep. 2013;5(Suppl 1):e6. https://doi.org/10.4081/idr.2013.s1.e6. Published 6 Jun 2013. https://www.ncbi.nlm.nih.gov/pmc/articles/PMC3892619/.
72. Centers for Disease Control and Prevention (CDC). HIV treatment overview. Updated 7 Jun 2022. https://www.hiv.gov/hiv-basics/staying-in-hiv-care/hiv-treatment/hiv-treatment-overview.
73. American Dental Association. Oral health topics, human immunodeficiency virus (HIV). Updated 26 Mar 2019. https://www.ada.org/en/member-center/oral-health-topics/hiv.

Overview of Infectious Diseases of Concern to Dental Practitioners: Other Viral Infections Airborne Pathogens

4

Sydnee Chavis and Erica Caffrey

4.1 Introduction

The nature of dentistry, working within the oral cavity in close proximity to patients and with instrumentation that causes aerosolization of pathogens, classifies dentistry as high risk for exposure to pathogens, especially ones that can be airborne and transmitted via aerosolization or droplets. It is important to understand which pathogens may be present within the oral cavity, as well as the method of infection and the virology of those pathogens.

Oral health providers should be aware and informed of the pathogens that can contribute to viral infections, as there is an inherent risk of airborne pathogens being transmitted to oral healthcare providers. Standard precautions, diligent use of personal protective equipment (PPE), and awareness of such pathogens can help mitigate the risks and concerns for transmission among oral health providers.

4.2 Pathogens of Concern

Viral pathogens are ubiquitous in the world around us, and some particularly thrive within the oral cavity, where they may be transmitted via aerosols or droplets produced from saliva and other intraoral fluids, such as mucous and blood [1]. Viral pathogens require a host to live as well as to be transmitted from person to person.

S. Chavis (✉)
Department of Oral-Maxillofacial Surgery, The University of Maryland School of Dentistry, Baltimore, MD, USA
e-mail: schavis@umaryland.edu

E. Caffrey
Department of Pediatric Dentistry, The University of Maryland School of Dentistry, Baltimore, MD, USA
e-mail: ecaffrey@umaryland.edu

L. DePaola et al. (eds.), *Infection Control in the Dental Office in the Era of COVID-19*, https://doi.org/10.1007/978-3-031-64611-9_4

Some viral pathogens are more prominently virulent, causing illness and clinical symptoms at the onset of infection. Some viral pathogens have an incubation period, in which the virus lingers within the host with a delay in clinical symptoms, and some viral pathogens may remain dormant within a host without causing clinical symptoms. Virulence of these pathogens may depend on the viral load, host immunity, and host vulnerability.

Generally, viruses are transmitted via respiratory secretions but may also be spread via other bodily fluids, such as blood. They may be passed from host to host via contact, droplets, or aerosolized secretions, all of which necessitate close proximity of an uninfected to infected person. While it is rare, some viruses can live outside of a host on a surface for a small amount of time and be transmitted via non-direct contact.

4.3 SARS-CoV-2

4.3.1 Description

Sars-Cov-2 is a coronavirus that causes COVID-19. It is a positive-sense single-stranded RNA virus which causes respiratory illness in humans [2]. The virus mutates easily, contributing to evolving variants that contribute to its persistent virulence. The SARS-CoV-2 coronavirus has a crown-like shape with glycoprotein spikes (Fig. 4.1). It is a zoonotic virus, meaning it can be transferred from animals to humans and between humans and animals.

4.3.2 Clinical Manifestations

SARS-Cov-2 causes respiratory symptoms and illness including fever, cough, sore throat, shortness of breath, fatigue and body aches, new loss of taste of smell, nausea and vomiting, and diarrhea. Symptoms and illness may range from mild to

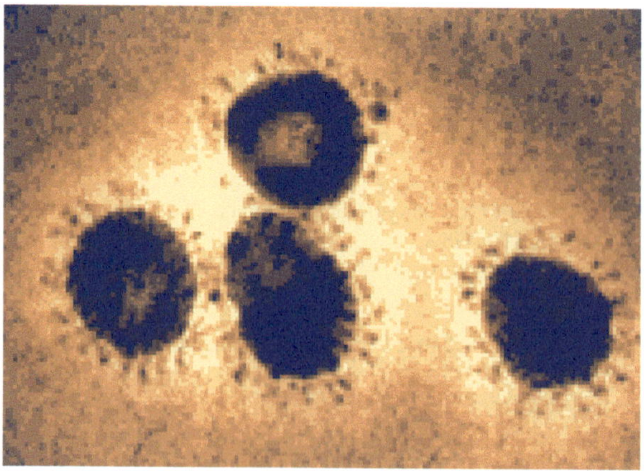

Fig. 4.1 Electron micrograph image of SARS-CoV-2 coronavirus. Notice the spike projections from the virus envelope that give the virus its crown-like appearance. (Source: CDC Image Library: https://www.cdc.gov/sars/lab/images/coronavirus.png)

severe illness and may be worse depending on a person's immune competency. Symptoms may appear 2 days to 14 days after exposure and last for a few days up to a few weeks, or possibly longer which has been termed "long COVID" [3]. Symptoms and illness may be self-limited; however, more severe symptoms may require medical intervention and/or hospitalization [2].

4.3.3 Pathogenesis/Transmission

SARS-Cov-2 is transmitted via respiratory droplets and particles that contain the virus. It is easily transmitted between people and can be very contagious especially within groups of people. SARS-CoV-2 can be spread even by people who have no symptoms but have been infected with the virus. Within dental settings, close proximity to the oral cavity and exposure to droplets and respiratory secretions and particles may expose providers to the virus. However PPE can help mitigate the risk of transmission, and with proper use of PPE, the risk of transmission in dental settings is low.

4.3.4 Treatment

For mild to moderate symptoms with SARS-Cov-2 infection and COVID-19, treatment may be supportive such as rest, fluids, over-the-counter fever-reducing medication, and prescription antiviral medications. For those with more severe illness and symptoms, treatment may include hospitalization with treatment therapies to support breathing and systemic effects and complications of COVID-19 and convalescent plasma [2, 4].

4.3.5 Prevention

Several vaccines have been developed to prevent the spread of SARS-Cov-2 and illness with COVID-19. A single dose or series of initial vaccinations have been approved for people ages 6 months and older for primary prophylaxis from severe SARS-CoV-2 infection. Several booster vaccines have been and are being developed to combat the spread of newer variants of the virus [5]. Due to the rapidly evolving and mutating nature of the virus, booster vaccines help to modulate immune response and build antibody resistance against new virus strains.

4.4 Herpes Simplex Virus (HSV)

Herpesviruses are a large family of viruses that contribute to a broad array of infections and diseases in humans and animals. Herpes simplex virus (HSV) is one of nine herpesviruses known to infect humans and contributes to diseases of oral and genital herpes, the clinical diagnoses of herpes simplex virus 1 and 2 [6]. HSV is a large, enveloped, double-stranded DNA virus. It is common in the United States, infecting 11.9% of people aged 14–49 years for HSV-2 infection [7, 8]. HSV-1 typically infects the oral cavity and has historically been acquired by those infected in childhood. HSV-2 usually presents as clinical genital herpes. However, the prevalence of HSV-1 infections has declined over the last few decades, which has contributed to HSV-1 contributing more to genital herpes.

4.4.1 HSV-1

Description

Herpes simplex virus 1 (HSV-1) is a DNA virus that causes oral and genital herpes. It is highly contagious and has historically been mostly acquired in childhood, though that trend is changing with decreased childhood acquisition but higher prevalence of infection in adulthood.

Clinical Manifestations

HSV-1 typically contributes to oral vesicles and ulcerations, sometimes referred to as "cold sores," but is contributing to genital blisters and lesions with increasing prevalence in recent years. These blisters may be erythematous and somewhat crusty in appearance. They appear as papular vesicles and may occur individually or in clusters (Fig. 4.2).

Pathogenesis/Transmission

HSV-1 can be transmitted through contact with saliva, active sores from an infected person, mucosal or skin contact, or oral sex from someone with active HSV-1 lesions. There does not have to be the presence of active lesions for the transmission of HSV-1, and the virus can be transmitted during viral shedding without the presence of lesions, which occurs approximately 10% of the time [9]. If a person has previously been infected with HSV-2, they can additionally be infected with HSV-1.

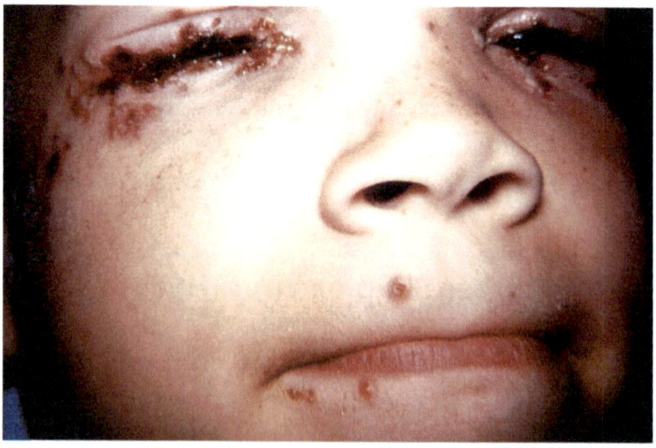

Fig. 4.2 Clinical photograph of a 7 year old child with HSV 1 infection orally and ocularly. (Source: CDC Image Library: https://phil.cdc.gov/Details.aspx?pid=6476)

Treatment and Prevention

There is no cure for herpes infection with HSV-1, but treatment with antiviral medications can help limit symptoms and reduce or prevent new outbreaks. Behavioral and sexual health counseling can be helpful for preventing the spread of herpes, especially among people who are at high risk or participate in risky behaviors, such as unprotected sex with multiple partners.

4.4.2 HSV-2

Description

Similar to HSV-1, HSV-2 is a large, enveloped double-stranded DNA virus that is highly contagious [8]. HSV-2 typically contributes to genital herpetic lesions and infections but can be transmitted to the oral cavity and contribute to oral infection via oral sex.

Clinical Manifestations

Similar to HSV-1, HSV-2 lesions occur as papular-vesicular lesions that typically occur in the genital region but may also present around the rectum or mouth, including oral mucosa, tongue, and the lips [6–8]. These lesions may be individual or clustered and consist of vesicles that rupture and become ulcerated and are painful. Lesions may take between 2 and 4 weeks to heal.

Pathogenesis/Transmission

HSV-2 is generally transmitted by people without active lesions during contact with oral or genital mucosa or skin. The virus can be transmitted without active lesions present when the virus is shedding. However, the most likely and common method of transmission is contact with an active lesion during a viral outbreak [7]. Viral shedding can take place among persons without any active lesions or symptoms approximately 10% of the time [7, 8]. Nonetheless, more likely modes of transmission are via contact with active lesions during symptomatic infection, both via oral contact and genital contact. If a person has previously been infected with HSV-1, they can still be infected with HSV-2, contributing to increased necessity for patient education and mitigation of risk transmission for persons with prior herpetic infections.

Treatment

While there is no cure for herpes, herpetic outbreaks may be limited or shortened by antiviral medications, especially if medications are taken before clinical symptoms occur. Treatment before lesions appear, or during prodromal symptoms, can help limit outbreak recurrences and reduce the duration of clinical symptoms [10]. For symptomatic outbreaks, which can be very painful and visually apparent, topical analgesics and antiviral medications can also help limit the duration and discomfort of outbreaks.

Prevention

There is no vaccine for HSV; however, prevention can be encouraged by patient education, limiting sexual contact with people known to be infected with HSV, as well as behavior counseling to limit sexually risky behaviors, especially among populations who may be at high risk for HSV exposure and infection [6, 11]. Similarly, patient education, awareness of risk factors, methods of transmission, and discussions of risky behaviors can help inform and encourage patients to limit their potential exposure and transmission of herpes viruses.

4.5 Varicella Zoster

4.5.1 Description

Varicella zoster is a type of DNA herpesvirus (known as human herpesvirus 3) that causes the clinical conditions of varicella (chickenpox) and herpes zoster (shingles) [12]. Initial infection with the varicella zoster virus causes the clinical condition of chickenpox, which presents as a pruritic, itchy rash. Following a primary infection with varicella zoster and initial presentation of chickenpox, the virus remains dormant in vitro and can re-present as zoster, or shingles infection. Shingles is an exquisitely painful condition that presents with a similarly pruritic rash along dermatomal planes [13]. While it usually impacts older adults, any person who has been infected with the varicella zoster virus can have a recurrence of herpes zoster and have clinical shingles.

4.5.2 Clinical Manifestations

The classic initial presentation of the varicella zoster virus is the emergency of a pruritic rash all over one's body. After an incubation period of approximately 14–16 days, with a total possible incubation range of 10–21 days, the rash will appear over a person's entire body. The rash is usually the first manifestation of varicella zoster (known as chicken pox), but a mild fever and prodromal symptoms, like malaise, may occur 1–2 days prior [12].

Lesions of the rash usually begin as erythematous macules before they turn to papules and then vesicular, after which point they tend to crust over. Lesions tend to appear first, and most, on the chest and back but do progress to covering the entire body. The rash and concomitant symptoms, including fever, malaise, and itching, last 4–7 days.

Breakthrough varicella, which can occur after vaccination, usually presents with very mild, if any, symptoms, and fewer than 50 macular skin lesions [12].

Herpes zoster, or shingles, presents initially with pain, tingling, or itching in the area, usually a dermatomal plane, where the rash will develop. This may begin up to several days before the rash appears. Some people may develop a fever prior to the rash as well [13].

The classic shingles rash consists of a stripe of a macular rash that will then become papular and vesicular and similarly crust over within about 7–10 days of the rash emergence. Shingles usually occurs in older adults but can affect any person who has had chickenpox. The rash usually occurs unilaterally but may occur on the face. A rash that occurs over the dermatome of the trigeminal nerve can affect the eyes and is considered an emergency, as it can contribute to eye damage and blindness. Shingles usually resolves within 2–4 weeks (Fig. 4.3).

4.5.3 Pathogenesis/Transmission

Varicella zoster is highly contagious and can be spread through respiratory droplets or aerosols from an infected person, direct contact with a vesicular lesion of an infected person, or inhalation of an aerosol or droplet from a vesicular lesion of an

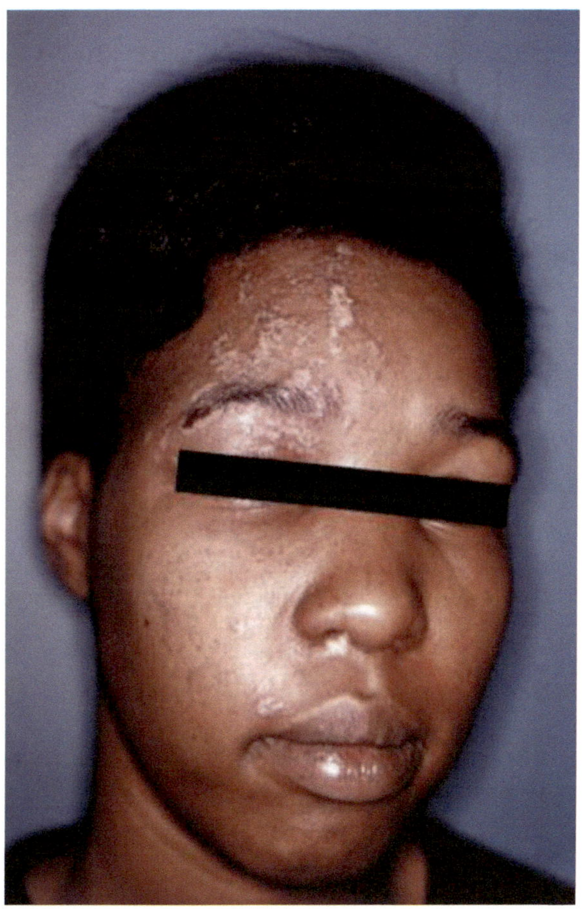

Fig. 4.3 The pustulovesicular rash on this African-American woman's face, represented a herpes outbreak, due to the varicella zoster virus (VZV) pathogen, also known as human herpesvirus 3 (HHV-3), which may lay dormant in the spinal nerve roots throughout a chickenpox-infected individual's life, only manifesting its presence through outbreaks, as shingles, or herpes zoster. It is caused by the *Herpesviridae* chickenpox virus. (Source: CDC, https://phil.cdc.gov/Details.aspx?pid=12621)

acutely infected person [12]. Varicella is contagious beginning 1–2 days before the rash appears and until the vesicular lesions have crusted over.

Similarly, zoster is contagious from contact or inhalation with vesicular fluid from the rash that develops. Unlike varicella (chickenpox), zoster (shingles) cannot be spread through respiratory droplets [13]. Zoster is only infectious once the rash appears, and it is no longer contagious once the rash scabs over. Those who do acquire varicella zoster from contacts with someone with shingles will likely develop chickenpox.

Varicella zoster is highly contagious, with 90% transmission rate when unvaccinated people are exposed to the virus by someone with acute varicella. Due to the longer incubation period of 10–21 days, exposure and illness are not immediately recognized [12].

Chickenpox can be very dangerous for people who have reduced immunity, such as premature babies, those who are immunocompromised, or people with HIV/AIDS.

4.5.4 Treatment

Varicella and zoster are both self-limiting. Treatment for varicella is usually for symptoms control and includes topical ointments, such as calamine lotion, for the itchiness of the rash, as well as cool baths with baking soda or oatmeal to soothe the itching of the full-body rash. Maintaining short fingernails can help mitigate scratching the rash and inflicting epidermal trauma. People, especially children, with chickenpox should not take aspirin as it can lead to an increased risk of Reye's syndrome, a condition which can cause swelling of the liver and brain and can lead to death, especially in children [12].

Antiviral medications may be prescribed for people with chickenpox who are more likely to develop serious and life-threatening diseases, such as pregnant people, people with chronic skin or lung disease, and people who are otherwise immunocompromised. Antiviral medications may also be recommended and prescribed for people who are over 12 and otherwise healthy [12].

Zoster can be treated with antiviral medications, such as acyclovir, valacyclovir, and famciclovir. While the medications do not cure zoster, taking an antiviral can limit the duration and severity of illness. It is best when a medication is started as soon as possible after the rash appears and symptoms begin. To prevent spread of the virus during an active infection of zoster, one should cover the rash [13].

4.5.5 Prevention

There are very safe and effective vaccines for both varicella and zoster. There are two options in the United States for varicella vaccination, Varivax, which contains only chickenpox vaccine, and ProQuad, which is a combination vaccine for measles, mumps, rubella, and varicella (MMR-V). Varivax is approved for people

12 months and older, and ProQuad is approved for children 12 months to 12 years old [14].

Varicella vaccination is recommended for children under 13 years old in a two-dose series. The first dose occurs at age 12–15 months, and the second dose occurs at 4–6 years. The second dose may be administered earlier, as long as it is given more than 3 months after the first dose [14].

For children 13 years and older who have never had chickenpox, vaccination can take place as a two-dose series, with the two doses being administered at least 28 days apart [14]. Varicella vaccination is especially recommended for those who work closely with people, including healthcare personnel; people who work with immunocompromised people; teachers; those who live in communal living environments, such as college dorms; and nonpregnant people of child-bearing age.

Those who are at high risk for chickenpox illness are immunocompromised, have cancer or are undergoing cancer treatment, or have had a recent transfusion of blood products should not be vaccinated.

For people with acute chickenpox, the best means of prevention is limiting contact in close proximity with other people and limiting physical contact with any rash lesions.

A vaccine for zoster, or shingles, is available for healthy adults aged 50 and older, as well as adults 19 years and older who are immunocompromised due to disease or therapy. Shingrix, the zoster vaccine, is recommended to be given in two doses among these populations [15].

4.6 Cytomegalovirus

4.6.1 Description

Cytomegalovirus (CMV) is a very common, widespread virus that can affect and infect people of all ages. It is a herpes virus (herpes virus Type 5) with which approximately 33% of children are infected with by age 5, and approximately 50% of people are infected with by age 40 [16]. Like other viruses, once infected with CMV, the virus remains within a person's body dormant and can reactivate later in life. However, most people infected with CMV have no symptoms and are not aware that they have been infected, as the competent immune system is very adept at managing the virus.

4.6.2 Clinical Manifestations

Most people infected with CMV have no symptoms or signs of infection. However, some people may develop flu-like symptoms upon infection with CMV, including fever, malaise, muscle aches, and a sore throat. CMV is most concerning for infection for people who are immunocompromised or pregnant women, as it can pose a risk to the baby. Congenital CMV is when a baby is born with a CMV infection, and it can present with a rash, jaundice, low birth weight, microcephaly, hearing deficits or loss in one or both ears, and problems with the eyes, liver, or spleen [16, 17].

4.6.3 Pathogenesis/Transmission

CMV is spread through close contact with bodily fluids, including saliva droplets or aerosolized respiratory particles, blood, breast milk, urine, feces, and through sexual contact. However, CMV can only be transmitted during active infection. It is highly transmissible but does not often cause clinical disease.

4.6.4 Treatment

CMV does not require treatment if it is not causing symptoms. Like most viral illnesses, there is no cure for CMV, but for individuals who are at high risk, including babies diagnosed with congenital CMV and those with weakened immune systems, antiviral medications can limit severity and duration of clinical CMV illness [16].

4.6.5 Prevention

Good hygiene practices and primary prevention of disease spread by diligent and frequent hand washing, avoiding close contact with many people, and avoiding prolonged times in crowded places can help limit the spread of CMV. It is always a good practice to avoid contact with people with symptoms of illness or to stay home and isolate if you have symptoms of any illness. There is no vaccine for CMV, but immunity from prior infection can help limit new disease and virus spread.

4.7 HIV/HIV-Associated Pathogens and Opportunistic Infections

4.7.1 Description

HIV (human immunodeficiency virus) is the viral pathogen that contributes to AIDS (acquired immunodeficiency syndrome). HIV is a lentivirus, which is a subgroup of retrovirus, meaning that it inserts the DNA for its RNA into a host cell to effectively take over the cell. HIV infects CD4 lymphocyte immune cells in humans which contributes to significant immune compromise and susceptibility to otherwise less virulent pathogens and clinical illnesses [18]. HIV advances to clinical AIDS when CD4 count drops below 200 cells/mm^3, which is measured via blood test. Most other viruses mentioned within this chapter can become more pathogenic and problematic for people with poorly managed HIV/AIDS, as well as other conditions such as Kaposi's sarcoma and common cold.

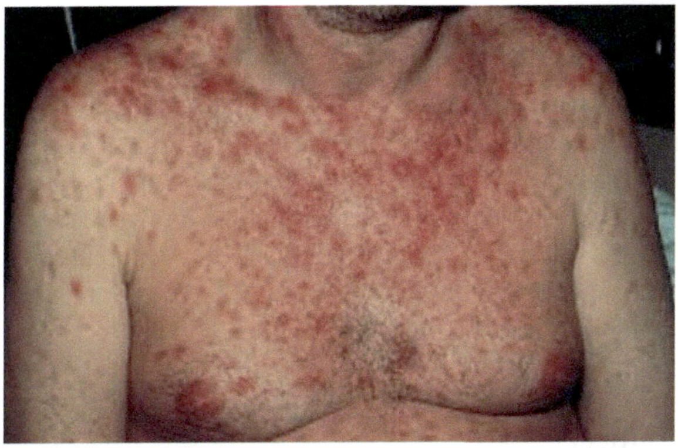

Fig. 4.4 Rash is a common symptom in early HIV, and it can cover the entire body, including the palms, soles, and scalp. The most commonly affected areas are the neck and chest. It is mildly itchy. Rash usually appears 48 hours after the onset of fever and self-resolves in a week's time. The rash usually consists of well-defined red or pink spots. (Source: Image source: U.S. National Library of Medicine/National Institutes of Health, https://stdcenterny.com/hiv-comparison.html)

4.7.2 Clinical Manifestations

Acute infection with HIV presents 2–4 weeks after initial exposure with flu-like symptoms, including malaise, fever, chills, fatigue, sore throat, and a nonspecific macular-papular rash, which may be difficult to differentiate from other viral infections (Fig. 4.4). The symptoms may last days to weeks, as HIV replicates most rapidly upon initial infection, and then replicates as slower rates as time proceeds.

Following the initial presentation of acute HIV, the symptoms diminish, but without appropriate treatment, HIV can progress to AIDS, which can manifest as significant and severe illness secondary to infection from most pathogens. Infection by opportunistic infections, such as CMV, candidiasis, HSV, and Kaposi's sarcoma, to name a few, can also be indications for the diagnosis of progression to AIDS.

4.7.3 Pathogenesis/Transmission

HIV is transmitted via contact with or exposure to blood and sexual fluids from an infected person. HIV is most commonly transmitted through anal or vaginal sex, as well as sharing needles, syringes, or other drug injection equipment. Receptive anal sex poses a 17 times higher risk of HIV transmission than receptive vaginal sex, though either partner can become infected with HIV via unprotected sex [18]. Oral sex carries little risk of HIV transmission. Other lesions, such as active HSV, cuts, or areas of skin abrasion, can lead to an increased risk of transmission. HIV is not transmitted via saliva, urine, or feces.

HIV can be transmitted from a mother to her baby during pregnancy, birth, or breastfeeding. However, with modern HIV treatment and management, the risk of transmission of HIV can be very low.

4.7.4 Treatment

Antiretroviral medications are very effective treatment for HIV and can lower HIV counts to be undetectable, as well as mitigate the progression to clinical AIDS [19]. There are several antiretroviral medications, and they may be administered as a pill or a shot, depending on the status of the infection and viral load or count. Depending on a person's viral load, status of infection, or health, different antiretrovirals may be recommended. There is no cure for HIV, but it is very manageable with current treatments and medications.

4.7.5 Prevention

The most effective ways to prevent the transmission of HIV are avoiding sharing needles and injection equipment, abstaining from sex, and/or practicing safe sex by using condoms and other physical barriers. Limiting sexual partners, practicing safe hygiene and equipment use, and never sharing needles for blood, drug, and injectable products can help mitigate risk of transmission. It is important for individuals to be aware of their HIV status so that they can appropriately assess and manage risk for themselves as well as partners and the community.

Medications can help prevent infection and exposure to HIV with pre-exposure prophylaxis (PrEP) as well as postexposure prophylaxis (PEP) PrEP can be taken routinely by people at high risk for transmission, while PEP must be started within 72 hours after possible exposure [20]. There are also several medical, social, and emotional resources that are widely available to the public to help support communities and individuals who might be at higher risk for HIV transmission and infection. The most important and effective prevention strategy to mitigate HIV transmission and infection is knowledge of how it is transmitted, as well as knowledge of your status [19].

4.8 Measles

4.8.1 Description

Measles (i.e., rubeola) is a RNA virus in the *Paramyxoviridae* family that is highly transmissible via respiratory droplets or direct contact with saliva or nasal secretions of an infected individual. The virus presents with characteristic rash and symptoms of fever, cough, runny nose, and conjunctivitis. Most individuals start to recover in one week's time, but complications in including pneumonia can follow. Fortunately, a vaccine for measles was developed in the 1960s and has prevented many populations from the sequelae of this virus. While measles prevalence in the United States is low due to high vaccination rates, there can be outbreaks due to under-immunized communities. In 2019, close to 1300 cases were reported in the United States. Since then, the number of cases has declined significantly, and only

121 cases were reported in 2022 [21]. Globally, many thousands of cases of measles were reported as part of outbreaks in 2023 [22].

4.8.2 Clinical Manifestations

- The measles virus commonly presents with:
- Acute fever
- The "3 C's": cough, coryza (runny nose), and conjunctivitis
- Koplik's spots: white/blue lesions that appear intraorally on red buccal mucosa (Fig. 4.5)
- An erythematous, flat, maculopapular rash

The measles rash will most often appear several days after the onset of fever, beginning with the face and postauricular area and then spreading to the trunk and extremities. Koplik's spots typically present several days after the onset of symptoms and are pathognomonic for measles (Fig. 4.6).

The duration of symptoms is approximately 1 week. Complications of the respiratory tract are most common, including pneumonia and croup [23]. The virus increases a person's susceptibility to secondary bacterial infections, which may manifest as severe diarrhea, otitis media, or keratoconjunctivitis. Ear involvement

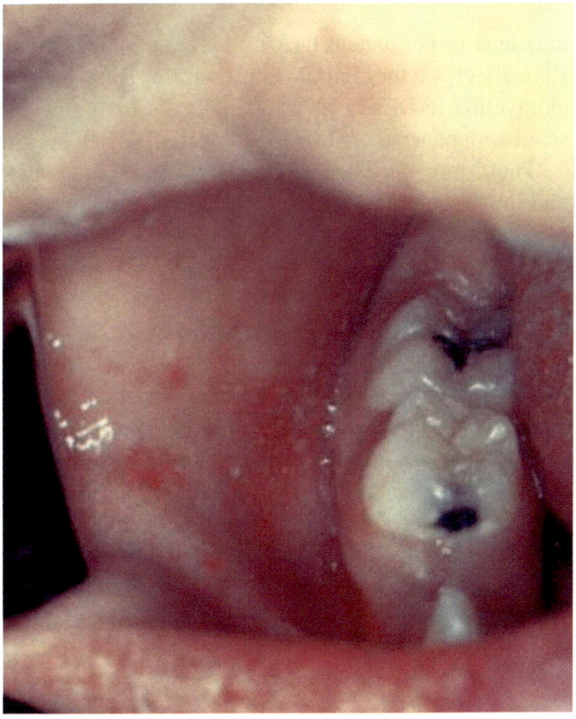

Fig. 4.5 Koplik's spots: white/blue lesions that appear intraorally on red buccal mucosa. (Source: CDC Image Library—https://www.cdc.gov/measles/symptoms/photos.html)

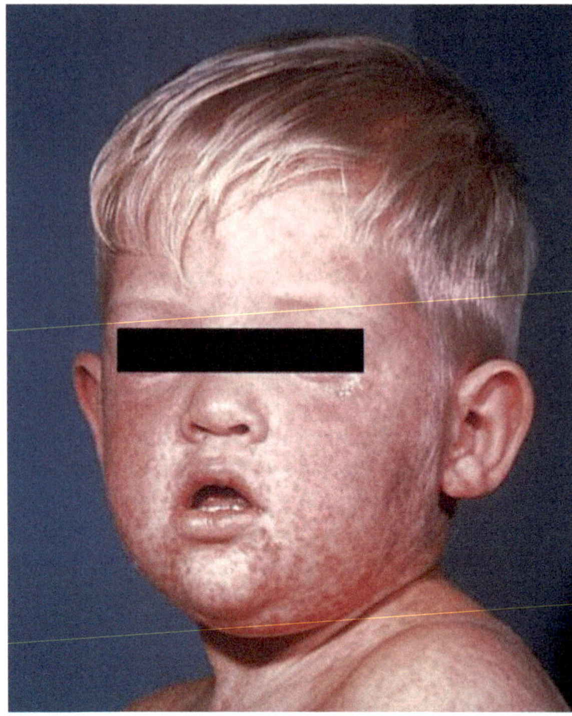

Fig. 4.6 Child with 3-day-old erythematous, flat, maculopapular rash as commonly seen with measles. (Source: CDC Image Library—https://www.cdc.gov/measles/symptoms/photos.html)

may lead to permanent hearing loss, and ocular involvement can cause blindness. Rare effects on the central nervous system may include acute disseminated encephalomyelitis (ADEM), measles inclusion body encephalitis (MIBE), and subacute sclerosing panencephalitis (SSPE), all of which are life-threatening [23].

Those most at risk for complications include very young children, the elderly, and immunocompromised individuals. Pregnant women are also at risk of premature labor and delivery of infants with low birth weight.

4.8.3 Transmission and Pathogenesis

Measles is carried only by humans and there is no asymptomatic carrier state. Transmission of the measles virus is through respiratory droplets that can travel short distances and aerosols that can survive in the air for close to 2 hours [23]. It is highly contagious and will cause infection in 90% of individuals exposed to the virus in a closed space [24]. Infection occurs via the virus' hemagglutinin protein, which binds to cell surface receptors on multiple immune cells including alveolar macrophages or dendritic cells in the respiratory tract. Fusion proteins then allow the virus to infect the host cell's cytoplasm, and these infected cells then carry the virus to lymphoid tissue and epithelial cells [23]. Viremia allows for infection across virtually every organ system in the body, with varying histologic findings including multinucleated cells with eosinophilic nuclear inclusions that are pathognomonic of measles [25].

The virus' incubation period is about 10 days prior to the onset of symptoms. Peak infectiousness occurs several days prior to and several days after a skin rash becomes apparent. Infection does not remain dormant and lifelong immunity follows infection and resolution.

4.8.4 Treatment

A blood test immunoassay to detect IgM antibodies is the most common method to confirm measles infection, although IgM antibodies may not be present in great enough numbers in the initial stages of infection and will only last 6–8 weeks. In the longer term, IgG antibodies are made and will confer immunity against further infection. A throat, nasal, or nasopharyngeal swab or urine sample can also be tested for viral RNA through PCR testing.

Management of measles is supportive and meant to address dehydration and vitamin deficiencies and to treat secondary infections. In children with severe cases of measles, vitamin A supplementation is recommended [26].

No specific measles antiviral medication has been developed, although some other antivirals such as ribavirin have been used to reduce symptom duration and mortality in severe cases [27].

4.8.5 Prevention

Vaccination for measles was introduced in 1963 and has successfully eradicated the virus in most developed countries. Isolated outbreaks occur, however, in unvaccinated communities and call attention to the need for continued awareness and recognition of the presentation of this illness by healthcare providers. The COVID-19 pandemic led to decrease in well-child visits for routine immunizations, which along with the spread of vaccine misinformation has led to the re-emergence of measles in the United States and the most recent measles outbreak in 2019 [28].

Available vaccines include the MMR (measles-mumps-rubella) vaccine and the MMR-V (measles-mumps-rubella-varicella) vaccine. MMR vaccination is recommended by the american academy of pediatrics (AAP) to be administered at age of 12–15 months, with a second dose at age 4–6 years. It is also recommended for adults born after 1957 who do not have evidence of previous vaccination or natural immunity. The MMR-V vaccine can also be given to children as young as 12 months of age and again at age 4–6 years [29]. The MMR-V vaccine should not be given to anyone older than 12 years of age.

4.9 HPV

4.9.1 Description

Human papillomavirus (HPV) is a double-stranded DNA virus that includes over 200 identified genotypes, a subset of which is described as low-risk or high-risk types according to their effect on mucosal epithelial cells. Many of these strains can be transmitted through sexual contact. Current data indicates that over 40 million Americans live with HPV infections, including 13 million adolescents who contract HPV annually [30]. HPV-6 and HPV-11 are known to cause benign mucosal lesions (e.g., respiratory tract papillomas, low-grade cervical cell abnormalities, anogenital warts) [31], whereas HPV-16 and HPV-18 are implicated in the epithelial lesions that lead to squamous cell carcinomas of the head, neck, and/or anogenital tract [32]. Additional strains (HPV-31, HPV-33, HPV-45, HPV-52, and HPV-58) can also be found in HPV-associated cancers. The most common site for HPV-associated cancer in the United States is the cervical, followed by the oropharynx [33]. Genital HPV is the most common sexually transmitted disease in the United States. HPV is responsible for the majority of anogenital cancers, and over 70% of oropharyngeal cancers. Cervical cancer is the fourth leading cause of death in women worldwide, with over 340,000 deaths reported in 2020 [34]. More than 50% of precancerous cervical lesions are attributable to HPV-16 or HPV-18. Comprehensive screening, care, and vaccination to prevent and treat HPV-related cancers are critical to ensure improved health outcomes. The majority of HPV cases, however, are asymptomatic and self-limiting.

4.9.2 Oral Manifestations

Benign oral manifestations:

- Benign squamous cell papillomas (Fig. 4.7).
- Oral condylomas: genital warts (condyloma acuminatum) may also affect oral mucosa, most often on keratinized tissue.

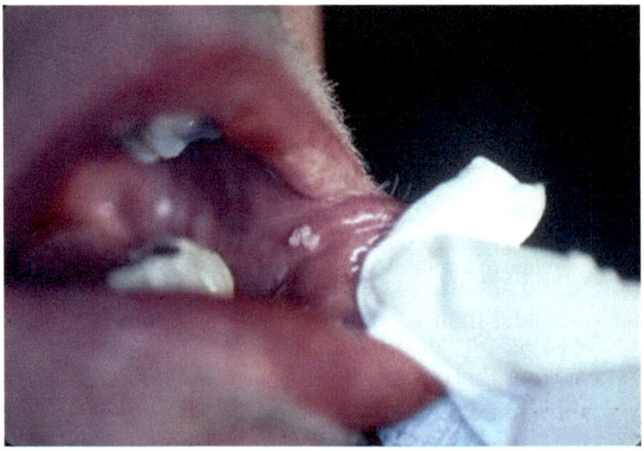

Fig. 4.7 Papilloma on mandibular labial mucosa; note cauliflower-like appearance. (Source: MAAETC, Module 6, Oral Lesions Associated with HIV Disease: Viral & Bacterial, Courtesy of Dr. Valli I. Meeks)

- Verruca vulgaris: lips, hard palate, gingiva.
- Heck's disease (focal epithelial hyperplasia): found in both children and adults, familial disorder with autosomal recessive inheritance.

Recurrent Respiratory Papillomatosis (RRP): Recurrent wart-like tumors occur at the airway, despite surgical excision. Perinatal HPV transmission can cause this presentation in children, leading to life-threatening respiratory sequelae.

Oral squamous cell carcinoma can present with symptoms of sore throat, hoarseness, earaches, lymphadenopathy, dysphagia, hemoptysis, and unexplained weight loss. In the oral cavity, the virus has a preference for the lymphoepithelial tissue found in the lingual and palatine tonsils. Vigilance in screening for symptoms can lead to timely referrals to health professionals to facilitate treatment.

4.9.3 Transmission

Transmission of HPV can occur through both sexual and nonsexual contact. Skin-to-skin, skin-to-mouth, oral sex, and sexual intercourse are all possible routes of transmission. Perinatal transmission is possible and may account for HPV infection in newborns [32]. While most oral HPV infections clear within 6 months and are undetectable within 2 years, the most commonly persistent strain in the oral and oropharynx is HPV-16. Smoking is a risk factor for persistence of oral HPV infection in men, and women with concurrent genital HPV infection may be more likely to have reduced oral clearance of the virus [32]. Additional at-risk populations include those with immunosuppression.

HPV infects the basal cells of epithelium through microabrasions or during wound healing; here, the virus can replicate and remain latent for years. Later, the viral particles are able to switch into a "packagable" state and move beyond the epithelium, where they can activate various growth factors, interfere with apoptosis, and evade the immune response. As the virus integrates into host cells, they can transform host cell chromosomes, causing dysregulation of oncogenes and carcinogenesis [32].

4.9.4 Treatment

Diagnosis of HPV requires testing of the lesion for viral DNA or RNA. Commercial kits are available to identify specific high-risk HPV strains in a biopsied sample.

Treatment of HPV depends on the lesion type and diagnosis. Benign oral lesions may be treated by simple excision. Squamous cell carcinomas may involve adjunctive chemotherapeutics or radiation. Proper clinical examination, thorough history-taking, and detailed histologic report will facilitate an accurate diagnosis and appropriate treatment protocol.

4.9.5 Prevention

An HPV vaccine (Gardasil 9) is available and recommended to prevent infection with high-risk HPV strains [31]. The vaccine is recommended for both males and females at age 11 or 12 years but can be started as early as age 9 years old and is recommended for anyone up through age 26.

A two-dose regimen is recommended for those under age 15 years; if administered at age 15 or beyond, three doses are recommended. It is important to note that the vaccine can prevent, but not treat, a patient currently infected with HPV. However, even in an individual currently carrying HPV infection, it can prevent infection by other strains in the future. Vaccination should be encouraged to prevent oropharyngeal cancer and anogenital cancers in both males and females before they have exposure to the virus and is especially helpful when administered prior to the time an individual becomes sexually active [35]. Use of condoms and other physical barriers during sexual intercourse can also help prevent transmission.

4.10 Monkeypox Virus (MPXV)

4.10.1 Description

MPXV is a double-stranded DNA virus, closely related to smallpox (variola). Monkeypox virus (MPXV) was first described in 1970 in the Democratic Republic of Congo and has historically been endemic to a subset of countries in West and Central Africa. There have been global outbreaks, however, including those in 2003 and again in 2022 in the United States in 2003. MPXV is zoonotic and can also transfer between humans via close contact or through aerosols [36].

4.10.2 Clinical Manifestations

MPXV has a 1- to 2-week incubation period. Symptoms include [37]:

- Fever (often the first symptom)
- Headache
- Muscle aches and body pain
- Lethargy
- Lymphadenopathy
- Skin rash

Lymphadenopathy is an important diagnostic fever that can help distinguish MPVX from other orthopoxviruses. A macular rash first presents on the face, palms, and soles of feet 1–3 days following the onset of fever [37, 38]. The mucosal membranes of the mouth, genitals, and eyes may also be involved. [36–38] The rash will become more papular, vesicular and pustular and may eventually crust over [38]. Most courses are benign, and symptoms typically resolve within 2–4 weeks [38].

Complications may occur and include encephalitis and nausea and vomiting leading to dehydration and electrolyte imbalances [38]. Scarring of lesions may occur, and corneal lesion scarring can cause blindness in rare cases [38]. Tonsillitis, pharyngitis, and bronchopneumonia are documented airway sequelae of monkeypox [36, 38]. Unvaccinated patients, immunosuppressed individuals, and children are more susceptible to severe complications [38]. The fatality rate is low in adults but can reach over 10% in children [39].

4.10.3 Transmission

Unlike smallpox, MPVX infection is zoonotic and can infect animals including rodents, squirrels, and monkeys. In humans, MPVX can be transmitted through contact with infected sores, including those that have crusted over, from inanimate objects such as shared clothes and bedding that has been used by someone with monkeypox, or through the bodily transfer of fluids [40]. The monkeypox virus enters the skin and infects keratinocytes, resulting in ballooning degeneration and inflammation. The virus can then travel to lymph nodes, where it replicates and further spreads to distant organs [36].

Additionally, transfer through aerosols and air-suspended viral particles is possible, and sharing a closed space with an infected individual for longer than 3 hours is a risk for transmission. Perinatal infection is possible, as the virus can pass through the placenta and puts the fetus at higher risk for spontaneous abortion or perinatal death. A recent outbreak among men who have sex with men (MSM) has raised concerns for a sexual mode of transmission as well.

4.10.4 Treatment

Diagnosis of MPXV can be made through a PCR test of a viral swab of vesicles or ulcers [36]. Other diagnostic techniques include cell cultures, electron microscopy, and serologic tests. Antiviral agents, while not specific for monkeypox virus, have shown promise and are effective against smallpox. These agents can decrease lesion formation and symptoms and reduce mortality rates: cidofovir, brincidofovir, and tecovirimat. Additionally, the vaccinia immune globulin (VIG), which uses plasma-derived smallpox antibodies, may be used to reduce viremia and mortality by neutralizing virus particles [40].

4.10.5 Prevention

Due to the risk of zoonotic infection, individuals should avoid direct contact with animals that may carry the virus. Additionally, they should refrain from touching objects that may have been in direct contact with infected animals [40].

Mass vaccination against monkeypox is not currently recommended, but vaccination is recommended for individuals at high risk for monkeypox infection. Two vaccines are currently Food and Drug Administration (FDA)-approved for orthopoxviruses (ACAM2000® and JYNNEOS™). In the clinical setting, contact with affected individuals should be avoided, and universal precautions, including hand washing and sanitization, should take place. The use of personal protective equipment and surface decontamination is essential. For those healthcare workers who must provide urgent care to infected patients, personal protective equipment is essential, and prophylactic vaccination is recommended. Postexposure prophylactic vaccination is recommended by the FDA and Centers for Disease Control and Prevention (CDC) if known exposure has occurred. This should occur within 4–14 days of exposure to avoid development of the disease [38]. Individuals infected with MPXV should remain in quarantine until the lesions have entirely resolved [38].

4.11 Respiratory Syncytial Virus

4.11.1 Description

Human respiratory syncytial virus (RSV) is a single-stranded RNA virus that belongs to the *Pneumoviridae* genus. The RSV virus invades epithelial cells of the respiratory tract, which can lead to a robust innate immune response. Most children have experienced at least one RSV infection by age 2 years [41]. The disease is seasonal, and peak onset and offset depend on geographic location and climate. RSV is the leading cause of lower respiratory tract infections (LRTI) in children under aged 2, and LRTI occurs in 15–50% of infants and young children; 1–3% are hospitalized annually [42, 43]. 80% of LRTIs in infants are due to RSV, and peak age of incidence is 2–3 months old [44].

4.11.2 Clinical Manifestations

Symptoms of RSV range from mild upper respiratory tract illness or otitis media to severe and potentially life-threatening lower respiratory tract involvement, including bronchiolitis, pneumonia, and croup [41]. There are multiple risk factors for severe RSV, of which age is the most significant. Infants and children have smaller airways and decreased respiratory capacity and reserve and are more vulnerable to obstruction than older children and adults [44]. Premature birth prevents transmission of maternal antibodies to the newborn, putting those youngest babies at higher risk for RSV severity. Prematurity of birth, airway anomalies, and comorbidities such as congenital heart defects predispose infected children to increased risk of hospital admission, increased duration of hospital stay, and need for mechanical ventilation [44]. Bronchiolitis in young children may include rhinorrhea, dry wheezy cough, tachypnea, dyspnea, and retractions. Fever may or may not occur. A wheeze and inspiratory crackles may be heard on auscultation [41]. Infants may present with lethargy, irritability, and poor feeding. A chest X-ray may reveal hyperinflation and patchy atelectasis [41]. With subsequent exposures, symptom severity typically decreases, and reinfections are common throughout life. Those children infected with RSV early on, however, are more vulnerable to future morbidities including wheezing, asthma, and increased allergies [42, 43, 45]. In older children and adults, symptoms may be confined to the upper respiratory tract infections (URTI) or absent altogether. Adults at risk for significant LRTI include immunocompromised patients, those with cardiopulmonary disease, neuromuscular conditions, and the elderly [41–43, 45].

4.11.3 Transmission

RSV is transmitted through droplets, often emitted through sneezes and coughs, that contact the eyes, nose or mouth. Auto-innoculation is possible through contact with contaminated objects or skin [44]. Contaminated nonporous surfaces can maintain viable RSV droplets for up to 6 hours [44]. The duration of aerosolized droplet viability is unknown, but transmission through aerosols is also possible. Symptoms are due to the immune response to the virus, which starts with binding of RSV to nasal epithelial host cells [43]. Alveolar macrophages and epithelial cells are activated to release cytokines that recruit additional immune cells (e.g., neutrophils, monocytes, and dendritic cells) to the lung. While essential for the immune response, neutrophils also degranulate and release proteolytic enzymes and reactive oxygen species and encourage mucus production [43]. Reinfections typically result in milder infection due to T cell-mediated responses.

4.11.4 Treatment

Treatment for RSV is palliative and based on symptoms. Analgesics and antipyretics including acetaminophen and ibuprofen are appropriate. Prevention of dehydration through fluid intake is important. Dyspnea or dehydration, particularly in infants and very young children, may require hospital admission for IV fluids, supplemental oxygen, or, in worse-case scenarios, intubation with mechanical ventilation.

4.11.5 Prevention

Universal precautions, proper environmental disinfection, and personal protective equipment are important to spread the risk of aerosol transmission. Anti-RSV antibodies can be passed through the placenta and through breastfeeding to a newborn. Breastfeeding is protective against RSV in infants due to the antibodies, immunomodulators, and anti-inflammatory components found in human milk. For very young children, who are at high risk for severe RSV, there are two monoclonal antibody products available to be administered by intramuscular injection. For children under 8 months, an RSV monoclonal antibody (nirsevimab) was approved by the US Food and Drug Administration (FDA) in 2023 to be administered during or right before infants experiencing their first RSV season. For children between 8 and 19 months of age, nirsevimab is recommended only for those who are at increased risk for severe RSV disease as they enter their second RSV season [46]. These children include those with chronic lung disease of prematurity, immunocompromised conditions, cystic fibrosis with severe lung disease, and/or American Indian and Alaska native children. If nirsevimab is not available, a different monoclonal antibody (palivizumab) may be administered monthly by intramuscular injection during RSV season. Palivizumab has been shown to significantly reduce RSV infection rates and severe respiratory manifestations in premature infants [42]. It is recommended that women in their 32–36th week of pregnancy receive an RSV vaccine right before or during RSV season. Adults above age 60 years are also eligible to receive an RSV vaccine [47].

4.12 Influenza

4.12.1 Description

Influenza is an orthomyxovirus classified according to four types (A, B, C, and D) which causes a contagious respiratory illness known as the flu and infects the nose, throat, and lungs. These viruses circulate in the United States most often in the late fall through early spring. Types A and B are the two most common types that cause seasonal flu in humans. Each type has multiple subtypes due to genetic diversity that leads to different antigenic characteristics and surface proteins (hemagglutinins (H) and neuraminidase (N)). There are currently 18 Type A influenza hemaggluttinin subtypes and 11 neuraminidase subtypes (H1–18 and N1–11), and new virulent strains of Type A are most often implicated in influenza pandemics. The subtypes vary in their infectivity, transmissibility, replication, duration, incubation, severity, mortality, and hospitalization rates. Antigenic shift occurs when two different types of influenza infect the same cell, resulting in a new subtype as occurred with the swine flu or Spanish flu [48]. Since the late 1800s, five antigenic shifts have led to pandemics including the 1918 Spanish flu and the 2009 H1N1 pandemic. Antigenic drift describes genetic mutations that occur in the viral genome over time and explains the need for frequent updating of vaccines to target the most current flu antigens. [48]

The flu is a not a reportable illness in the United States, and the exact prevalence is unknown [49]. Most infected individuals recover without serious complications. Those at risk for severe illness include very young children, pregnant women, those with chronic medical conditions, and the elderly [50]. Estimates from the CDC are that about 8% of Americans get sick from the flu each season [51]. An estimated average of 37,463 flu-associated deaths have occurred annually in the United States between 2010 and 2022 [49].

4.12.2 Clinical Manifestations

Symptoms of the flu include sore throat, runny nose, fever, cough, muscle/body aches, headaches, fatigue, and, in some cases, vomiting and diarrhea [51].

Complications of the flu include moderate sequelae such as sinusitis and otitis media. Severe complications include pneumonia (primary or via secondary bacterial infection), exacerbations of underlying respiratory conditions such as asthma or bronchitis, and death. While pulmonary complications are most common, there can be renal, cardiac, and neurologic sequelae as well. Myocarditis, encephalitis, myositis, and kidney failure are examples, and extreme inflammatory responses can lead to sepsis.

4.12.3 Pathogenesis/Transmission

Influenza is transmitted via respiratory droplets, aerosols, or contaminated objects that are touched prior to touching one's eyes, nose, or mouth. In humans, the flu virus enters the epithelium of the respiratory tract and replicates, destroying host cells. Virus is shed in respiratory secretions for 5–10 days, with a peak contagiousness at days 1–3 [52]. The incubation period for influenza is 1–4 days prior to symptom onset.

4.12.4 Treatment

Diagnosis of influenza virus is based on a PCR test or viral culture of throat secretions. While rapid tests are available, they may have limited sensitivity, and false negatives are common [53]. Antiviral medications are available to treat the flu, either by blocking neuraminidase activity or by impeding viral replication. These drugs, oseltamivir phosphate, zanamivir, peramivir, and baloxavir marboxil, can decrease the duration of flu symptoms and lower the likelihood of pneumonia. These drugs work best when started within a few days of symptoms [53]. Palliative treatment is recommended including analgesics, hydration, and rest. The CDC recommends isolation for at least 24 hours after fever has resolved without the need for antipyretics.

4.12.5 Prevention

Flu vaccines are the best source of prevention. Three influenza vaccine types are currently available in the United States (inactivated influenza vaccine; live, attenuated influenza vaccine; recombinant influenza vaccine). Vaccination is recommended for all persons aged 6 months and older. These vaccines are administered annually to combat decline in antibodies over time and antigenic drift. Vaccination can reduce the risk of flu-related illness by 40–60% in the overall population [52]. Efficacy of flu vaccination is limited by imperfect perfect alignment between the vaccine formulation and the antigen makeup of the current flu strain, previous flu immunity, age, weight, biological sex, and immune status.

4.13 Mumps

4.13.1 Description

Mumps is a paramyxovirus RNA virus that presents with parotid gland pain and swelling. While vaccination has reduced the incidence and severity of symptoms associated with the disease, there are occasional outbreaks even in countries with high vaccination rates. This suggests waning immunity and decreases in antibody production over time and changes in vaccine coverage according to dose and strain used in the formulation [54].

4.13.2 Clinical Manifestations

About one half of individuals remain asymptomatic or have mild respiratory symptoms or fever [54]. Unilateral or bilateral parotitis is a classic sign of mumps infection. There is less commonly swelling of the submandibular or sublingual gland. Other symptoms may include headaches, muscle aches, fatigue, and loss of appetite [55], and these symptoms may precede the parotitis by 3–4 days. Recovery usually occurs in a few weeks, but there are possible sequelae including encephalitis, seizures, cranial nerve palsies, meningitis, hydrocephalus, orchitis, myocarditis, pancreatitis, nephritis, and deafness that can complicate the course of the disease. Orchitis, which occurs in 30% of unvaccinated males and 6% of vaccinated males, can lead to hypofertility and testicular atrophy [56]. The other complications listed above are rare, and there have been no mumps-related deaths reported in recent outbreaks [56].

4.13.3 Pathogenesis/Transmission

Mumps is transmitted in humans via respiratory droplets or oral secretions. The incubation period for mumps ranges from 12 to 25 days postexposure, and parotitis typically occurs 16–18 days after exposure [54]. The virus can be found in the saliva of an infected individual from 7 days before and 8 days after the onset of symptoms [54]. Mumps enters the upper respiratory tract epithelium and grows in glandular epithelium, shedding in saliva. The virus can then spread systemically to other organs.

4.13.4 Treatment

Diagnosis of mumps is made via RT-PCR testing of buccal swabs and viral cultures. Blood testing for IgM antibodies can also be useful to confirm mumps infection. Treatment is palliative to address symptoms. Management includes analgesics, hydration, soft foods, and warm/cool compresses to the face to alleviate painful parotid gland involvement.

4.13.5 Prevention

Mumps vaccination is currently administered in the combination measles-mumps-rubella vaccine and the measles-mumps-rubella-varicella vaccine. Vaccination has significantly reduced the incidence of mumps as well as its complications. After the two-dose MMR vaccine became standard, cases decreased by 99% in the United States [57]. Of the cases that are reported in the United States annually, most occur in vaccinated people. Reinfection is therefore possible, but symptoms are typically milder and shorter in duration in vaccinated individuals. Those diagnosed with mumps should stay isolated until at least 5 days after the onset of parotitis [58].

4.14 Rubella

4.14.1 Description

Rubella, also known as "German measles" is a contagious virus that often causes mild symptoms but can lead to serious birth defects when a pregnant woman becomes infected. Vaccination is available and has largely led to the eradication of rubella in the United States. Lack of worldwide vaccination against rubella, however, has led to its persistence in many other countries and has contributed to the ongoing global burden of this disease.

4.14.2 Clinical Manifestations

25–50% of people with rubella will be asymptomatic [59]. The most common symptom is a characteristic rash that starts on face and spreads to rest of the body, lasting about 3 days. Prodromal symptoms may include fever, headache, conjunctivitis, lymphadenopathy, cough, and coryza [59]. In females, arthritis is a common complication of rubella. Other more rare complications include brain infections and bleeding problems. More concerning are the teratogenic effects of rubella. Rubella is associated with spontaneous abortion and congenital defects including cardiac problems, vision loss, hearing loss, intellectual disability, and liver or spleen damage [60].

4.14.3 Transmission/Pathology

Transmission is via respiratory droplets or perinatally. Individuals are contagious 1 week prior to and after the development of rash. Asymptomatic carriers can still transmit rubella to others.

4.14.4 Treatment

There are no antivirals currently available for treatment of rubella. Treatment is palliative to manage hydration, pain, and fever.

4.14.5 Prevention

Rubella vaccination is currently administered in the combination measles-mumps-rubella vaccine and the measles-mumps-rubella-varicella vaccine. One dose of the MMR vaccine is 97% effective in preventing rubella [61]. Thanks to vaccination, rubella has been eradicated in the United States.

References

1. Kutter JS, Spronken MI, Fraaij PL, Fouchier RA, Herfst S. Transmission routes of respiratory viruses among humans. Curr Opin Virol. 2018;28:142–51. https://doi.org/10.1016/j.coviro.2018.01.001.
2. Centers for Disease Control and Prevention. About COVID-19. Updated 10 Jul 2023. https://www.cdc.gov/coronavirus/2019-ncov/your-health/about-covid-19.html. Accessed 15 Oct 2023.
3. Centers for Disease Control and Prevention: symptoms of COVID-19. Updated 26 Oct 2022. https://www.cdc.gov/coronavirus/2019-ncov/symptoms-testing/symptoms.html. Accessed 1 Nov 2023.
4. Centers for Disease Control and Prevention. COVID-19 treatments and medications. Updated 4 Oct 2023. https://www.cdc.gov/coronavirus/2019-ncov/your-health/treatments-for-severe-illness.html. Accessed 1 Nov 2023.
5. Centers for Disease Control and Prevention. SARS-CoV-2 variant classifications and definitions. Updated 1 Sept 2023. https://www.cdc.gov/coronavirus/2019-ncov/variants/variant-classifications.html#anchor_1632237683347. Accessed 23 Oct 2023.
6. Centers for Disease Control and Prevention. Genital herpes—CDC detailed fact sheet. https://www.cdc.gov/std/herpes/stdfact-herpes-detailed.htm. Accessed 10 Oct 2023.
7. McQuillan G, Kruszon-Moran D, Flagg EW, Paulose-Ram R. Prevalence of herpes simplex virus type 1 and type 2 in persons aged 14–49: United States, 2015–2016. NCHS data brief, no 304. Hyattsville: National Center for Health Statistics; 2018.
8. Cliffe A, Chang L, Colgrove R, Knipe DM. Herpes simplex virus. In: Reference module in biomedical sciences. Waltham: Elsevier; 2014. https://doi.org/10.1016/B978-0-12-801238-3.00080-5.
9. Mertz GJ. Asymptomatic shedding of herpes simplex virus 1 and 2: implications for prevention of transmission. J Infect Dis. 2008;198(8):1098–100.
10. Centers for Disease Control and Prevention. Genital herpes treatment and care. Updated 8 Dec 2021. https://www.cdc.gov/std/herpes/treatment.htm. Accessed 21 Oct 2023.
11. Centers for Disease Control and Prevention. Clinical prevention guidance. Updated 22 Jul 2021. https://www.cdc.gov/std/treatment-guidelines/clinical.htm. Accessed 23 Oct 2023.
12. Centers for Disease Control and Prevention. Chickenpox (varicella). Updated 21 Oct 2022. https://www.cdc.gov/chickenpox/hcp/index.html. Accessed 10 Oct 2023.
13. Centers for Disease Control and Prevention. Shingles (herpes zoster). Updated 10 May 2023. https://www.cdc.gov/shingles/about/symptoms.html. Accessed 10 Oct 2023.

14. Centers for Disease Control and Prevention. Chickenpox (varicella)- prevention and treatment. Updated 28 Apr 2021. https://www.cdc.gov/chickenpox/about/prevention-treatment.html. Accessed 11 Nov 2023.
15. Centers for Disease Control and Prevention. Shingles (herpes zoster)—prevention and treatment. Updated 10 May 2023. https://www.cdc.gov/shingles/about/treatment.html. Accessed 11 Nov 2023.
16. Kaye KM. Cytomegalovirus (CMV) infection. Merck manual. Published September 2022. https://www.merckmanuals.com/professional/infectious-diseases/herpesviruses/cytomegalovirus-cmv-infection?query=Cytomegalovirus%20(CMV)%20Infection
17. Cytomegalovirus. NHS. Published 20 Jul 2023. Accessed 1 Nov 2023. https://www.nhs.uk/conditions/cytomegalovirus-cmv/
18. CDC: HIV. Updated 30 Jun 2022. https://www.cdc.gov/hiv/basics/whatishiv.html. Accessed 3 Nov 2023.
19. HIV and AIDS: the basics. NIH. Updated 25 Jul 2023. https://Hivinfo.Nih.Gov/Understanding-Hiv/Fact-Sheets/Hiv-and-Aids-Basics. Accessed 3 Nov 2023.
20. Centers for Disease Control and Prevention. HIV—other HIV prevention methods. Updated 13 May 2021. https://Www.Cdc.Gov/Hiv/Basics/Hiv-Prevention/Other-Methods.Html. Accessed 1 Nov 2023.
21. Centers for Disease Control and Prevention. Measles cases and outbreaks. Centers for Disease Control and Prevention, 3 Nov 2023. https://www.cdc.gov/measles/cases-outbreaks.html. Accessed 14 Nov 2023.
22. Centers for Disease Control and Prevention. Global measles outbreaks. Centers for Disease Control and Prevention, 19 Oct 2023. https://www.cdc.gov/globalhealth/measles/data/global-measles-outbreaks.html
23. Moss WJ. Measles. Lancet. 2017;390(10111):2490–502. https://doi.org/10.1016/S0140-6736(17)31463-0.
24. Pinkbook: Measles | CDC. 21 Sept 2022. https://www.cdc.gov/vaccines/pubs/pinkbook/meas.html
25. Klassen-Fischer MK, et al. The reemergence of measles. Am J Clin Pathol. 2023;159(1):81–8. https://doi.org/10.1093/ajcp/aqac124.
26. Stinchfield PA, Orenstein WA. Vitamin A for the management of measles in the United States. Infect Dis Clin Pract. 2020;28:181. https://api.semanticscholar.org/CorpusID:225564081
27. Bichon A, et al. Case report: ribavirin and vitamin A in a severe case of measles. Medicine. 2017;96(50):e9154. https://doi.org/10.1097/MD.0000000000009154.
28. Hübschen JM, et al. Measles. Lancet. 2022;399(10325):678–90. https://doi.org/10.1016/S0140-6736(21)02004-3.
29. https://publications.aap.org/redbook/pages/Immunization-Schedules. Accessed 14 Nov 2023.
30. Centers for Disease Control and Prevention. Human papillomavirus (HPV) infection. Centers for Disease Control and Prevention, 10 Feb 2023. https://www.cdc.gov/hpv/parents/about-hpv.html
31. Pinkbook | HPV | Epidemiology of vaccine preventable diseases | CDC. 21 Sept 2022. https://www.cdc.gov/vaccines/pubs/pinkbook/hpv.html
32. Syrjänen S. Oral manifestations of human papillomavirus infections. Eur J Oral Sci. 2018;126(S1):49–66. https://doi.org/10.1111/eos.12538.
33. Cleveland JL, et al. The connection between human papillomavirus and oropharyngeal squamous cell carcinomas in the United States. J Am Dent Assoc. 2011;142(8):915–24. https://doi.org/10.14219/jada.archive.2011.0298.
34. Human papillomavirus (HPV). https://www.who.int/teams/health-product-policy-and-standards/standards-and-specifications/vaccine-standardization/human-papillomavirus. Accessed 14 Nov 2023.
35. Guadiana D, et al. Oral health care professionals recommending and administering the HPV vaccine: understanding the strengths and assessing the barriers. PLoS One, edited by Giovanni Delli Carpini. 2021;16(3):e0248047. https://doi.org/10.1371/journal.pone.0248047.

36. Hamdana AH, et al. Monkeypox virus and other emerging outbreaks: an overview and future perspective. Inquiry. 2023;60:004695802311754. https://doi.org/10.1177/00469580231175437.
37. Sookaromdee P, Wiwanitkit V. Mouth sores and monkeypox: a consideration. J Stomatol Oral Maxillofac Surg. 2022;123(6):593–4. https://doi.org/10.1016/j.jormas.2022.06.020.
38. Ghazanfar A. Epidemiology, clinical features, diagnosis and management of monkeypox virus: a clinical review article. Cureus. 2022;14(8):e28598.
39. Farasani A. Monkeypox virus: future role in human population. J Infect Public Health. 2022;15(11):1270–5. https://doi.org/10.1016/j.jiph.2022.10.002.
40. Malik S, et al. Recent developments in Mpox prevention and treatment options. Vaccine. 2023;11(3):500. https://doi.org/10.3390/vaccines11030500.
41. Borchers AT, et al. Respiratory syncytial virus—a comprehensive review. Clin Rev Allergy Immunol. 2013;45(3):331–79. https://doi.org/10.1007/s12016-013-8368-9.
42. Messina A, et al. New strategies for the prevention of respiratory syncytial virus (RSV). Early Hum Dev. 2022;174:105666. https://doi.org/10.1016/j.earlhumdev.2022.105666.
43. Langedijk AC, Bont LJ. Respiratory syncytial virus infection and novel interventions. Nat Rev Microbiol. 2023;21(11):734–49. https://doi.org/10.1038/s41579-023-00919-w.
44. Kaler J, et al. Respiratory syncytial virus: a comprehensive review of transmission, pathophysiology, and manifestation. Cureus. 2023;15:e36342. https://doi.org/10.7759/cureus.36342.
45. Bozzola E, et al. Respiratory syncytial virus pediatric hospitalization in the COVID-19 era. Int J Environ Res Public Health. 2022;19(23):15455. https://doi.org/10.3390/ijerph192315455.
46. Nirsevimab Administration. https://www.aap.org/en/patient-care/respiratory-syncytial-virus-rsv-prevention/nirsevimab-administration/. Accessed 14 Nov 2023.
47. RSV vaccine information statement | CDC. 19 Oct 2023. https://www.cdc.gov/vaccines/hcp/vis/vis-statements/rsv.html
48. CDC. How flu viruses can change. Centers for Disease Control and Prevention, 12 Dec 2022. https://www.cdc.gov/flu/about/viruses/change.htm
49. CDC. Burden of influenza. Centers for Disease Control and Prevention, 4 Oct 2022. https://www.cdc.gov/flu/about/burden/index.html
50. Grohskopf LA. Prevention and control of seasonal influenza with vaccines: recommendations of the advisory committee on immunization practices—United States, 2023–24 influenza season. MMWR Recomm Rep. 2023;72:1. https://doi.org/10.15585/mmwr.rr7202a. www.cdc.gov
51. CDC. Key facts about influenza (flu). Centers for Disease Control and Prevention, 2 May 2023. https://www.cdc.gov/flu/about/keyfacts.htm
52. Pinkbook: Influenza | CDC. 22 Sept 2022. https://www.cdc.gov/vaccines/pubs/pinkbook/flu.html
53. Diagnosing flu | CDC. 3 Oct 2022. https://www.cdc.gov/flu/symptoms/testing.htm
54. Su S-B, et al. Current status of mumps virus infection: epidemiology, pathogenesis, and vaccine. Int J Environ Res Public Health. 2020;17(5):1686. https://doi.org/10.3390/ijerph17051686.
55. Centers for Disease Control and Prevention. Mumps | Signs and symptoms | CDC. Centers for Disease Control and Prevention, 8 Mar 2021. https://www.cdc.gov/mumps/about/signs-symptoms.html
56. Centers for Disease Control and Prevention. Mumps complications | CDC. Centers for Disease Control and Prevention, 8 Mar 2021. https://www.cdc.gov/mumps/about/complications.html
57. Centers for Disease Control and Prevention. Mumps | For healthcare providers | CDC. Centers for Disease Control and Prevention, 9 Sept 2021. https://www.cdc.gov/mumps/hcp.html
58. Centers for Disease Control and Prevention. Mumps | Transmission | CDC. Centers for Disease Control and Prevention, 8 Mar 2021. https://www.cdc.gov/mumps/about/transmission.html
59. Rubella signs and symptoms | CDC. 20 Jul 2021. https://www.cdc.gov/rubella/about/symptoms.html
60. Rubella complications | CDC. 23 Nov 2022. https://www.cdc.gov/rubella/about/complications.html
61. Centers for Disease Control and Prevention. Rubella vaccination | CDC. 8 Sept 2022. https://www.cdc

Standard, Contact, Droplet, and Airborne

5

Patricia E. Meehan and Oksana Mishler

5.1 Introduction

For an infection to occur, an infectious agent, a susceptible individual, and a route of transmission *all* must be in place. There are numerous ways to transmit a pathogen to a susceptible host (Fig. 5.1). Considering that infections can be spread by touch, spraying or splashing, inhaling, or sharp injuries, the most common paths of transmission in dental settings are via contact with contaminated environmental surfaces, including dental equipment and instruments, aerosolization, and direct contact with contaminated water and bodily fluids [1].

To minimize the spread of infections in healthcare settings in general and dental settings in particular, two tiers of precautions have been established: Standard Precautions and Transmission-Based Precautions (Fig. 5.2) [2]. Standard Precautions, as the name suggests, are used for *all* patients, symptomatic or asymptomatic. Transmission-Based Precautions are used in addition to Standard Precautions for patients with known or suspected infections [2].

5.2 Standard Precautions

5.2.1 Evolution

Standard Precautions is a relatively new concept in the realm of infection control practices. Although it was first introduced in 1996, the predecessor to Standard Precautions, the *Isolation Technique for Use in Hospitals* documents, dates back to

P. E. Meehan · O. Mishler (✉)
Department of Advanced Oral Sciences and Therapeutics, The University of Maryland School of Dentistry, Baltimore, MD, USA
e-mail: PMeehan@umaryland.edu; OMishler@umaryland.edu

L. DePaola et al. (eds.), *Infection Control in the Dental Office in the Era of COVID-19*, https://doi.org/10.1007/978-3-031-64611-9_5

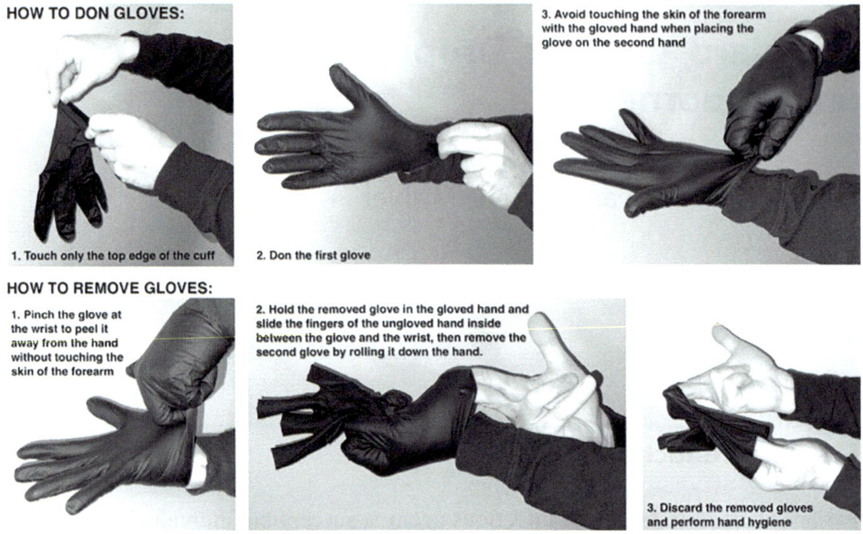

Fig. 5.1 Routes of transmission. Centers for Disease Control and Prevention. (Adapted from *Infection control in the dental office: a global perspective* (DePaola and Grant, November 2019))

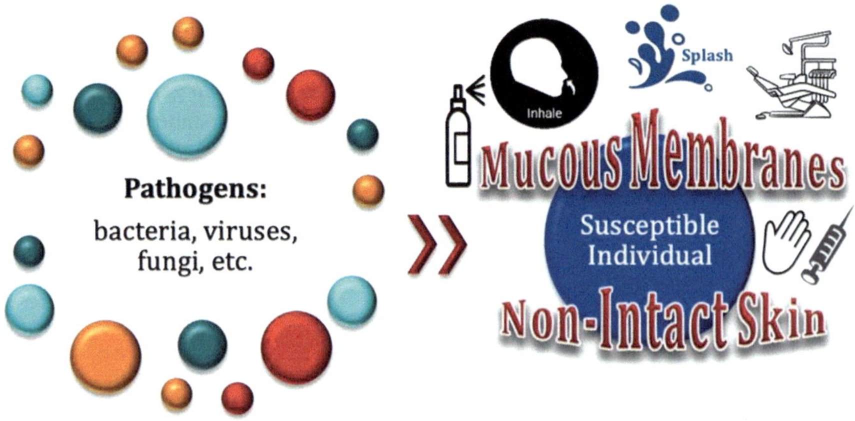

Fig. 5.2 Two tiers of infection control. Centers for Disease Control and Prevention. (Adapted from Infection control in the dental office: a global perspective (DePaola and Grant, November 2019))

1970s [3]. These documents introduced the system of isolation precautions, with each category containing a specific set of recommendations as determined by the route of transmission (Fig. 5.3):

- Strict isolation
- Respiratory isolation

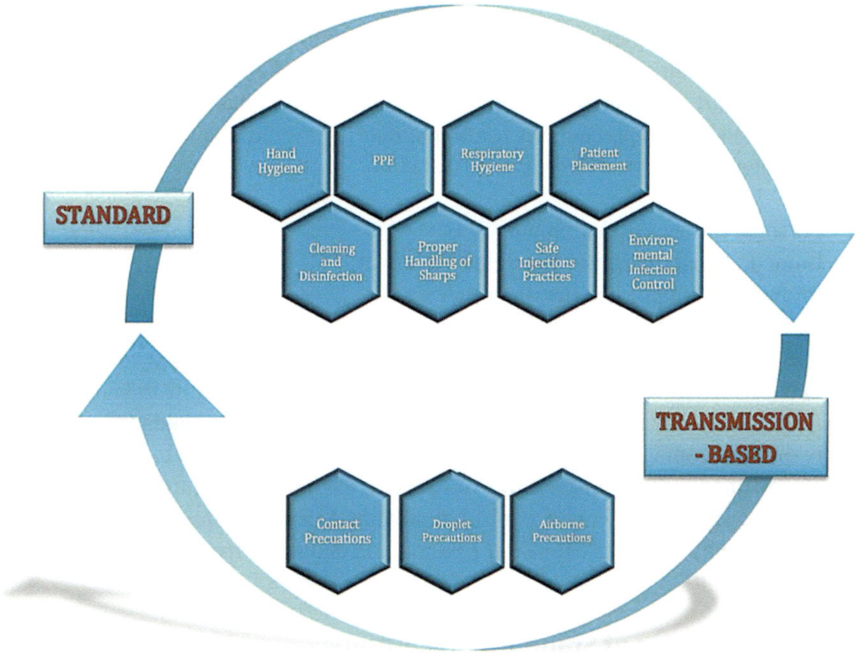

Fig. 5.3 Evolution of standard precautions. Centers for Disease Control and Prevention. (Adapted from *Infection control in the dental office: a global perspective* (DePaola and Grant, November 2019))

- Enteric isolation
- Protective isolation
- Wound and skin precautions
- Discharge precautions
- Blood precautions [3].

It was not until 1983 when the first official *CDC Guideline for Isolation Precautions in Hospitals* emerged, grouping isolation precautions into category-specific and disease-specific procedures [3]. Unlike the 1970s document, this guideline emphasized decision-making by healthcare providers and updated isolation precautions categories:

- Strict isolation
- Respiratory isolation
- Enteric isolation
- AFB
- Contact
- Drainage/secretion
- Blood and body fluids [3]

Discovery of the acquired immune deficiency syndrome (AIDS) in early 1980s posed some new challenges to the ongoing evolution of the infection control practices and procedures. With disease etiology in mind, the CDC published the new infection control standards, *Universal Precautions*, to emphasize the application of blood and body fluid precautions for *all* patients [3]. Additional safety practices that were added to *Universal Precautions* were:

- Personal protective equipment (PPE)
- Immediate handwashing after glove removal
- Proper handling of needles and other sharps

Even though *Universal Precautions* dictated application of blood and body fluid precautions regardless of patient's infectious status, it was not until 1987—when the *body substance isolation* precautions emerged—that *all* bodily fluids, except sweat, were deemed contagious regardless of presence of blood [3]. And in 1996, applying emerging knowledge of disease transmission to the infection control and prevention guidelines, the new infection control standards, known as *Standard Precautions*, were formed by merging *Universal Precautions* and the *body substance isolation*.

5.2.2 Principles of Standard Precautions

Standard Precautions is a set of safe practices that aim to prevent pathogens from reaching a susceptible individual. These safe practices, listed below, are required at a minimum in every clinical situation at all times during patient care:

- *Hand Hygiene* to remove dirt, organic materials, or microorganisms [4]
- *Personal Protective Equipment* to cover one's clothes, skin, or mucous membranes [5]
- *Respiratory Hygiene* to prevent dispersing potentially infectious secretions into the air via coughs and sneezes
- *Patient Placement* to isolate individuals with known or suspected infection
- *Cleaning and Disinfection* of surfaces, equipment, and instruments
- *Proper Handling of Sharps* to prevent related injuries
- *Safe Injection Practices* to protect patients and providers
- *Environmental Infection Control* to prevent the spread of infection outside of a healthcare facility

5.2.3 Hand Hygiene

Considering that the most common mode of transmission of pathogens to a susceptible individual is hands, hand hygiene is one of the most effective ways to prevent the spread of diseases [6]. Hand hygiene is an umbrella term for handwashing, use of alcohol-based hand rub, and surgical hand hygiene antisepsis.

Specific to handwashing, it should be noted that the soap—either regular or antimicrobial—must be applied to *wet* hands and scrubbed for 15–20 seconds before rinsing off under clean, running water [6]. For best handwashing practices, all surfaces—the backs of the hands, between the fingers, and under the nails—should be thoroughly cleaned and well dried, as pathogens can be transmitted more easily to and from wet hands [7]. In healthcare settings, it is recommended to dry hands with disposable towels and avoid adding soap to partially empty refillable soap dispensers to prevent bacterial contamination, as refillable soap dispensers are prone to extrinsic bacterial contamination [8]. Relevant to dental settings, all jewelry, including watches, must be removed prior to handwashing, and providers' fingernails should be trimmed to approximately 1/4 inch and filed to eliminate sharp edges [9].

When soap and water are not readily available, alcohol-based hand rubs—containing at least 60% alcohol—may be used. Although, easily accessible and conveniently located, it is important to note that hand rubs may not remove all pathogens and are less effective when hands are visibly soiled [6]. Therefore, for effective disease prevention practices, visibly soiled hands must be washed with soap and water. Figure 5.4 summarizes the recommendations for performing hand hygiene in dental settings.

It is important to note that the abovementioned general guidelines and dentistry-specific recommendations for hand hygiene are relevant to routine dental procedures. Additional steps and specific modifications must be incorporated into hand hygiene practices prior to surgical procedures. A step-by-step surgical hand antisepsis is summarized in Fig. 5.5, along with the recommended technique for routine hand hygiene. One of the most notable differences in performing routine handwashing, as compared to surgical hand antisepsis, is the selection of soap. For routine handwashing either regular or antimicrobial soap is acceptable. For surgical hand antisepsis, however, providers must use *antimicrobial* soap, with a longer contact time [10].

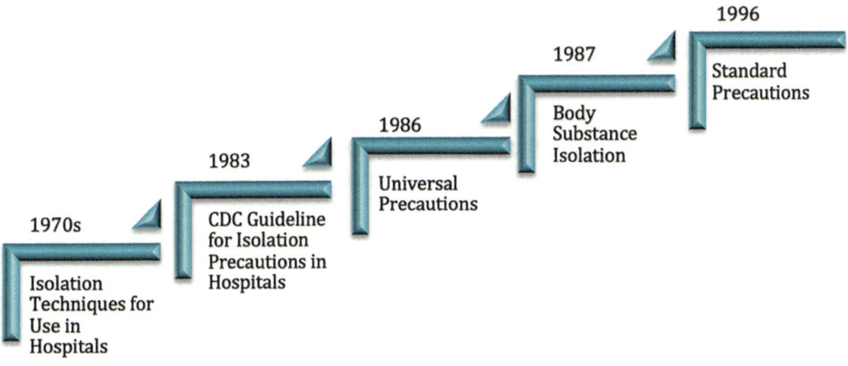

Fig. 5.4 Hand hygiene in dental settings. Centers for Disease Control and Prevention. (Adapted from *Infection control in the dental office: a global perspective* (DePaola and Grant, November 2019))

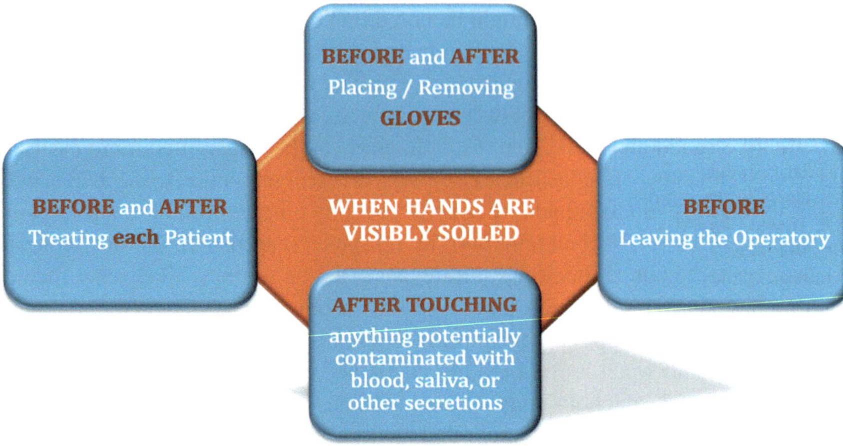

Fig. 5.5 Hand hygiene technique. Centers for Disease Control and Prevention. (Adapted from *Infection control in the dental office: a global perspective* (DePaola and Grant, November 2019))

Although hand hygiene is imperative for disease control and prevention, frequent handwashing or use of antiseptics can contribute to developing dry skin, can cause severe skin reactions, and can lead to irritant contact dermatitis [11]. To avoid these unfortunate consequences, without compromising adequate hand hygiene practices, it is important to incorporate hand lotions or creams into daily routine.

There are other aspects of hand hygiene that must be considered for preventing the transmission of infectious agents in healthcare settings: gloves and fingernails. As previously mentioned, for the best infection control practices, fingernails should be kept short, and healthcare provider involved in direct patient care with patients at high risk should avoid wearing artificial nails or extensions and be mindful of nail polish. As evidence suggests, chipped nail polish or artificial nails can harbor pathogens that cannot be effectively removed by handwashing [12].

Even though the literature is lacking evidence regarding wearing rings in healthcare settings, it seems logical to assume that hand and wrist jewelry could potentially compromise the structural integrity of gloves, putting both, patients and providers, at risk for disease transmission. It seems common knowledge to change gloves between patients and not wash gloves between uses. However, healthcare providers should be reminded that they must also change gloves during patient care when moving from a contaminated site to a clean site within the same patient or environment [4].

5.2.4 Personal Protective Equipment

Taking into consideration the close proximity between dental providers and patients during dental treatments and the fact that dental services take place within the oral cavity, both, dental providers and dental patients are at high risk for transmitting *and* acquiring harmful pathogens. To prevent the spread of infections in dental settings, dental providers can take extra precautions to protect themselves and their patients from infectious agents. By covering their skin, airways, mucous membranes, and clothing, dental providers can reduce the risk of transmitting pathogens to and from patients and other individuals in dental settings.

The barriers that are used to protect healthcare providers' skin, mucous membranes, airways, and clothing are defined as personal protective equipment (PPE). In dental settings, the most common PPE include:

- Gloves
- Face masks
- Protective eyewear
- Face shields
- Protective clothing [13]

Gloves

The types of gloves that are most frequently used in dental settings are:

- Non-sterile examination gloves for nonsurgical procedures
- Sterile surgical gloves
- Heavy-duty utility gloves for handling used instruments as part of cleaning and disinfection

In addition to direct patient care, gloves should be worn during situations when in contact with non-intact skin, mucous membranes, blood or bodily fluids, or other potentially infectious materials—such as removable dental prostheses—which is anticipated [13]. Wearing gloves can prevent transmission between providers and patients. It can also reduce the risk of pathogen dissemination outside of dental settings and thereby environmental contamination. Although effective in preventing the spread of infections, gloves do not provide complete protection against hand contamination [14]. Harmful pathogens can gain access to provider's hands via small defects in gloves or during improper glove removal. Thus, providers should perform hand hygiene *immediately* after removing used gloves and avoid touching the outside surface of the glove with bare hands during removal. Similarly, when putting on gloves, providers should avoid contact with the skin by touching *only* the top edge of the glove cuff [14]. Please refer to Diagram 5.1 for proper donning and doffing of gloves.

Face Masks/Respirators

While the purpose for using masks in healthcare settings remains the same—to protect provider's nasal and oral cavities from harmful pathogens—the types of masks deemed safe in dental settings underwent multiple modifications during and immediately after the COVID-19 pandemic. Although the CDC recommendations can change as new scientific evidence emerge, the current recommendation

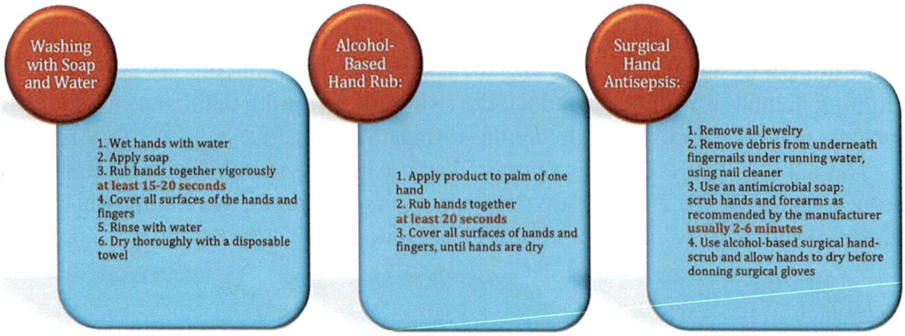

Diagram 5.1 Donning on and doffing off non-sterile exam gloves. (Courtesy of Okasan Mishler, Oksana P. Mishler, RDH, MS, DHS; School of Dentistry University of Maryland)

regarding masks and respirators suggests wearing the most protective, well-fitted yet comfortable mask or respirator during patient care [15].

When considering which type of mask or respirator to wear, healthcare providers should take into consideration the level of protection. As a general rule, KN95 provides more protection than surgical masks, with National Institute for Occupational Safety and Health (NIOSH)-approved respirators, inclusive of N95, providing the highest level of protection [15]. While masks and respirators offer a different level of protection, masks are intended to *contain* droplets and particles, and respirator—additionally—to *filter out* particles, proper fit remains the most important criteria. Ensuring that your mask or respirator fits closely on the face will provide additional level of protection against pathogens and prevent the spread of infections [15].

Protective Eyewear/Face Protection

For continuous protection of mucous membranes, especially during aerosol-generated procedures or situations when splashes or sprays of blood or other potentially infectious materials are anticipated, eye protection is strongly recommended [16]. There is a wide variety of protective eyewear: safety glasses, goggles, face shields, and full-face respirators. While full-face respirators are least common in dental settings, let us review the advantages and drawbacks of safety glasses, goggles, and face shields.

Safety glasses are the most common terminology used in dental settings in reference to protective eyewear. However, safety glasses, unlike appropriately fitted goggles, do not provide the same level of splash or droplet protection and should not be used alone for infection purposes [16]. Properly fitted goggles with a manufacturer's antifog coating are the most reliable eyewear against splashes, sprays, and respiratory droplets. For the best eye protection, goggles must fit snugly, especially from the corners of the eyes across the eyebrow [16].

Face Shields

While face shields have always been part of the recommended PPE in dental settings, their use has noticeably increased since the COVID-19 pandemic. Although face shields are commonly considered as an alternative to goggles, unlike goggles, face shields protect other areas of the face from splashes and sprays [16]. When healthcare providers are performing procedures that may result in face coverings become wet or soiled—which ultimately reduces the ability to provide adequate protection to oral and nasal cavities—face shields should be added as an *additional* layer of protection, not to replace face covering. It should also be noted that not all face shields provide the same level of protection. For optimal infection control practices, face shields should be chin length, have crown, and wrap around the entire face, from ear to ear [16].

Protective Clothing

In the same realm of disease prevention, to disrupt the spread of infections inside and outside of dental settings, protective clothing should be worn in situations when contact with blood, bodily fluids, or other potentially infectious materials is anticipated [13]. Protective garments should cover personal clothing and skin that cannot be covered with other PPE. Protective gowns or jackets should be fully buttoned from neck to the mid-thigh, with sleeves long enough to cover the forearms [17]. While they can be disposable or reusable, protective clothing must be changed when visibly soiled and removed before leaving the work area.

Additional Considerations for Use of PPE

Placing and removing PPE should be done in a sequence to prevent the further spread of potentially infectious pathogens or materials (Fig. 5.6).

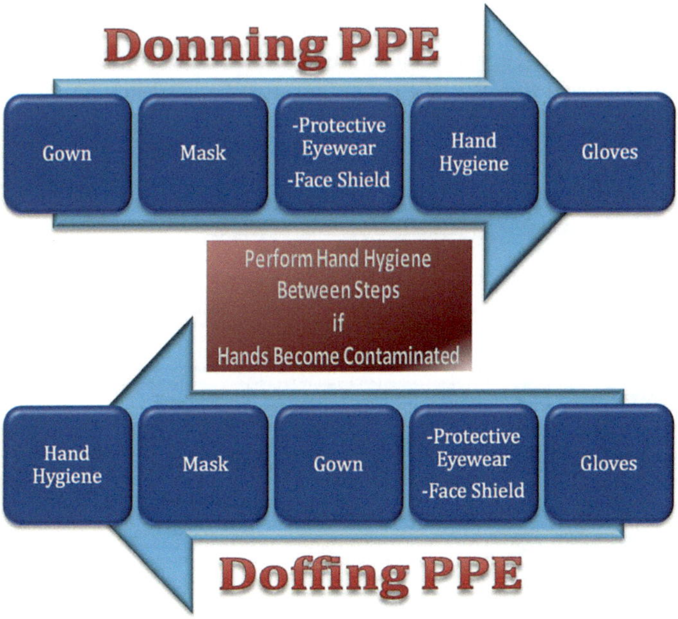

Fig. 5.6 Sequence of placing and removing PPE (CDC, n.d.). (Adapted from *Infection control in the dental office: a global perspective* (DePaola and Grant, November 2019))

Additional precautions that dental providers should keep in mind when wearing PPE:

- Keep hands away from face.
- Avoid touching surfaces.
- Work from "clean" to "dirty."
- Provide protective eyewear for patients.

5.2.5 Other Dentistry-Specific Considerations

Although the CDC has developed the *Summary of Infection Prevention Practices in Dental Settings*, this document was not intended to replace the existing principles of *Standard Precautions* in dental settings; rather it aimed to summarize the basic expectations of infection control relevant to dentistry [18]. Considering that *Hand Hygiene* and *PPE* have been discussed at length, Fig. 5.7 summarizes the remaining principles of *Standard Precautions* specific to dental settings.

5.2.6 Transmission-Based Precautions and COVID-19

For patients with known or suspected infection(s), *Standard Precautions* should be supplemented with *Transmission-Based Precautions*. *Transmission-Based Precautions* target a specific route of disease transmission that *Standard Precautions* alone cannot disrupt and consist of the following categories: Contact Precautions, Droplet Precautions, and Airborne Precautions [19].

Specific to COVID-19, which has multiple routes of transmission, more than one category of *Transmission-Based Precautions* may be used in addition to *Standard Precautions*:

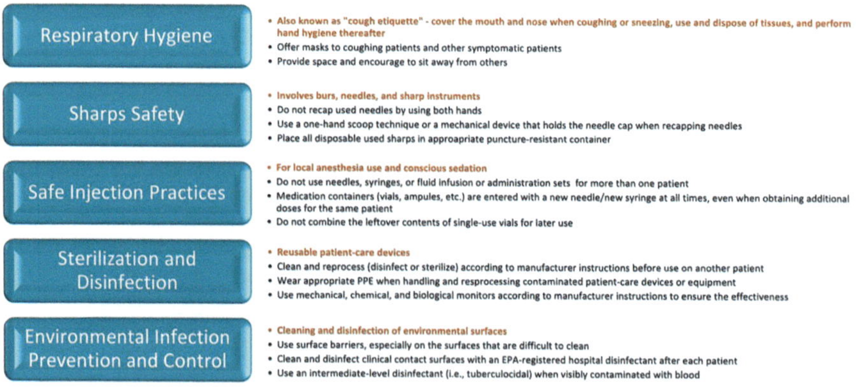

Fig. 5.7 Summary of infection prevention practices in dental settings. Centers for Disease Control and Prevention

- Contact and Droplet Precautions.
- Airborne Precautions for aerosol-generated procedures [20, 21].

Contact and Droplet Precautions

Contact transmission may occur through direct physical contact with an infected individual or indirectly through a contaminated surface, object, or person. Droplets—particles that are larger than 5 microns—are generated by coughing, sneezing, or simply talking. Droplets can be transmitted directly from a respiratory tract to mucous surface or indirectly through hands [22].

To disrupt transmission by contact and droplets, a patient with suspected or confirmed COVID-19 infection, when possible, should be isolated. Providers involved in patient care must don the following PPE *prior* to entering the room of suspected or confirmed COVID-19 patient:

- Long-sleeved protective gown
- Eye protection
- Medical mask
- Medical gloves [23]

Respirators could also be considered instead of medical masks even if aerosol-generating procedures are not performed [21, 22]. The potentially infected surfaces must be thoroughly and frequently cleaned and disinfected [23].

Airborne Precautions

Unlike droplets, aerosols are smaller than 5 microns particles. They remain infective over time, can be dispersed over long distances through ventilation or air-conditioning systems, and inhaled without direct contact with an infected individual [17]. Thus, healthcare providers that are involved in aerosol-generating procedures, which are routine in dental settings, should wear surgical N95 respirator as opposed to medical mask [23]. It is also recommended to perform aerosol-generating procedures in adequately ventilated rooms [21].

5.3 Summary and Conclusion

As demonstrated by the recent COVID-19 pandemic, infection control standards continue to evolve. As healthcare providers, we have professional obligation to implement appropriate infection control measures to protect ourselves, our patients, our colleagues, and the general public from disease-causing pathogens. Most likely the current infection control guidelines will undergo yet another evolution, as new pathogens emerge and continuously mutate. Until then, *Standard Precautions* supplemented with *Transmission-Based Precautions* are the standard of care for *all* healthcare settings.

References

1. Upendran A, Gupta R, Geiger Z. Dental infection control. National Library of Medicine. National Center for Biotechnology Information; 8 Aug 2023. Retrieved from: https://www.ncbi.nlm.nih.gov/books/NBK470356/
2. Centers for Disease Control and Prevention. Infection control basics; 5 Jan 2016. Retrieved from: https://www.cdc.gov/infectioncontrol/basics/index.html
3. Centers for Disease Control and Prevention. History of guidelines for isolation precautions in hospitals; 5 Nov 2015. Retrieved from: https://www.cdc.gov/infectioncontrol/guidelines/isolation/appendix/history.html
4. World Health Organization. Hand hygiene: why, how & when? August 2009. Retrieved from https://cdn.who.int/media/docs/default-source/documents/health-topics/hand-hygiene-why-how-and-when-brochure.pdf
5. Occupational Safety and Health Administration. Personal protective equipment; 2023. Retrieved from: https://www.osha.gov/sites/default/files/publications/osha3151.pdf
6. Centers for Disease Control and Prevention. When and how to wash your hands. Handwashing in communities: clean hands save lives; 15 Nov 2022. Retrieved from: https://www.cdc.gov/handwashing/when-how-handwashing.html#:~:text=Washing%20your%20hands%20is%20easy,%2C%20schools%2C%20and%20childcare%20facilities
7. Centers for Disease Control and Prevention. Show me the science—how to wash your hands. Handwashing in communities: clean hands save lives; 10 Aug 2021. Retrieved from: https://www.cdc.gov/handwashing/show-me-the-science-handwashing.html
8. Centers for Disease Control and Prevention. Hand hygiene. Oral Health; 1 Mar 2016. Retrieved from: https://www.cdc.gov/oralhealth/infectioncontrol/faqs/hand-hygiene.html
9. American Dental Association. Hand hygiene for the dental team. Dental practice success; n.d. Retrieved from: https://www.ada.org/en/publications/dental-practice-success/hand-hygiene-for-the-dental-team
10. Centers for Disease Control and Prevention. Healthcare providers. Hand hygiene in healthcare settings; 8 Jan 2021. Retrieved from: https://www.cdc.gov/handhygiene/providers/
11. Centers for Disease Control and Prevention. Guideline for hand hygiene in health-care settings: recommendations of the Healthcare Infection Control Practices Advisory Committee and the HICPAC/SHEA/APIC/IDSA Hand Hygiene Task Force. Morb Mortal Wkly Rep; 25 Oct 2002. Retrieved from: https://www.cdc.gov/mmwr/preview/mmwrhtml/rr5116a1.htm
12. The Joint Commission. CDC or WHO—artificial nails and gels. National Patient Safety Goals NPSG; 11 Apr 2016. Retrieved from: https://www.jointcommission.org/standards/standard-faqs/ambulatory/national-patient-safety-goals-npsg/000001558/
13. Centers for Disease Control and Prevention. Personal protective equipment. Standard precautions. Oral Health; 18 Jun 2018. Retrieved from: https://www.cdc.gov/oralhealth/infectioncontrol/summary-infection-prevention-practices/standard-precautions.html/#PPE
14. World Health Organization. Glove use information leaflet; August 2009. Retrieved from: https://cdn.who.int/media/docs/default-source/integrated-health-services-(ihs)/infection-prevention-and-control/hand-hygiene/tools/glove-use-information-leaflet.pdf?sfvrsn=13670aa_10
15. Centers for Disease Control and Prevention. Use and care of masks. COVID-19; 11 May 2023. Retrieved from: https://www.cdc.gov/coronavirus/2019-ncov/prevent-getting-sick/about-face-coverings.html
16. Centers for Disease Control and Prevention. Eye safety—eye protection for infection control. The National Institute for Occupational Safety and Health (NIOSH); 29 Jul 2013. Retrieved from: https://www.cdc.gov/niosh/topics/eye/eye-infectious.html
17. Siegel JD, Rhinehart E, Jackson M, Chiarello L, The Healthcare Infection Control Practices Advisory Committee. 2007 guideline for isolation precautions: preventing transmission of infectious agents in healthcare settings; 2007. Retrieved from: https://www.cdc.gov/niosh/docket/archive/pdfs/niosh-219/0219-010107-siegel.pdf

18. Centers for Disease Control and Prevention. Summary of infection prevention practices in dental settings: basic expectations for safe care; October 2016). Retrieved from: https://www.cdc.gov/oralhealth/infectioncontrol/pdf/safe-care2.pdf
19. Centers for Disease Control and Prevention. Transmission-based precautions. Infection control; 7 Jan 2016. Retrieved from: https://www.cdc.gov/infectioncontrol/basics/transmission-based-precautions.html
20. Centers for Disease Control and Prevention. COVID-19 transmission-based precautions. COVID-19; 27 Oct 2023. Retrieved from: https://www.cdc.gov/coronavirus/2019-ncov/hcp/non-us-settings/overview/index.html#:~:text=Current%20WHO%20guidance%20for%20healthcare,case%20airborne%20precautions%20are%20needed
21. World Health Organization. Infection prevention and control during health care when coronavirus disease (COVID-19) is suspected or confirmed. Interim guidance; 12 Jul 2021. Retrieved from: https://iris.who.int/bitstream/handle/10665/342620/WHO-2019-nCoV-IPC-2021.1-eng.pdf?sequence=1
22. Occupational Safety and Health Administration. Infectious diseases. Healthcare; n.d. Retrieved from: https://www.osha.gov/healthcare/infectious-diseases/
23. Centers for Disease Control and Prevention. COVID-19 overview and infection prevention and control priorities in non-U.S. healthcare settings. COVID-19; 29 Nov 2021. Retrieved from: https://www.cdc.gov/coronavirus/2019-ncov/hcp/non-us-settings/overview/index.html

Aerosols in Dentistry

6

Robert Windsor, Erica Caffrey, and Nisha Ganesh

6.1 Introduction

The outbreak of the COVID-19 pandemic created the need for a re-evaluation of techniques and practices in the dental office. Most dental procedures create an aerosol plume. This plume contains the microbes present in the normal flora of the oral cavity. More importantly, the plume also contains infectious agents for a variety of respiratory infections.

The most common respiratory infections include respiratory syncytial virus (RSV), influenza, and pneumococcus. In March of 2020, the landscape of respiratory diseases irrevocably changed [1–4]. The World Health Organization first reported on January 31, 2019, that a pneumonia of unknown cause was detected in Wuhan. The outbreak was declared a Public Health Emergency of International Concern on January 30, 2020. On February 11, 2020, the WHO announced a name for the new coronavirus disease 2019 (COVID-19). Worldwide cases of COVID-19 soared, and the WHO declared COVID-19 a pandemic on March 11, 2020 (Table 6.1) [5, 6].

The American Dental Association responded to this problem with the March 16, 2020, recommendation instructing dentists to postpone all treatment except urgent/

R. Windsor (✉) · N. Ganesh
Department of Comprehensive Dentistry, The University of Maryland School of Dentistry, Baltimore, MD, USA
e-mail: rwindsor@umaryland.edu; nganesh@umaryland.edu

E. Caffrey
Department of Pediatric Dentistry, The University of Maryland School of Dentistry, Baltimore, MD, USA
e-mail: ecaffrey@umaryland.edu

L. DePaola et al. (eds.), *Infection Control in the Dental Office in the Era of COVID-19*, https://doi.org/10.1007/978-3-031-64611-9_6

Table 6.1 Most common respiratory diseases in the twenty-first century

Respiratory syncytial virus (RSV) [1–3]	Virus	100–500 deaths in children under the age of 5 estimated per year	Estimated 14,000 deaths annually in adults aged 65 and older
Influenza [4]	Virus	Kills ~400,000 annually	
Pneumococcus [5]	Bacteria	740,180 children under age 5 died	2.5 million people total died worldwide in 2019
SARS-CoV-2 (COVID-19) [6]	Virus	6,932,395 deaths to date (October 28, 2023)	

emergency procedures. Almost simultaneously, other worldwide dental agencies developed similar recommendations. Two days later an official ADA definition of emergency care was updated [7]:

Dental emergencies are potentially life-threatening and require immediate treatment to stop ongoing tissue bleeding, alleviate severe pain or infection, and include:

- Uncontrolled bleeding.
- Cellulitis or a diffuse soft tissue bacterial infection with intraoral or extraoral swelling that can potentially compromise the patient's airway.
- Trauma involving facial bones, potentially compromising the patient's airway [7].

With oral healthcare in the United States and many other developed countries essentially on hold, the true threat of COVID-19 in the dental office demanded immediate and thorough evaluation. The aerosol inherent to most dental procedures would require control to permit a safe return to dental care. The Centers for Disease Control and Prevention (CDC) in conjunction with key professional organizations assessed current infection control protocol, personal protective equipment, and facility engineering changes. The primary goal was to minimize the impact of the viral load present in the aerosol plume.

6.2 SARS-CoV-2

SARS-CoV-2 is a respiratory disease. It is easily transmitted by respiratory droplets. Common respiratory diseases include asthma, the common cold, influenza, respiratory syncytial virus (RSV), and COVID-19. Other respiratory diseases include chronic pulmonary disease, cystic fibrosis, lung cancer, tuberculosis, pneumonia, and emphysema. These diseases affect the respiratory tissues and organs that facilitate the oxygenation of blood and the exhalation of carbon dioxide [8].

6.3 Aerosols in Dentistry

Dentistry facilitates the transmission of aerosols procedurally. The high-speed handpiece is designed to create a water spray to cool the heat created by friction of the bur against tooth structure [9] (Fig. 6.1). The ultrasonic scaler also creates a water spray to rinse the area and mitigate heat production [10] (Fig. 6.2).

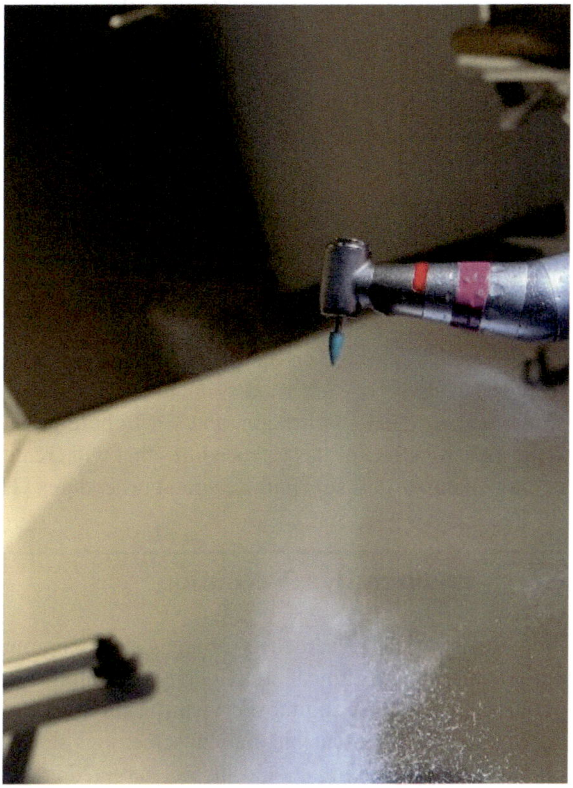

Fig. 6.1 Aerosol generated from the high-speed handpiece. (Image courtesy of Dr. Robert Windsor)

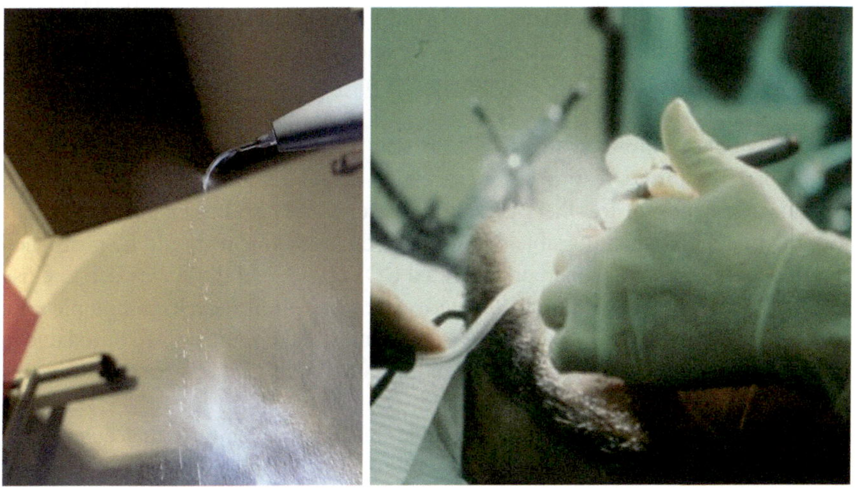

Fig. 6.2 Aerosol generated from the ultrasonic scaler. (Images courtesy of Dr. Robert Windsor and Dr. Louis G. DePaola)

The three-way syringe is used to rinse the work area, spray the area to dislodge materials, and dry the work area. High-volume evacuation creates an airflow of the aerosol. Surgical sterile irrigation and lasers employ water during use. These processes create an aerosol that will contain microbial load from the oral cavity.

The control of the aerosol can be approached in two ways, prevention, and management. This chapter will study methods of prevention including pre-op screening and testing, operator position, and pre-procedural oral rinses. Prevention techniques focus on reducing the potential exposure by controlling the source of possible transmission.

Management of the aerosol can be accomplished in several ways. Dental dam isolation, effective high-volume evacuation suction, and extraoral suction devices can be employed to lessen the pathogen load in the aerosol. Engineering controls include negative pressure rooms, air filtration systems employing high-efficiency particulate air (HEPA) filtration, and UV light to process the air in the operatory. It is the additive effect of these procedures that will create a safe working environment to allow dentists to resume all treatment procedures [11].

6.4 Preoperative Precautions

Individuals should be screened for signs and symptoms of communicable diseases before entering the clinical area. Ideally, screenings should be conducted through a phone interview or a digital pre-visit questionnaire within 24 hours of scheduled appointments. If not feasible, patient screenings should be completed at the time of check-in. The screening should include targeted questions about any recent travel, symptoms, known exposures due to close contact with someone with a confirmed case, and positive laboratory markers for the disease of concern [12]. Commonly reported symptoms of COVID-19 include fever or chills, cough, shortness of breath, fatigue, muscle aches or headaches, loss of smell or taste, sore throat, congestion, runny nose, and diarrhea [13]. A thermometer may be employed to quickly identify those with pyrexia.

Any patient exhibiting signs of COVID-19 or other concerning contagions should undergo further testing before receiving dental treatment, both to reduce the potential for exposure to others present in the operatory and to enable more comfortable treatment when possible. Nonurgent dental treatment should be postponed for all patients with confirmed or suspected COVID-19, and those exposed to close contacts with COVID-19 should likewise defer care until they have completed a recommended isolation period [14]. When urgent dental treatment is required due to trauma, infection, or severe pain, precautions should be taken as described in this chapter.

Rapid testing for COVID-19 is available through antigen tests that detect viral structural proteins. Antigen tests do not require special laboratory equipment and can easily be carried out through a simple nasopharyngeal or nasal swab, with results typically ready after 15 minutes [15]. Though antigen tests are generally less sensitive than polymerase chain reaction (PCR)-based tests for detection of

COVID-19, their use as a screening tool in the dental setting during periods of high community transmission should be considered.

Thoughtful planning can reduce the possibility of aerosol transmission in the waiting room. Posters that educate viewers on proper hand hygiene, coughing/sneezing etiquette, masking, and signs and symptoms of COVID-19 will help inform patients of concerning symptoms and mitigation strategies. Disposable tissues, hand sanitizer, and disposable masks should be made readily available. Patient families should be seated at least 1 meter (3.28 feet) apart in the waiting area and the registration line [16]. Adequate ventilation, including mechanical ventilation, open windows, or portable air purifier units, can reduce transmission of droplet-based airborne diseases [17].

6.5 Interventions to Reduce Aerosols in the Dental Setting

6.5.1 Pre-procedural Oral Rinses

Oral antiseptics may be used to reduce patient bacterial and viral load prior to the commencement of dental procedures [18]. Coronaviruses possess spike proteins and viral envelope proteins that target angiotensin-converting enzyme 2 (ACE2) and transmembrane serine protease-2 (TMPRSS2) receptors, both of which are found in epithelial cells of the tongue, gingiva, oral mucosa, taste buds, and salivary gland tissues of the oral cavity [19]. Oral rinses generally work through disruption of the viral envelope and prevention of the SARS-CoV-2 spike glycoprotein insertion [20]. Available oral rinses currently include solutions of ethanol, essential oils, chlorhexidine (0.12–0.2%), cetylpyridinum chloride, hypochlorous acid, hydrogen peroxide (1%), and povidone-iodine (1–5%) [21–23]. It should be noted that these mouth rinses may decrease viral, fungal, and bacterial load temporarily, but that rinsing does not permanently reduce infectivity and that intraoral load will rise again through viral replication and physical actions such as coughing. Furthermore, these rinses are not considered as part of the treatment regimen for the disease. Rather, a protocol in which patients rinse with one of the abovementioned solutions for approximately 30 seconds may mitigate the risk of aerosol transmission by reducing viral load for the length of time necessary to complete a dental appointment [22].

6.5.2 Isolation and Suction

Intraoral isolation is necessary to prevent contamination of restorative work with saliva and blood. Dental dams, saliva ejectors, and high-volume evacuation are also helpful in limiting the spread of aerosolized microbes in the dental operatory, both alone or in combination [12, 24–26]. Likewise, extraoral suction units can reduce spatter of aerosolizing droplets [27]. Extraoral suction units are generally flexible in positioning and can be adjusted to appropriate levels for ease of use. Measures to decrease aerosol generation through isolation and suction will help to reduce droplet settling on the patient, dental provider, and surrounding operatory equipment.

6.5.3 Avoidance of Aerosol-Generating Procedures

Providers may choose to limit the use of rotary handpieces, air-water syringes, ultrasonic devices, air polishers, and/or air abrasion during periods when aerosol transmission is a concern [28]. Such oscillating instruments are known to generate both spatter and aerosols, in part due to their air-water coolant, which will settle on both individuals and inanimate objects in the operatory even at a distance of multiple feet [24, 29]. Alternative procedures may be appropriate when necessary to reduce transmission, including interim therapeutic restorations, antibiotic therapy, atraumatic restorative treatment, hand scaling, and extractions [30, 31].

6.6 Management of Dental Unit Water Lines

Dental unit waterlines supply all instruments attached to the dental chair unit, including handpieces, water syringes, and ultrasonic scalers. Lack of proper maintenance, stagnant water, low flow rates, mechanical failure, or use of non-sterile water can cause contamination with bacterial microbes including *Legionella, Pseudomonas,* and *Mycobacteria* [32, 33]. Dental procedures using water coolant from dental waterline units can subsequently generate aerosols containing microbial droplets that contaminate the air and operatory surfaces. Viruses are typically smaller and can reach further than bacteria and remain airborne for hours [34]. Careful monitoring of dental waterline units is essential to prevent possible transmission of contaminated water to individuals via aerosol-generating procedures. Nonsurgical dental procedures should maintain water that aligns with the standards for drinking water (<500 colony forming units/mL of heterotrophic water bacteria is what is required in the United States). Addition of antiseptics (e.g., hydrogen peroxide) to dental unit waterline units may be considered for use with aerosol-generating procedures [35]. Providers should consult with the manufacturers regarding the best ways to implement and monitor the dental water in their units. Surgical procedures should use sterile saline or sterile water in bulb syringes, single-use containers, or systems that bypass dental units and use sterilizable tubing, since it is not possible to fully decontaminate conventional dental unit water reservoirs [33].

6.7 Management of Aerosols in a Dental Setting

6.7.1 Personal Protective Equipment

Personal protective equipment, including gowns, gloves, masks, face shields, eyewear (i.e., goggles), and caps, are critical in reducing the transmission of infections in a dental setting. These items act as physical barriers to prevent direct contact exposure to pathogens. Relatedly, any protective item is susceptible to contamination via blood, saliva, and/or droplets. For this reason, disposable items should be switched upon completion of treatment of each patient, and correct donning and

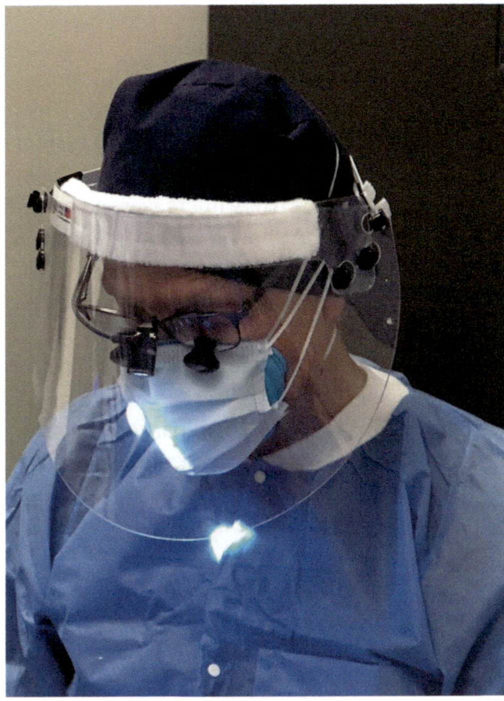

Fig. 6.3 A fit-tested N95 respirator or the equivalent provides maximal respiratory protection during outbreaks of respiratory diseases. (Image courtesy of Dr. Louis Depaola)

doffing procedures should be followed. Masks have the additional function of filtering out droplets and are particularly important to protect pathogens from entering the respiratory tract via the nasal passages and oral cavity. Mask filtration is dependent on multiple factors including tightness of mask fit, duration of wear, moisture, production quality, and the droplet and aerosol particle size [36].

Surgical masks can provide partial coverage against splatter, sprays, and large droplets but lack the ability to filter out smaller particles and are prone to leakage due to a loose fit over the nose and mouth. N95 respirators are regulated medical devices that have the benefit of a tighter fit and higher filtration of very small droplets. N95 respirators are reported to filter out 95% of airborne particles that are as small as 300 nm [37]. A tight seal is important to prevent leakage, and healthcare workers should undergo a fit test annually to ensure that they wear a properly sized device (Fig. 6.3) [38].

6.8 Management in the Era of COVID-19

It is not possible to eliminate all viral particles from aerosol-generating dental procedures. Engineering controls to help manage the particulate matter in the air are necessary to provide a safe environment for the dental healthcare worker. There are several levels of engineering control that might be employed.

6.8.1 Positive Airflow

Positive airflow is defined as positive air pressure created in a space to push air out of the area by increasing the rate of flow. This functionality can be added to a heating ventilation air conditioning (HVAC) system in a dental office. The use of a high-efficiency particulate air (HEPA) filter in the system removes particles down to 0.3 micron in size. The HEPA filters were first used in the 1940s to contain radioactive dust particles [39]. Although HEPA filters are effective, there are several limitations to consider. Volatile organic compounds (VOCs), ozone, and certain allergens are not managed at 100% efficiency.

- *VOCs*: volatile organic compounds—airborne chemicals that are well-known carcinogens [40].
- *Ozone*: This is a very small particle that does not stick to the HEPA filter. Ozone is unhealthy to breathe and can react with VOCs to produce very small particles that can enter the bloodstream through penetration into the lungs [40].
- *Allergens*: Most can be trapped by the HEPA filter, but some are small enough to penetrate [40].

Activated carbon is often included as part of the HEPA filter system. This can help with VOCs and ozone [40].

6.8.2 Room-Sized Filtration Systems

Room-sized filtration systems are another engineering control for the bioaerosol. These systems utilize positive airflow on a smaller scale. They use the HEPA-RX filters and UV-C lamp. According to Philip Tierno, PhD, a clinical professor in the Department of Pathology at New York University Langone Medical Center, "the UV-C light has a range of effectiveness which interferes and disrupts the nucleic acids of bacteria and other microbes" including SARS-CoV-2. The UV-C light will also disrupt proteins in the microbes by killing certain amino acids. These filtration systems augment the positive airflow through building an HVAC system [41].

6.8.3 Extraoral Evaluation Systems

The use of dental aspiration units (intraoral suction units) has been an essential component of the armamentarium since 1961 when Durr Dental introduced the first of its kind [42] (Fig. 6.4). Extraoral evacuation systems are an engineering control employed chairside in the dental operatory. This system employs the HEPA filter and UV-C light to disinfect and purify the air. This suction system is placed in close proximity to the patient oral cavity to remove most of the bioaerosol that escapes the

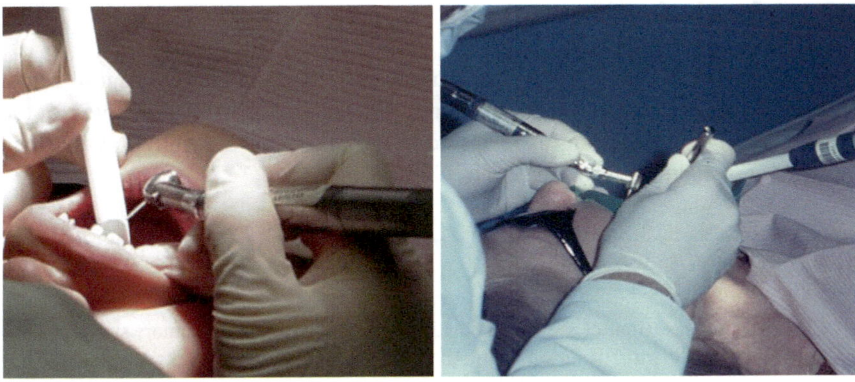

Fig. 6.4 HVE (high-volume evacuator) has the capacity to remove100 cu feet of air per minute. A minimum of HVE is recommended for any aerosoling procedure. (Images courtesy of Dr. Louis Depaola)

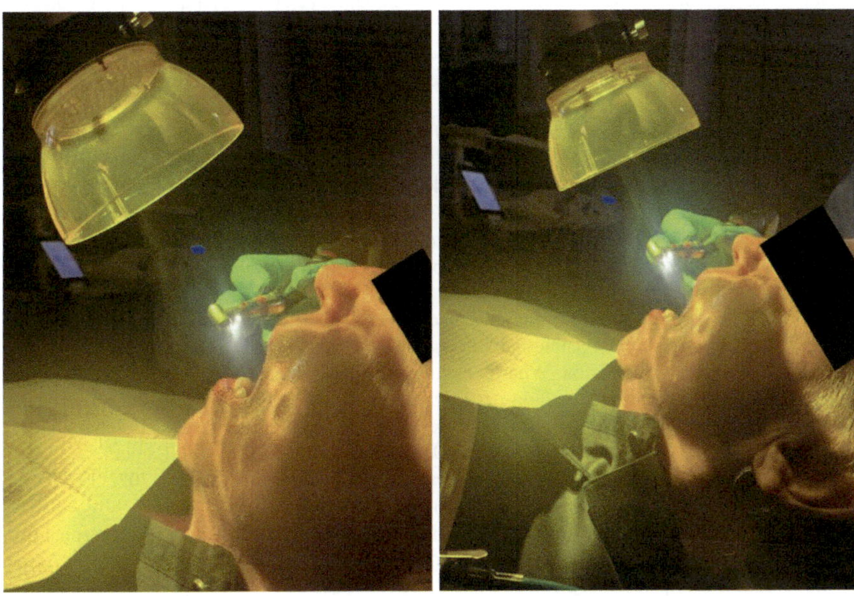

Fig. 6.5 Extraoral suction: 1000 cu feet per minute (4-inch diameter) which is a tenfold increase from just using HVE. Note the aerosol plume being sucked up by this device. (Courtesy of Dr. Robert Windsor)

high-volume evacuation suction [27, 43]. The extraoral suction units are an effective method of reducing droplet spatter during operative dental procedures and can be useful in helping reduce risk of experiencing COVID-19 spread during dental procedures [35, 42] (Fig. 6.5).

6.9 Conclusions

The emergence of COVID-19 has brought the importance of management of dental aerosols to the forefront of infection control. When adhering to the principles for the control of airborne infections as reviewed in this chapter, oral health providers can safely treat dental patients in the era of COVID-19.

References

1. Centers for Disease Control and Prevention. Increased interseasonal respiratory syncytial virus (RSV) activity in parts of the southern United States. https://emergency.cdc.gov/han/2021/han00443.asp. Accessed 29 Jun 2022.
2. Falsey AR, Hennessey PA, Formica MA, Cox C, Walsh EE. Respiratory syncytial virus infection in elderly and high-risk adults. N Engl J Med. 2005;352(17):1749–59. https://doi.org/10.1056/NEJMoa043951.
3. Thompson WW, Shay DK, Weintraub E, et al. Mortality associated with influenza and respiratory syncytial virus in the United States. JAMA. 2003;289(2):179–86. https://doi.org/10.1001/jama.289.2.179.
4. Iuliano AD, Roguski KM, Chang HH, Muscatello DJ, Palekar R, Tempia S, Cohen C, Gran JM, Schanzer D, Cowling BJ, Wu P, Kyncl J, Ang LW, Park M, Redlberger-Fritz M, Yu H, Espenhain L, Krishnan A, Emukule G, van Asten L, Pereira Da Silva S, Aungkulanon S, Buchholz U, Widdowson MA, Bresee JS. Global seasonal influenza-associated mortality collaborator network. Lancet. 2018;391(10127):1285–300. https://doi.org/10.1016/S0140-6736(17)33293-2. Epub 2017 Dec 14.
5. Centers for Disease Control and Prevention. CDC museum COVID-19 timeline. Last reviewed: 15 Mar 2023. https://www.cdc.gov/museum/timeline/covid19.html#:~:text=December%2031%2C%202019,the%20Huanan%20Seafood%20Wholesale%20Market. Accessed 29 Jun 2022.
6. World Health Organization. Coronavirus disease (COVID-19) pandemic—COVID-19. https://www.who.int/europe/emergencies/situations/covid-19. Accessed 18 Nov 2023.
7. American Dental Association. What constitutes a dental emergency?, 18 Mar 2020. https://www.ada.org/-/media/project/ada-organization/ada/ada-org/files/resources/coronavirus/covid-19-practice-resources/ada_covid19_dental_emergency_dds.pdf?rev=51b8c64b2b6e45f1a7edca6343be8985&hash=DB74D9EA759D90C491B3B0EE7D934A88Lamers
8. Lamers MM, Haagmans BL. SARS-CoV-2 pathogenesis. Nat Rev Microbiol. 2022;20:270–84. https://doi.org/10.1038/s41579-022-00713-0.
9. Ionescu AC, Brambilla E, Manzoli L, Orsini G, Gentili V, Rizzo R. Efficacy of personal protective equipment against coronavirus transmission via dental handpieces. J Am Dent Assoc. 2021;152:631. https://doi.org/10.1016/j.adaj.2021.03.007.
10. Ibiyemi O, Taiwo J, Oke GA. Improvised source of water coolant for ultrasonic scaler: an appropriate technology in underserved communities. Rural Remote Health. 2012;12:2260. https://doi.org/10.22605/RRH2260.
11. Geisinger ML. Aerosols in the dental office: best practices for patient and practitioner safety. Proctor & Gamble CE course 619.
12. Ge ZY, Yang LM, Xia JJ, Fu XH, Zhang YZ. Possible aerosol transmission of COVID-19 and special precautions in dentistry. J Zhejiang Univ Sci B. 2020;21(5):361–8.
13. Centers for Disease Control and Prevention. COVID-19 and your health. Centers for Disease Control and Prevention, 11 Feb 2020. https://www.cdc.gov/coronavirus/2019-ncov/symptoms-testing/symptoms.html

14. Centers for Disease Control and Prevention. Isolation. Centers for Disease Control and Prevention, 11 May 2023. https://www.cdc.gov/coronavirus/2019-ncov/your-health/isolation.html
15. Shirazi S, Stanford CM, Cooper LF. Testing for COVID-19 in dental offices: mechanism of action, application, and interpretation of laboratory and point-of-care screening tests. J Am Dent Assoc. 2021;152(7):514–525.e8.
16. Chu DK, Akl EA, Duda S, Solo K, Yaacoub S, Schünemann HJ, COVID-19 Systematic Urgent Review Group Effort (SURGE) Study Authors. Physical distancing, face masks, and eye protection to prevent person-to-person transmission of SARS-CoV-2 and COVID-19: a systematic review and meta-analysis. Lancet. 2020;395(10242):1973–87.
17. Salmonsmith J, Ducci A, Balachandran R, Guo L, Torii R, Houlihan C, Epstein R, Rubin J, Tiwari MK, Lovat LB. Use of portable air purifiers to reduce aerosols in hospital settings and cut down the clinical backlog. Epidemiol Infect. 2023 Jan;18(151):e21.
18. Meethil AP, et al. Sources of SARS-CoV-2 and other microorganisms in dental aerosols. J Dent Res. 2021;100:817. https://doi.org/10.1177/00220345211015948.
19. Guerrero Bernal CG, et al. Oral antiseptics against SARS-CoV-2: a literature review. Int J Environ Res Public Health. 2022;19(14):8768.
20. Ting M, Dahlkemper A, Schwartz JJ, Woodfork M, Suzuki JB. Preprocedural viral load effects of oral antiseptics on SARS-CoV-2 in patients with COVID-19: a systematic review. Biomedicines. 2023;11(6):1694.
21. Idrees M, McGowan B, Fawzy A, Abuderman AA, Balasubramaniam R, Kujan O. Efficacy of mouth rinses and nasal spray in the inactivation of SARS-CoV-2: a systematic review and meta-analysis of in vitro and in vivo studies. Int J Environ Res Public Health. 2022;19(19):12148.
22. Mesiter TL, et al. Virucidal efficacy of different oral rinses against severe acute respiratory syndrome coronavirus 2. J Infect Dis. 2020;222(8):1289–92.
23. Weber J, et al. Preprocedural mouthwashes for infection control in dentistry-an update. Clin Oral Investig. 2023;27(Suppl 1):33–44.
24. Harrel SK, Molinari J. Aerosols and splatter in dentistry: a brief review of the literature and infection control implications. J Am Dent Assoc. 2004;135(4):429–37.
25. Suprono MS, Won J, Savignano R, Zhong Z, Ahmed A, Roque-Torres G, Zhang W, Oyoyo U, Richardson P, Caruso J, Handysides R, Li Y. A clinical investigation of dental evacuation systems in reducing aerosols. J Am Dent Assoc. 2021;152(6):455–62.
26. Kumbargere Nagraj S, Eachempati P, Paisi M, Nasser M, Sivaramakrishnan G, Verbeek JH. Interventions to reduce contaminated aerosols produced during dental procedures for preventing infectious diseases. Cochrane Database Syst Rev. 2020;10(10):CD013686.
27. Chavis SE, Hines SE, Dyalram D, Wilken NC, Dalby RN. Can extraoral suction units minimize droplet spatter during a simulated dental procedure? J Am Dent Assoc. 2021;152(2):157–65.
28. Ionescu AC, Cagetti MG, Ferracane JL, Garcia-Godoy F, Brambilla E. Topographic aspects of airborne contamination caused by the use of dental handpieces in the operative environment. J Am Dent Assoc. 2020;151(9):660–7.
29. Ahmed MA, Jouhar R. Dissemination of aerosol and splatter in clinical environment during cavity preparation: an in vitro study. Int J Environ Res Public Health. 2021;18:3773.
30. Benzian H, Niederman R. A dental response to the COVID-19 pandemic-SAFER aerosol-free emergent (SAFER) dentistry. Front Med (Lausanne). 2020;7:520.
31. Deana NF, Seiffert A, Aravena-Rivas Y, Alonso-Coello P, Muñoz-Millán P, Espinoza-Espinoza G, Pineda P, Zaror C. Recommendations for safe dental care: a systematic review of clinical practice guidelines in the first year of the COVID-19 pandemic. Int J Environ Res Public Health. 2021;18(19):10059.
32. Chang SP, Jiang HL, Wang YC, Chao HC, Lee JJ, Chung HC, Wang LS, Ding DC. A program to improve the quality of dental unit water in a medical center. Medicine (Baltimore). 2021;100(47):e28019.
33. Centers for Disease Control and Prevention. Dental unit water quality | FAQs | Infection control | Division of Oral Health | CDC. 31 Oct 2022. https://www.cdc.gov/oralhealth/infectioncontrol/faqs/dental-unit-water-quality.html

34. Zemouri C, et al. Dental aerosols: microbial composition and spatial distribution. J Oral Microbiol. 2020;12(1):1762040.
35. Roy T, Damoulakis G, Komperda J, Mashayek F, Cooper LF, Rowan SA, Megaridis CM. Effect of H2O2 antiseptic on dispersal of cavitation-induced microdroplets. J Dent Res. 2021;100(11):1258–64.
36. Gund MP, Naim J, Rupf S, Gärtner B, Hannig M. Bacterial contamination potential of personal protective equipment itself in dental aerosol-producing treatments. Odontology. 2023;112:309.
37. Alkhalaf A, Aljaroudi E, Al-Hulami M, Gaffar B, Almas K. Efficacy of surgical masks versus N95 respirators for the prevention of COVID-19 in dental settings: a systematic review. Cureus. 2023;15(4):e37631.
38. Krah J, Shamblin M, Shaffer R. Filtering out confusion: frequently asked questions about respiratory protection, user seal check. U.S. Department of Health and Human Services, Centers for Disease Control and Prevention, National Institute for Occupational Safety and Health, DHHS (NIOSH) Publication 2018-130; 2018.
39. Centers for Disease Control and Prevention. Guidelines for environmental infection control in health-care facilities. Updated July 2019. https://www.cdc.gov/infectioncontrol/pdf/guidelines/environmental-guidelines-P.pdf
40. King H. HEPA filters—preclinical testing on HEPA and PECO: what can destruction add to air purification? MoLEKULE blog, 26 Jul 2023.
41. Tierno PM Jr, Lifshitz MS. UV-C light information—Henry's clinical diagnosis and management by laboratory methods. 21st ed. Philadelphia: Saunders-Elsevier; 2007. p. 133–43. (4478)
42. Choi JJE, Chen J, Choi YJ, Moffat SM, Duncan WJ, Waddell JN, Jermy M. Dental high-speed handpiece and ultrasonic scaler aerosol generation levels and the effect of suction and air supply. Infect Control Hosp Epidemiol. MID: 35938186 PMCID: PMC10262170. 44:926. https://doi.org/10.1017/ice.2022.196.
43. Zhu M, Medina M, Nalliah R, Boehman A, Capecelatro J, Wooldridge M. Experimental evaluation of aerosol mitigation strategies in large open-plan dental clinics. J Am Dent Assoc. 2022;153:208. https://doi.org/10.1016/j.adaj.2021.07.030.

Vaccines, Vaccinations, and the Re-emergence of and Vaccine-Preventable Diseases

7

Martina Majstorovic and Darien Weatherspoon

7.1 Introduction

Vaccines are recommended and commonly used to reduce the risk of spreading infection, thus, protecting populations against diseases that may have serious and detrimental consequences to overall health. Timely receipt of vaccines is based on suggested public health guidelines. These guidelines are based on recommendations that have been developed by the Centers for Disease Control and Prevention (CDC), which is a public health agency under the US Department of Health and Human Services. Recommendations provided by the CDC are in accordance with those promoted by the World Health Organization (WHO). The same standards apply to the European Center for Disease Control (EU CDC).

However, in developing and implementing vaccination protocols, minor differences between the US, European, and British health standards are noted due to differences in social, economic, cultural, religious, and other factors relevant to the specific population and its region. Additionally, constant fluctuation in immigration, climate challenges, and consequential re-emergence of certain diseases revealed the need to reassess and constantly monitor for potential outbreaks of certain vaccine-preventable diseases.

The aim of this chapter is to summarize and give current prospectives for the most common vaccines as they relate to vaccine-preventable diseases in the United

M. Majstorovic (✉)
Department of Pediatric Dentistry, The University of Maryland School of Dentistry, Baltimore, MD, USA
e-mail: mmajstorovic@umaryland.edu

D. Weatherspoon
Department of Dental Public Health, The University of Maryland School of Dentistry, Baltimore, MD, USA
e-mail: dweatherspoon@umaryland.edu

L. DePaola et al. (eds.), *Infection Control in the Dental Office in the Era of COVID-19*, https://doi.org/10.1007/978-3-031-64611-9_7

States based on the most recent CDC guidelines. This chapter will also present a brief overview of the European and British vaccine standards, as they pertain to the current US standards and global standards.

7.2 Vaccines

7.2.1 Definition and Overview

Vaccines are biological preparations that are used for the primary prevention of disease in a population [1]. Vaccines are prepared using multiple components, with the principal component being the antigen of the pathogen for which the vaccine protects against [2, 3]. Other important components include adjuvants, used to improve the immune system response; preservatives, used to prevent external pathogens from disrupting the vaccine; and stabilizers, used to stabilize the vaccine during storage and transportation [2, 3]. Vaccines are administered into the body primarily through intramuscular or subcutaneous injections, although they can less frequently be delivered through other routes, such as orally and intranasally [4].

Vaccines work by priming and stimulating the body's immune system [5]. The immune system contains white blood cells, such as macrophages, B-lymphocytes, and T-lymphocytes, which respond to and protect against pathogens attempting to infect the body [5]. Vaccines stimulate the immune system by mimicking an infection in a way that doesn't cause illness but, rather, produces antibodies and "memory cells" (T-lymphocytes) which allows the immune system to recognize and remember how to respond to a specific infection in the future [5, 6].

Vaccines can differ in how they are prepared and designed to help stimulate the body's immune system. They can be categorized into six major vaccine types based on their preparation (Table 7.1) [5, 7].

Table 7.1 Categories of vaccines and how they are prepared

Vaccine type	How vaccine is prepared
Inactivate vaccines	These vaccines are prepared by using an inactivated or dead version of the pathogen
Live, attenuated vaccines	These vaccines are prepared by using a weakened or attenuated version of the pathogen
Subunit, recombinant, polysaccharide, and conjugate vaccines	These vaccines are prepared by using a specific portion of the pathogen, including a subunit, protein, polysaccharide, or capsid
Toxoid vaccines	These vaccines are prepared by using a weakened toxoid of a pathogen
Viral vector vaccines	These vaccines are prepared by using a modified version of a different pathogen that is used as a vector
Messenger RNA (mRNA) vaccines	These vaccines are prepared by using mRNA of a pathogen

Source:
Centers for Disease Control and Prevention [5]
U.S. Department of Health and Human Services [7]

7.2.2 Re-emergence of Vaccine-Preventable Diseases

Over time, the United States and many other developed countries have experienced a precipitous decline in infectious diseases, resulting in an increase in chronic disease prevalence [8]. While there are several factors that have contributed to this trend of declining infectious diseases, public health preventive measures, including vaccinations, have played a key role [8].

Vaccination is the process of administering a vaccine into the body [9]. Immunization is the resulting process by which a person becomes immune to a given disease after receiving a vaccination [9]. Although the terms vaccination and immunization are slightly different, they are often used interchangeably. Vaccination has become an integral component of public health in the United States with most states having established laws that require vaccines in order to attend public schools and day care centers [10]. They are important for public health because they not only help to confer immunity to the individual that is vaccinated, but they can also protect at a community level when enough people get vaccinated by slowing down the spread of an infectious agent and protecting those who are unable to get vaccinated, a concept referred to as "herd immunity" [11].

Vaccine-preventable diseases are those diseases for which a vaccine is available that is effective at preventing the disease. These diseases include [12] dengue, diphtheria, *Haemophilus influenzae* type b (Hib), hepatitis A, hepatitis B, herpes zoster (HZ), human papillomavirus (HPV)-related cancers, influenza, measles, meningococcal disease, mumps, pertussis, pneumonia, polio (poliomyelitis), rotavirus diseases, rubella, tetanus, and varicella. Vaccine-preventable diseases that are less common in the United States include adenovirus illnesses, anthrax, cholera, Japanese encephalitis, rabies, smallpox, tuberculosis, typhoid fever, and yellow fever.

While vaccines have been integral in curtailing disease, surveillance has identified a re-emergence of some vaccine-preventable diseases in the United States during recent time periods, including measles, mumps, and pertussis [13, 14]. Factors contributing to the observed increase in vaccine-preventable disease include parents refusing or delaying vaccination for their children, which can result in in undervaccination and less herd immunity [13]. Waning immunity and less effective vaccines have also been attributed to the re-emergence of vaccine-preventable diseases [13]. Additionally, the increase in international travel has increased the risk of these diseases spreading globally, including to the United States [13, 15]. The risk of re-emergence is likely to persist with the recent COVID-19 pandemic since vaccination rates decreased significantly during the pandemic and have not yet returned to pre-pandemic levels [16].

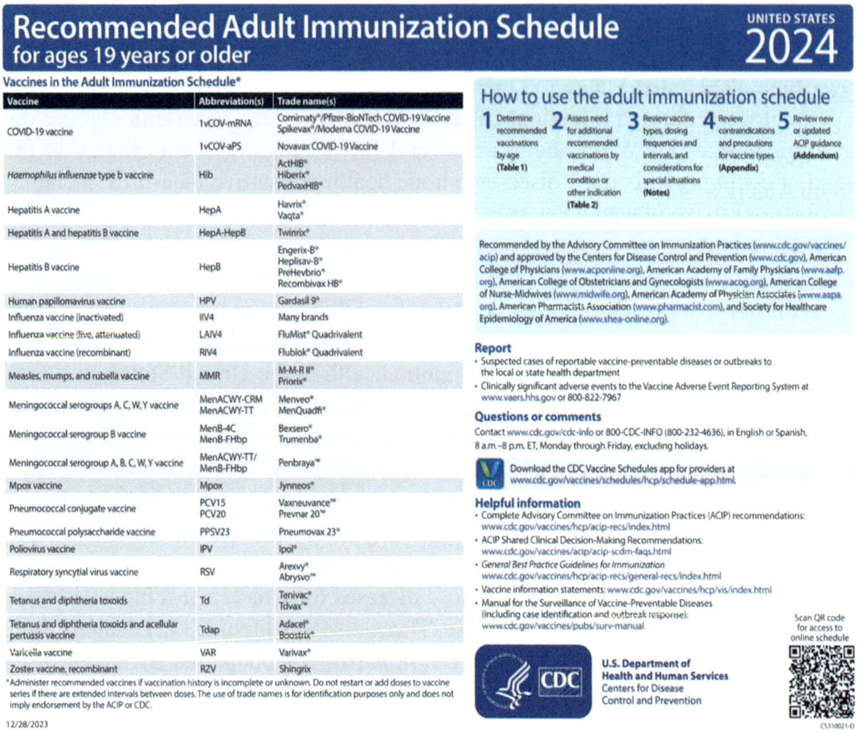

Recommended Adult Immunization Schedule
for ages 19 years or older

UNITED STATES 2024

Vaccines in the Adult Immunization Schedule*

Vaccine	Abbreviation(s)	Trade name(s)
COVID-19 vaccine	1vCOV-mRNA	Comirnaty®/Pfizer-BioNTech COVID-19 Vaccine Spikevax®/Moderna COVID-19 Vaccine
	1vCOV-aPS	Novavax COVID-19 Vaccine
Haemophilus influenzae type b vaccine	Hib	ActHIB® Hiberix® PedvaxHIB®
Hepatitis A vaccine	HepA	Havrix® Vaqta®
Hepatitis A and hepatitis B vaccine	HepA-HepB	Twinrix®
Hepatitis B vaccine	HepB	Engerix-B® Heplisav-B® PreHevbrio® Recombivax HB®
Human papillomavirus vaccine	HPV	Gardasil 9®
Influenza vaccine (inactivated)	IIV4	Many brands
Influenza vaccine (live, attenuated)	LAIV4	FluMist® Quadrivalent
Influenza vaccine (recombinant)	RIV4	Flublok® Quadrivalent
Measles, mumps, and rubella vaccine	MMR	M-M-R II® Priorix®
Meningococcal serogroups A, C, W, Y vaccine	MenACWY-CRM MenACWY-TT	Menveo® MenQuadfi®
Meningococcal serogroup B vaccine	MenB-4C MenB-FHbp	Bexsero® Trumenba®
Meningococcal serogroup A, B, C, W, Y vaccine	MenACWY-TT/ MenB-FHbp	Penbraya™
Mpox vaccine	Mpox	Jynneos®
Pneumococcal conjugate vaccine	PCV15 PCV20	Vaxneuvance™ Prevnar 20™
Pneumococcal polysaccharide vaccine	PPSV23	Pneumovax 23®
Poliovirus vaccine	IPV	Ipol®
Respiratory syncytial virus vaccine	RSV	Arexvy® Abrysvo™
Tetanus and diphtheria toxoids	Td	Tenivac® Tdvax™
Tetanus and diphtheria toxoids and acellular pertussis vaccine	Tdap	Adacel® Boostrix®
Varicella vaccine	VAR	Varivax®
Zoster vaccine, recombinant	RZV	Shingrix

*Administer recommended vaccines if vaccination history is incomplete or unknown. Do not restart or add doses to vaccine series if there are extended intervals between doses. The use of trade names is for identification purposes only and does not imply endorsement by the ACIP or CDC.

12/28/2023

How to use the adult immunization schedule

1. Determine recommended vaccinations by age **(Table 1)**
2. Assess need for additional recommended vaccinations by medical condition or other indication **(Table 2)**
3. Review vaccine types, dosing frequencies and intervals, and considerations for special situations **(Notes)**
4. Review contraindications and precautions for vaccine types **(Appendix)**
5. Review new or updated ACIP guidance **(Addendum)**

Recommended by the Advisory Committee on Immunization Practices (www.cdc.gov/vaccines/acip) and approved by the Centers for Disease Control and Prevention (www.cdc.gov), American College of Physicians (www.acponline.org), American Academy of Family Physicians (www.aafp.org), American College of Obstetricians and Gynecologists (www.acog.org), American College of Nurse-Midwives (www.midwife.org), American Academy of Physician Associates (www.aapa.org), American Pharmacists Association (www.pharmacist.com), and Society for Healthcare Epidemiology of America (www.shea-online.org).

Report

- Suspected cases of reportable vaccine-preventable diseases or outbreaks to the local or state health department
- Clinically significant adverse events to the Vaccine Adverse Event Reporting System at www.vaers.hhs.gov or 800-822-7967

Questions or comments

Contact www.cdc.gov/cdc-info or 800-CDC-INFO (800-232-4636), in English or Spanish, 8 a.m.–8 p.m. ET, Monday through Friday, excluding holidays.

Download the CDC Vaccine Schedules app for providers at www.cdc.gov/vaccines/schedules/hcp/schedule-app.html.

Helpful information

- Complete Advisory Committee on Immunization Practices (ACIP) recommendations: www.cdc.gov/vaccines/hcp/acip-recs/index.html
- ACIP Shared Clinical Decision-Making Recommendations: www.cdc.gov/vaccines/acip/acip-scdm-faqs.html
- *General Best Practice Guidelines for Immunization* www.cdc.gov/vaccines/hcp/acip-recs/general-recs/index.html
- Vaccine information statements: www.cdc.gov/vaccines/hcp/vis/index.html
- Manual for the Surveillance of Vaccine-Preventable Diseases (including case identification and outbreak response): www.cdc.gov/vaccines/pubs/surv-manual

U.S. Department of Health and Human Services
Centers for Disease Control and Prevention

Scan QR code for access to online schedule

CS310021-D

Fig. 7.1 Recommended Adult Immunization Schedule for Ages 19 years or older (Image source: https://www.cdc.gov/vaccines/hcp/imz-schedules/downloads/adult/adult-combined-schedule.pdf)

7.2.3 Vaccine Recommendations

To promote public health, the Centers for Disease Control and Prevention has recommended vaccines for both children and adults (Figs. 7.1 and 7.2). This section provides pertinent information on the most common vaccines and the diseases for which they protect against.

While these are the recommendations for the United States, each country will have specific recommendations for the various vaccination schedules. Approved vaccines may differ as well. Although most countries have similar recommendations, there will be some differences, and dental practitioners should be knowledgeable about the recommended vaccination schedules in their countries as well as the approved vaccines for administration.

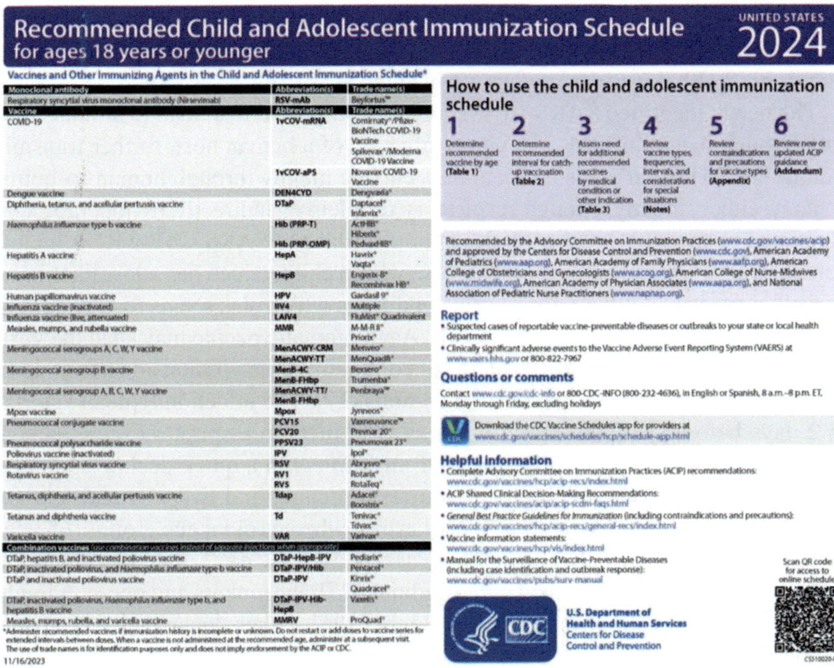

Recommended Child and Adolescent Immunization Schedule
for ages 18 years or younger

UNITED STATES
2024

Vaccines and Other Immunizing Agents in the Child and Adolescent Immunization Schedule*

Monoclonal antibody	Abbreviation(s)	Trade name(s)
Respiratory syncytial virus monoclonal antibody (Nirsevimab)	RSV-mAb	Beyfortus™
Vaccine	**Abbreviation(s)**	**Trade name(s)**
COVID-19	1vCOV-mRNA	Comirnaty®/Pfizer-BioNTech COVID-19 Vaccine Spikevax®/Moderna COVID-19 Vaccine
	1vCOV-aPS	Novavax COVID-19 Vaccine
Dengue vaccine	DEN4CYD	Dengvaxia®
Diphtheria, tetanus, and acellular pertussis vaccine	DTaP	Daptacel® Infanrix®
Haemophilus influenzae type b vaccine	Hib (PRP-T)	ActHIB® Hiberix®
	Hib (PRP-OMP)	PedvaxHIB®
Hepatitis A vaccine	HepA	Havrix® Vaqta®
Hepatitis B vaccine	HepB	Engerix-B® Recombivax HB®
Human papillomavirus vaccine	HPV	Gardasil 9®
Influenza vaccine (inactivated)	IIV4	Multiple
Influenza vaccine (live, attenuated)	LAIV4	FluMist® Quadrivalent
Measles, mumps, and rubella vaccine	MMR	M-M-R II® Priorix®
Meningococcal serogroups A, C, W, Y vaccine	MenACWY-CRM	Menveo®
	MenACWY-TT	MenQuadfi®
Meningococcal serogroup B vaccine	MenB-4C	Bexsero®
	MenB-FHbp	Trumenba®
Meningococcal serogroup A, B, C, W, Y vaccine	MenACWY-TT/ MenB-FHbp	Penbraya™
Mpox vaccine	Mpox	Jynneos®
Pneumococcal conjugate vaccine	PCV15	Vaxneuvance™
	PCV20	Prevnar 20®
Pneumococcal polysaccharide vaccine	PPSV23	Pneumovax 23®
Poliovirus vaccine (inactivated)	IPV	Ipol®
Respiratory syncytial virus vaccine	RSV	Abrysvo™
Rotavirus vaccine	RV1	Rotarix®
	RV5	RotaTeq®
Tetanus, diphtheria, and acellular pertussis vaccine	Tdap	Adacel® Boostrix®
Tetanus and diphtheria vaccine	Td	Tenivac® Tdvax™
Varicella vaccine	VAR	Varivax®
Combination vaccines *(use combination vaccines instead of separate injections when appropriate)*		
DTaP, hepatitis B, and inactivated poliovirus vaccine	DTaP-HepB-IPV	Pediarix®
DTaP, inactivated poliovirus, and *Haemophilus influenzae* type b vaccine	DTaP-IPV/Hib	Pentacel®
DTaP and inactivated poliovirus vaccine	DTaP-IPV	Kinrix® Quadracel®
DTaP, inactivated poliovirus, *Haemophilus influenzae* type b, and hepatitis B vaccine	DTaP-IPV-Hib-HepB	Vaxelis®
Measles, mumps, rubella, and varicella vaccine	MMRV	ProQuad®

*Administer recommended vaccines if immunization history is incomplete or unknown. Do not restart or add doses to vaccine series for extended intervals between doses. When a vaccine is not administered at the recommended age, administer at a subsequent visit. The use of trade names is for identification purposes only and does not imply endorsement by the ACIP or CDC.

11/16/2023

How to use the child and adolescent immunization schedule

1 Determine recommended vaccine by age **(Table 1)**

2 Determine recommended interval for catch-up vaccination **(Table 2)**

3 Assess need for additional recommended vaccines by medical condition or other indication **(Table 3)**

4 Review vaccine types, frequencies, intervals, and considerations for special situations **(Notes)**

5 Review contraindications and precautions for vaccine types **(Appendix)**

6 Review new or updated ACIP guidance **(Addendum)**

Recommended by the Advisory Committee on Immunization Practices (www.cdc.gov/vaccines/acip) and approved by the Centers for Disease Control and Prevention (www.cdc.gov), American Academy of Pediatrics (www.aap.org), American Academy of Family Physicians (www.aafp.org), American College of Obstetricians and Gynecologists (www.acog.org), American College of Nurse-Midwives (www.midwife.org), American Academy of Physician Associates (www.aapa.org), and National Association of Pediatric Nurse Practitioners (www.napnap.org).

Report
- Suspected cases of reportable vaccine-preventable diseases or outbreaks to your state or local health department
- Clinically significant adverse events to the Vaccine Adverse Event Reporting System (VAERS) at www.vaers.hhs.gov or 800-822-7967

Questions or comments

Contact www.cdc.gov/cdc-info or 800-CDC-INFO (800-232-4636), in English or Spanish, 8 a.m.–8 p.m. ET, Monday through Friday, excluding holidays

Download the CDC Vaccine Schedules app for providers at www.cdc.gov/vaccines/schedules/hcp/schedule-app.html

Helpful information
- Complete Advisory Committee on Immunization Practices (ACIP) recommendations: www.cdc.gov/vaccines/hcp/acip-recs/index.html
- ACIP Shared Clinical Decision-Making Recommendations: www.cdc.gov/vaccines/acip/acip-scdm-faqs.html
- *General Best Practice Guidelines for Immunization* (including contraindications and precautions): www.cdc.gov/vaccines/hcp/acip-recs/general-recs/index.html
- Vaccine information statements: www.cdc.gov/vaccines/hcp/vis/index.html
- Manual for the Surveillance of Vaccine-Preventable Diseases (including case identification and outbreak response): www.cdc.gov/vaccines/pubs/surv-manual

Scan QR code for access to online schedule

U.S. Department of Health and Human Services
Centers for Disease Control and Prevention

CS310020-D

Fig. 7.2 Recommended Child and Adolescent Immunization Schedule for ages 18 years or younger (Image source: https://www.cdc.gov/vaccines/hcp/imz-schedules/downloads/child/0-18yrs-child-combined-schedule.pdf)

7.3 CDC Vaccine Recommendations, 2023 (Children and Adults)

7.3.1 COVID-19

Cov (coronavirus) is a group of viruses belonging to the *Nidovirales* order, which comprises of *Coronaviridae*, *Roniviridae*, and *Arteriviridae* families. Crucial features imply that they are enveloped, non-segmented positive-sense RNA viruses.

In 2019, a novel Cov, named as severe acute respiratory syndrome coronavirus-2 (SARS-CoV-2) (the International Committee on Taxonomy of Viruses) emerged causing a worldwide pandemic. The virus is known to belong to the genus beta-CoV, which comprises of the severe acute respiratory syndrome CoV (SARS-CoV), and Middle Eastern respiratory syndrome CoV (MERS-CoV) [17].

Mortality rate of SARS-CoV-2 is lower than SARS-CoV and MERS-CoV; however, it is transmitted much more quickly and widely [18].

On February 11, 2020, the World Health Organization (WHO) announced a new name for a disease caused by SARS-CoV-2: CoV disease (COVID-19), and on March 11, 2020, it was declared as a pandemic [17–19].

The newly identified SARS-CoV-2 has been suspected to extend to humans from bats through pangolins [20, 21]. Upon infection of a human host, further transmission of the SARS-CoV-2 is horizontal, occurring mainly through human-to-human contact, either directly through respiratory droplets or indirectly by touching contaminated surfaces [21]. Other modes of transmission of SARS-CoV-2 RNA include vertical transmission from a mother to a newborn child, which has a low likelihood, as well as presence of the virus in urine and feces which also seems to play a minor role in transmission of infection [21–23]. Asymptomatic people may shed the virus, which may represent a major problem for continuous transmission and accounts for approximately 25–50% of total new infections [17]. The infection typically starts 1 to 2 days before symptom onset, whereas viral titers in respiratory secretions are noted to be highest in the early stages of infection with a quick decline soon after [24]. The most common complaints are fever, cough, and dyspnea and less frequently gastrointestinal symptoms like diarrhea, whereas older age groups (65 years or older) are at higher risk of developing severe SARS-CoV-2 infection because of higher proportion of established comorbidities [25]. In smokers and obese individuals, the severity of the disease may be higher [26]. Other documented symptoms include taste alterations and olfactory disturbances during the earlier course of the disease [27]; cutaneous manifestations such as erythematous rashes and urticaria [28]; neurological manifestations such as headache, altered conscious state, dizziness, and acute cerebrovascular disease that have also been exhibited by patients [29]; liver injury; venous and arterial thrombotic events and pulmonary embolisms (PEs) [30]; and ophthalmological issues, such as ocular pain, redness, and follicular conjunctivitis [31]. In children, SARS-CoV-2-induced inflammation disease has been documented as multisystem inflammatory syndrome in children (MIS-C) [32, 33]. Ever since the onset of the pandemic, collaborative efforts among the pharmaceutical companies, the WHO, the and scientific society have been done worldwide to develop the COVID-19 vaccine. Eight vaccines have been approved for Emergency Use Authorization (EUA) and should be considered depending on age. These belong to four different groups based on their mode of action, which include mRNA-based vaccine, inactivated vaccine, non-replicating viral vector vaccine, and peptide vaccine. Two the mRNA-based vaccines developed by Pfizer-BioNTech and Moderna have gained popularity owing to their approval in multiple countries [17].

Vaccines available in the United States are two types of COVID-19 vaccines are [34]:

1. mRNA vaccines

   Moderna Vaccine: Moderna COVID-19 vaccine (2023–2024 formula) is authorized for children ages 6 months–11 years. SPIKEVAX is the licensed Moderna product for people ages 12 years and older.

   Pfizer-BioNTech COVID-19 vaccine (2023–2024 formula) is authorized for children ages 6 months–11 years. COMIRNATY is the licensed Pfizer-BioNTech product for people ages 12 years and older.

2. Protein subunit vaccine

   Novavax COVID-19 vaccine, adjuvanted, is authorized for individuals ages 12 years and older for primary vaccination and, in limited situations, as a booster dose in people ages 18 years and older.

As per CDC initial guidelines, the following vaccination schedule is recommended [35]:

- Children aged 5 years and older are recommended to receive one dose of updated (2023–2024 Formula) mRNA COVID-19 vaccine.
- Children ages 6 months–4 years.
  - Initial vaccination: either two doses of updated (2023–2024 formula) Moderna or three doses of updated (2023–2024 formula) Pfizer-BioNTech COVID-19 vaccine
  - Received previous mRNA doses: one or two doses of updated (2023–2024 formula) Moderna or updated (2023–2024 formula) Pfizer-BioNTech COVID-19 vaccine/depending on the number of prior doses
- Moderately or severely immunocompromised individuals:
  - Initial vaccination: three-dose series of updated (2023–2024 formula) Moderna or updated (2023–2024 formula) Pfizer-BioNTech COVID-19 vaccine
  - Received previous mRNA doses: one or two doses of updated (2023–2024 formula) Moderna or updated (2023–2024 formula) Pfizer-BioNTech COVID-19 vaccine/depending on the number of prior doses
  - May receive one or more additional updated (2023–2024 formula) mRNA COVID-19 vaccine doses

Individuals with moderate or severe immunocompromised status undergo some specific adjustments in their vaccination schedule [36]:

- 6 months–4 years: three-dose series at 0, 4, and 8 weeks (Moderna) or three-dose series at 0, 3, and 11 weeks (Pfizer-BioNTech)
- 5–11 years: three-dose series at 0, 4, and 8 weeks (Moderna) or three-dose series at 0, 3, and 7 weeks (Pfizer-BioNTech)
- 12–18 years: three-dose series at 0, 4, and 8 weeks (Moderna) or two-dose series at 0 and 3 weeks (Novavax) or three-dose series at 0, 3, and 7 weeks (Pfizer-BioNTech).

And finally, the most recent adjustments to Moderna and Pfizer-BioNTech COVID-19 vaccine recommendations in the United States included children and newborns [37].

The last formulated CDC policy as of September 12, 2023, recommended monovalent XBB containing COVID-19 vaccines, authorized under emergency authorization use (EUA) or approved by Biologic License Application (BLA), to be used in individuals ≥6 months of age. As per the above-mentioned updates, CDC recommends the following vaccination schedule of primary series of either Moderna or Pfizer-BioNTech COVID-19 vaccines [37, 38]:

- Age 6 months–4 years: two-dose series at 0 and 4–8 weeks (Moderna) or three-dose series at 0, 3–8, and 11–16 weeks (Pfizer-BioNTech)
- Age 5–11 years: two-dose series at 0 and 4–8 weeks (Moderna) or two-dose series at 0 and 3–8 weeks (Pfizer-BioNTech)
- Age 12–18 years: two-dose series at 0 and 4–8 weeks (Moderna) or two-dose series at 0 and 3–8 weeks (Novavax, Pfizer-BioNTech)

Bivalent mRNA COVID-19 vaccines have been the most recent vaccines authorized in the United States to simplify the vaccination schedule for most individuals [39].

As to primary series vaccination by using either mRNA COVID-19 vaccine (Moderna and Pfizer-BioNTech), or Novavax (protein subunit), an 8-week interval is recommended between the first and the second doses to minimize a potential risk of myocarditis and pericarditis. This extended interval applies to children ages 6 months–4 years and individuals aged 12 years and older receiving Novavax vaccine, depending on their vaccination history [40].

No major concerns have been documented with respect to COVID-19 vaccines; however, as with every vaccine, it takes time to establish routine approach and make the public aware of the necessary steps in preventing the spread of the virus. However, syncope (fainting) may occur with any injectable vaccine, particularly in young adults or needle-phobia patients, but anaphylactic reaction has been reported rarely [41].

7.3.2 Influenza

Influenza (flu) is a contagious respiratory disease caused by two main types of influenza viruses (types A and B), which typically spread mostly during the fall and winter seasons reaching the peak between December and February. However, since the COVID pandemic, the duration and activity of flu have become unpredictable. The overall impact on health is documented by CDC reports on distribution of infection and occurrence of hospitalizations and deaths.

Influenza can be prevented by following everyday measures of precaution, and we can minimize the risk of spreading the virus by washing hands, avoiding contacts with contagious individuals, disinfecting potentially contagious surfaces, etc. Adjusted vaccine effectiveness estimates for influenza seasons from 2004 to 2023 are available on the CDC website [42].

Seasonal flu vaccines are designed to protect against the influenza viruses. All flu vaccines in the United States are "quadrivalent" vaccines, which means they protect against four different flu viruses: an influenza A(H1N1) virus, an influenza A(H3N2) virus, and two influenza B viruses [43].

Of utmost importance is the time of vaccination and an individual risk for developing severe symptoms and consequent medical complications. Vaccination is scheduled starting September, prior to flu season, and it takes approximately 2 weeks for protection to develop. Recommendations are age-appropriate and depend on an individual health status for a single flu season. Children 6 months through 8 years are recommended to get two doses per flu season [44].

Priority is given to a population considered to be at high risk, either due to their age or due to overall condition (which may lead to medical complications, particularly if severe symptoms develop) [45].

Individuals due to an elevated risk of developing severe symptoms due to influenza are highly considered for influenza vaccination [46].

As per CDC, the high-risk population are the following individuals [47]:

- Children aged 6 through 59 months and population aged ≥50 years
- Adults and children who have chronic pulmonary (including asthma), cardiovascular (excluding isolated hypertension), renal, hepatic, neurologic, hematologic, or metabolic disorders (including diabetes mellitus)
- Persons who are immunocompromised due to any cause (including but not limited to immunosuppression caused by medications or HIV infection)
- Persons who are or will be pregnant during the influenza season
- Children and adolescents (aged 6 months through 18 years) who are receiving aspirin- or salicylate-containing medications and who might be at risk for experiencing Reye syndrome after influenza virus infection
- Residents of nursing homes and other long-term care facilities
- American Indian or Alaska natives
- Persons who are extremely obese (body mass index ≥40 for adults)

In children, the following time frame schedule should be used, depending on a child's age and vaccine status (Fig. 7.3) [48]:

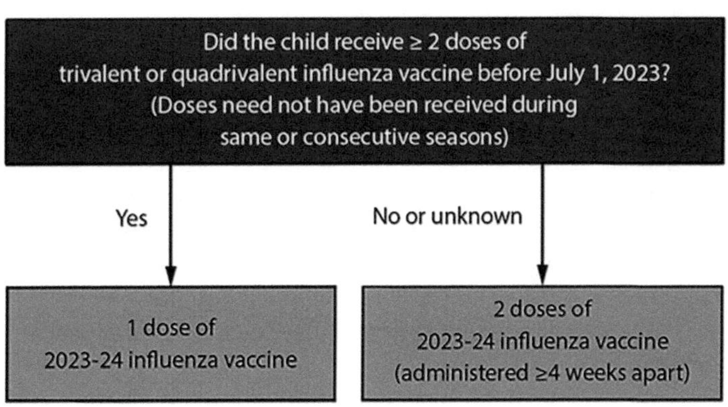

Fig. 7.3 Prevention and control of seasonal influenza with vaccines: recommendation of the Advisory Committee on Immunization Practices (ACIP)-United States, 2023–2024. (Courtesy of CDC)

Table 7.2 Currently available age-related influenza vaccine types and recommended doses (Courtesy of CDC)

Vaccine, approved ages & dose volume		
Vaccine	Approved ages	Dose volume (mL)
Afluria Quadrivalent	6 through 35 months	0.25
	≥3 years	0.5
Fluarix Quadrivalent	≥6 months	0.5
FluLaval Quadrivalent	≥6 months	0.5
Fluzone Quadrivalent	6 through 35 months	0.5 (see below)
	≥3 years	0.5
Flucelvax Quadrivalent	≥6 months	0.5
Flublok Quadrivalent	≥18 years	0.5
Fluzone high-dose Quadrivalent	≥65 years	0.7
Fluad Quadrivalent	≥65 years	0.5

Source:
Center for Disease Control and Prevention [50]

- Two doses, at least 4 weeks apart
  - For children 6 months–8 years who have received fewer than two influenza vaccine doses before July 1, 2022, or whose influenza vaccination history is unknown, administer dose 2 even if the child turns 9 between receipt of dose 1 and dose 2
- One dose for children 6 months–8 years who have received at least two influenza vaccine doses before July 1, 2022
- One dose for all individuals 9 years or older

In adults aged ≥65 years, either quadrivalent high-dose inactivated influenza vaccine (HD-IIV4), quadrivalent recombinant influenza vaccine (RIV4), or quadrivalent adjuvanted inactivated influenza vaccine (aIIV4) are used [49].

As per the most recent CDC 2023–2024 influenza vaccine recommendations, two types of influenza vaccines are prioritized: inactivated influenza virus-quadrivalent virus (IIV-4s) or recombinant influenza virus-quadrivalent virus (RIV-4) (Table 7.2) [50].

7.3.3 Tetanus, Diphtheria, and Pertussis (Tdap or Td)

Tetanus is a serious disease caused by a gram-positive bacteria *Clostridium tetani* which is ubiquitous, particularly in soil, dust, and dirt. It mostly affects the nervous system, causing painful muscular spasms that affect the nervous system. Tetanus is a leading cause for neonatal death in the developing world [51].

Tetanus is still prevalent in many developing countries, but it can be prevented through vaccination.

Diphtheria is a disease of the upper respiratory tract and sometimes skin, caused by toxigenic strains of *Corynebacterium diphtheriae* biotype mitis, gravis, intermedius, or belfant. It is also preventable through vaccination.

Pertussis—"whooping cough," caused by *Bordetella pertussis*—can be a life-threatening disease in infants with small airways. It has been reported as endemic worldwide, including the United States and other countries, with high vaccination rates. In adults, it is represented by protracted cough with paroxysms that may be followed by vomiting.

Due to a vaccination program, the disease has been successfully prevented; however, outbreaks have been reported in recent years [52–56].

The tetanus toxoid (TT) vaccines were first introduced in the United States in the mid-1940s. After that, the incidence of reported tetanus declined by >98% [53].

Currently, two types of Tdap vaccines are licensed for use in the United States (CDC recommendations: https://www.cdc.gov/vaccines/acip/recs/grade/tdap-etr.html:

1. Boostrix (GlaxoSmithKline), which has been approved for a single dose in persons aged ≥10 years.
2. Adacel (Sanofi Pasteur), which has been approved for persons aged 10–64 years.

In the United States, diphtheria-tetanus-acellular pertussis (DTaP) vaccine is routinely administered to children at 2, 4, and 6 months, followed by boosters at 15–18 months and 4–6 years. A single booster dose of a vaccine containing tetanus toxoid reduced diphtheria toxoid, and acellular pertussis (Tdap) is recommended for 11- to 12-year-olds and every 10 years after that. In 2020, Advisory Committee on Immunization Practices (ACIP) released new recommendations allowing either Tdap or Td to be used as the booster or for wound management while previously only Td was recommended [53, 57].

In 2005, a single booster dose of Tdap has been recommended for children and adolescents aged 11–18 years and adults aged 19–64 years to increase protection against tetanus, diphtheria, and pertussis [56, 58].

Booster doses are recommended every 10 years or when indicated for wound management, in individuals who had previously received Tdap, if multiple doses in the immunization schedule are required for individuals aged ≥7 years who have unknown or unclear vaccination history.

In 2019, the Advisory Committee on Immunization Practices (ACIP) accepted either Td vaccine (tetanus and diphtheria toxoid) or Tdap vaccine (tetanus toxoid, reduced diphtheria toxoid, and acellular pertussis) as booster doses recommended every 10 years [59].

General recommendations are based on CDC recommendations [60, 61].

As per the most recent guidelines, the vaccination is as follows [62]:

- Age 11–18 years: A single dose of Tdap (at the preventive visit at age 11–12 years): one booster dose of either Td or Tdap should be further readministered every 10 years throughout life.
- Age ≥ 19 years: Individuals who have never received a dose of Tdap should receive one dose of Tdap and those individuals who received it previously, regardless of the interval since their last tetanus or diphtheria toxoid-containing vaccine; ensure continued protection against tetanus and diphtheria; one booster

dose of either Td or Tdap should be further readministered every 10 years throughout life.
- Pregnant women: One dose of Tdap during each pregnancy, irrespective of their history of receiving the vaccine. Recommended timing is at the 27–36 weeks of gestation (preferably during the earlier part of this period); however, it may be administered at any time during pregnancy.

In general, individuals receiving the vaccine for the first time, or those with unknown vaccination status, as well as pregnant women, would receive Tdap (tetanus toxoid, reduced diphtheria toxoid, and acellular pertussis) [57].

However, certain situations require special precaution and a modified approach [57].

These specific situations include [57]:

1. Individuals aged 7–18 years who previously did not receive primary vaccination series for tetanus, diphtheria, or pertussis, who should then receive the vaccine as follows:
   - One dose of Tdap (first dose) followed by one dose Td or Tdap at least 4 weeks later (second dose).
   - Td or Tdap 6 to 12 months after the second dose (Tdap can be substituted for any Td dose but preferred as first dose).
   - Td or Tdap every 10 years thereafter, to increase the existing immunity.
2. Individuals aged 7–18 years who are not fully immunized against tetanus and diphtheria and who should then receive one dose of Tdap, preferably as the first dose in the catch-up series. (The vaccination series doesn't need to be restarted, regardless of the time elapsed).

Special precaution is required for wound management. In managing wounds, Tdap or Td is required if more than 10 years since last dose of tetanus-toxoid-containing vaccine (only clear wounds), and in all other cases of wound management, the vaccine is required if >5 years have passed since the last tetanus toxoid-containing vaccine dose [57].

7.3.4 Measles, Mumps, Rubella (MMR)

Measles, mumps, rubella, and varicella (chickenpox) are serious and highly contagious diseases that can lead to serious complications, disability, and death [63–65]. Measles, also called rubeola, and mumps are caused by paramyxovirus, whereas chickenpox is caused by the varicella-zoster virus (VZV). Measles appears to be the most contagious infection among humans and mortality for mumps is less than that for measles. However, consequent complications may result in orchitis, meningitis, encephalitis, and death [66]. Measles (also called rubeola) is an acute viral respiratory illness, caused by a single-stranded RNA virus of the genus *Morbillivirus* and the family *Paramyxoviridae*. It is characterized by a prodrome presenting with a high fever (up to 105 °F) and overall symptoms of malaise, cough, coryza, and conjunctivitis, including pathognomonic enanthema (Koplik spots), followed by a maculopapular rash. The rash usually appears 14 days upon exposure, spreading from the head to the trunk and lower extremities. Infected individuals are considered to be contagious from 4 days before to 4 days after the rash appears. Rubella infection presents as relatively mild disease for children but in pregnant women, particularly during early stages, may lead to miscarriage, fetal death, or congenital rubella syndrome [64].

Mumps is a contagious viral illness and at one time was a very common childhood disease prior to introduction of vaccine. The trivalent infection can be prevented through vaccination, although some controversies regarding safety vs. effectiveness still exist. However, despite controversy, the recommended vaccine provides safe and effective protection against these three viral diseases—measles, mumps, and rubella.

Two MMR vaccines available for use in the United States are M-M-R II and PRIORIX and can be used interchangeably [65].

As an alternative, MMRV vaccine (against measles, mumps, rubella, and varicella/chickenpox) can be administered in children aged 12 months through age 12 [66].

Children should get two doses of MMR vaccine, starting with the first dose at 12 to 15 months of age and the second dose at 4 through 6 years of age. Teens and adults should also be up to date on their MMR vaccination. Adult individuals, i.e., teenagers and adults, expected to be exposed to infection should consider receiving two doses which should be administered 28 days apart [67].

As per general recommendations, routine vaccination requiring one dose of MMR vaccine is required in individuals with no evidence of immunity to measles, mumps, or rubella and individuals who have evidence of immunity and born before 1957 (healthcare personnel) with laboratory evidence of immunity or documented receipt of MMR vaccine [68].

Adjustments to the routine MMR vaccine schedule is required in specific situations [69]:

- Nonpregnant individuals of childbearing age with no evidence of immunity to rubella (one dose MMR).
- Pregnant women with no evidence of immunity to rubella (one dose MMR).
- Note: MMR is contraindicated during pregnancy and immediately after pregnancy, i.e., before discharge from healthcare facility.
- HIV infection with CD4 percentages ≥15% and CD4 count ≥200 cells/mm3 for at least 6 months and no evidence of immunity to measles, mumps, or rubella (two-dose series at least 4 weeks apart).
- Note: MMR contraindicated for HIV infection with CD4 percentage < 15% or CD4 count <200 cells/mm^3 and in severe immunocompromising conditions.
- Students in postsecondary educational institutions, international travelers, and household or close personal contacts of immunocompromised persons with no evidence of immunity to measles, mumps, or rubella (two-dose series at least

4 weeks apart if previously did not receive any doses of MMR or one dose if previously received one-dose MMR).
- In mumps outbreak settings, two-dose series, with an additional third dose of MMR.

As to healthcare professionals, the following recommendations should be considered [69]:

- Healthcare personnel:
  - Born before 1957 with no evidence of immunity to measles, mumps, or rubella: two-dose series at least 4 weeks apart for protection against measles or mumps or one dose for protection against rubella
  - Born in 1957 or later with no evidence of immunity to measles, mumps, or rubella: two-dose series at least 4 weeks apart for protection against measles or mumps or at least one dose for protection against rubella

7.3.5 Varicella

The *varicella-zoster* virus (VZV) or human herpes virus 3 is a neurotropic human alpha herpes virus that causes chickenpox/varicella and shingles/*herpes zoster* [70]. Varicella is acquired through respiratory droplets or smears from vesicular varicella lesions and, besides measles, is considered one of the most contagious human infections, with the highest likelihood of appearance during childhood. Following airway infection, viremia occurs, which results in appearance of cutaneous vesicular eruptions. These lesions are present through different stages, from early vesiculation to crusted lesions and eventually crusted lesions and scars. The incubation period for varicella varies between 10 and 21 days. Varicella is contagious from 1 to 4 days before the cutaneous rash and until all vesicular cutaneous lesions have dried up [71]. In the acute eruptive phase after infection with VZV, clinical symptoms present with multiple umbilicated and painful vesicles which burst, ulcerate, and eventually dry out. This is the most contagious stage. Pain may be often severe and unresponsive to nonsteroidal pain medications. The acute infectious stage represented with eruptive lesions may last 2–4 weeks, whereas pain can continue longer. Varicella infection in pregnancy can spread via the placenta [72]. The varicella vaccine provides protection against a highly contagious virus known as varicella-zoster virus (VZV). However, herpes zoster is uncommon in children, and varicella vaccination does not appear to be effective in preventing herpes zoster infection later in life [73]. Therefore, further vaccination for herpes zoster is recommended later in life (see zoster recombinant vaccine).

The following are attenuated varicella-zoster virus-containing vaccines available in the United States for prevention of varicella [74]:

1. VARIVAX® (Merck & Co., Inc., Whitehouse Station, New Jersey), a single-antigen varicella vaccine which was licensed in the United States in 1995 for use among healthy children aged ≥12 months, adolescents, and adults.
2. ProQuad® (Merck & Co., Inc., Whitehouse Station, New Jersey), a combination measles, mumps, rubella, and varicella vaccine which was licensed in the United States in 2005 for use among healthy children aged 12 months–12 years.
3. In addition and as per the most recent updates, VARIZIG (Cangene Corporation, Winnipeg, Canada) is the only varicella-zoster immune globulin preparation available in the United States for postexposure prophylaxis of varicella in persons at high risk for severe disease who lack evidence of immunity to varicella and are ineligible for varicella vaccine [75].

As per CDC recommendation, the following routine vaccination schedule should be used for prevention of varicella [74]:

Routine two-dose vaccination schedule for prevention of varicella [76]

- first dose at age 12 through 15 months; second dose at age 4 through 6 years.
- *If the second dose is administered after the seventh birthday, the minimum interval between doses is 3 months for children age < 13 years and 4 weeks for persons age ≥ 13 years.
- Adolescents and adults (≥ age 13 years) without other evidence of immunity: two doses 4 to 8 weeks apart.

  *If it has been more than 8 weeks since the first dose, the second dose may be given without restarting the schedule.

Special consideration should be given in the following situations [72]

- Age 50 years or older: Two-dose series recombinant zoster vaccine (RZV, Shingrix), regardless of previous herpes zoster or history of zoster vaccine live (ZVL, Zostavax) vaccination, 2–6 months apart (at minimum is 4 weeks apart)/repeat dose if administered too soon).
- Pregnancy: Consider delaying RZV until after pregnancy.
- Immunocompromising conditions (including persons with HIV regardless of CD4 count): two-dose series recombinant zoster vaccine (RZV, Shingrix), regardless of previous herpes zoster or history of zoster vaccine live (ZVL, Zostavax) vaccination, 2–6 months apart (at minimum is 4 weeks apart)/repeat dose if administered too soon.

7.3.6 Zoster Recombinant

Herpes zoster (HZ) is an infection that appears secondary to varicella; therefore, incidence increases with age and compromised immunity. After primary infection, the varicella-zoster virus (VZV) becomes latent in nerval tissue and reactivates due to compromised immunity. Children and youngsters with metabolic and neoplastic disorders, as well as adults, under stress, immunocompromised, or associated with comorbidities (AIDS or COVID-19), are more prone to developing zoster symptoms. Clinical symptoms present with burning and pain within the affected dermatome minimally 2 days prior to cutaneous infection. Non-cutaneous symptoms such as headaches, general malaise, and photophobia may occur as well [77, 78]. Other complications relevant to herpes zoster infection may include vasculitis (associated with morbidity and mortality) and renal and gastrointestinal complications. Chronic herpes zoster infection is characterized by severe pain that lasts for months, most likely >4 weeks. Patients experience dysesthesias, paresthesia, and sometimes shock-like sensations.

Shingrix (recombinant zoster vaccine) provides strong protection showing more than 90% effectiveness against shingles and postherpetic neuralgia (PHN) in adults 50 years and older who have healthy immune systems [79]. Immunity stays strong for minimally 7 years after vaccination; in adults with weakened immune systems, studies show that Shingrix is effective in preventing shingles, depending on the condition that affects the immune system [79]:

Shingrix vaccine is recommended in the following situations:

- Received Zostavax.
- Received varicella (chickenpox) vaccine (chickenpox and shingles are related because they are caused by the same virus, which is known as varicella-zoster virus).
- Previous history of shingles (no specific length of time is required after recovering from previous shingle infection; however, it should be given after completely recovering from the shingle rash).

The CDC provides general recommendations for the prevention of herpes zoster (shingles) [80].

As per ACIP recommendations, two doses of RZV/recombinant zoster vaccine (Shingrix) are required regardless of previous history of shingles or previous receipt of zoster vaccine live (ZVL, Zostavax) to prevent shingles and related complications in adults aged ≥19 years who are or will be immunodeficient or immunosuppressed because of disease or therapy, with the second dose of RZV typically given 2–6 months after the first. There is no maximum age for getting Shingrix [81].

In immunodeficient or immunosuppressed individuals, the second dose can be administered 1–2 months after the first to facilitate avoiding vaccination during periods of more intense immunosuppression. However, if the second dose of RZV is given less than 4 weeks apart, the second dose should be repeated at least 4 weeks after the first dose that was given too early. The vaccine series does not need to be restarted if more than 6 months have elapsed since the first dose [81].

Clinical considerations for use of recombinant zoster vaccine (RZV, Shingrix) in immunocompromised adults aged ≥19 years have been provided by the CDC [82].

7.3.7 Human Papillomavirus (HPV)

Human papillomavirus (HPV) is the most common sexually transmitted infection in the United States [83, 84]. The Centers for Disease Control and Prevention (CDC) estimate that nearly 13 million people in the United States are infected by HPV annually and that nearly 85% of unvaccinated, sexually active individuals will be infected by the virus at some point during their lifetime [85].

Although the vast majority of HPV infections clear on their own, not all do, and HPV infection is associated with nearly 37,000 cervical, vulval, vaginal, penile, anal, and oropharyngeal cancer cases annually [86]. Among women, cervical cancer is the most common HPV-related cancer, while oropharyngeal cancer is the most common HPV-related cancer among men [86].

HPV vaccination is highly effective at preventing HPV-related cancers that can occur later in life [85]. The CDC recommends that all children receive the HPV vaccine at the ages of 11–12 years [87]. Importantly, this age is recommended because the vaccine works by preventing infection before being exposed to the virus [87]. The HPV vaccine is given in two doses, with the first dose given at the age 11–12 years and the second dose given 6–12 months after the first dose [87]. Adults through the age of 26 years are recommended to receive the HPV vaccine if they have not yet been fully vaccinated [87]. Additionally, while it is not recommended, adults ages 27–45 years are eligible to receive the HPV vaccine after speaking with their physician to determine whether the benefits of vaccination outweigh any risks [87].

7.3.8 Hepatitis A

Hepatitis A is an infection resulting in the inflammation of the liver due to the hepatitis A virus [88, 89]. In 2021, there were an estimated 5728 incident (new) cases of hepatitis A and nearly 11,500 total infections [90, 91]. Although the rate of infections has been declining recently, there were nearly four times as many Hep A cases in 2021 as compared to 2015 [90, 91]. The hepatitis A virus can be transmitted from person to person through the fecal-oral route or by consuming food or water that has been contaminated [90, 91]. Certain demographic groups are at greater risk for being infected, including international travelers, those with occupational risks, and the immunocompromised [90]. The virus typically results in an acute infection with symptoms usually lasting no more than 2 months after infection [90]. These symptoms can include fever, fatigue, nausea, vomiting, diarrhea, abdominal pain, and jaundice [90, 91].

Being vaccinated with the hepatitis A vaccine is the primary method of preventing hepatitis A infection [90]. The CDC recommends the hepatitis A vaccine for children at the ages of 12–23 months [90, 92]. It is a two-dose vaccine with the second dose given between 6 and 18 months after the first dose [90, 92]. Children and adolescents up to age 18 are also recommended to receive the vaccine if they did not previously receive it during the recommended age window [90, 92].

Individuals over the age of 18 are able to receive the hepatitis A vaccine, and it is recommended for those who are at greater risk for hepatitis A infection [90, 92]. For those ages 18 years and older, a hepatitis A and hepatitis B combination vaccine is available as a three-dose vaccine given over a 6-month window [90, 92].

7.3.9 Hepatitis B

Hepatitis B is also an infection that results in inflammation of the liver caused by the hepatitis B virus, another type of hepatitis virus [93]. While hepatitis B can be an acute infection, it can also be a chronic infection and result in serious conditions such as cirrhosis, damage to the liver, cancer, or even death [93]. It is estimated that nearly 880,000 individuals are living with chronic hepatitis B, with approximately 14,000 incident cases of acute hepatitis B estimated to have occurred in 2020 [93]. Acute hepatitis B does not always cause symptoms, but when it does, they can include [93] fever, fatigue, loss of appetite, nausea, vomiting, abdominal pain, dark urine, clay-colored bowel movements, joint pain, and jaundice. Hepatitis B can be transmitted through sex, needlestick injuries, contaminated needles or objects, or other exposures to infected blood [93].

Being vaccinated with the hepatitis B vaccine is the primary method of preventing hepatitis B infection [93]. The CDC recommends the hepatitis B vaccine be given to infants within 24 hours after birth if they are medically stable [93]. It is normally a three-dose vaccine with the second dose recommended at age 1–2 months and the third dose given at age 6–18 months [93]. Children and adolescents up to age 18 are also recommended to receive the vaccine if they did not previously receive it during the recommended age window [93]. Adults over the age of 18 up to the age of 59 are also recommended to receive the vaccine [93]. The vaccine is also recommended for adults ages 60 and older if they are at risk for hepatitis B infection [93]. For those ages 18 years and older, a hepatitis A and hepatitis B combination vaccine is available as a three-dose vaccine given over a 6-month window [93].

7.3.10 Pneumococcal Disease

Pneumococcal disease is an infection caused by the bacteria *Streptococcus pneumoniae* [94]. The disease can be characterized by several different types of infections depending on where it occurs, including [95] pneumonia, meningitis, otitis media, sinusitis, or bacteremia. Individuals at greatest risk for pneumococcal disease include children under the age of 5 years and older adults of ages 65 years and older [96]. Pneumococcal disease is transmitted through respiratory secretions [96]. The specific symptoms of pneumococcal disease will vary depending on the specific infection but can include [97] headaches, fever or chills, cough, sore throat, chest pain, stiff neck, difficulty breathing, confusion, sensitivity to light, and ear pain. While symptoms are typically mild, death can occur with infection [97].

Receiving the pneumococcal vaccine can be effective at preventing pneumococcal disease, as it protects against many common types of pneumococcal bacteria [98]. The CDC recommends pneumococcal vaccination for all children younger than 5 years of age and for adults ages 65 years and older [98]. The vaccine is a four-dose series with the first dose typically given at 2 months and the remaining doses given at 4 months, 6 months, and 12–15 months [98]. For adults ages 65 years and older, the vaccine is given as a single dose. The vaccine is recommended by the CDC for individuals between the ages of 5 through 64 years if they are at increased risk for pneumococcal disease [98].

7.3.11 Meningococcal Disease

Meningococcal disease is an infection caused by the bacteria *Neisseria meningitidis* [99]. Meningococcal meningitis and meningococcemia are the most common types of meningococcal infections [100]. The disease is transmitted through respiratory and throat secretions [100]. Meningococcal meningitis results from an infection of the brain and spinal cord, and common symptoms include [100] fever, headache, stiff neck, nausea, vomiting, increased sensitivity to light, and confusion. Meningococcemia results from an infection of the bloodstream, and common symptoms include [100] fever and chills, fatigue, vomiting, cold hands and feet, aches or pain, rapid breathing, diarrhea, and a dark purple rash.

Receiving the meningococcal vaccine can be effective at preventing meningococcal disease [99]. The vaccine is recommended by the CDC as a two-dose vaccine for all individuals ages 11 to 12 years (initial dose), with a booster dose at age 16 years [99]. The vaccine is also recommended for older children and adults who are at increased risk for meningococcal disease [99]. For older adults, the number of doses varies depending on the specific meningococcal vaccine and the indication [99].

7.3.12 Haemophilus influenzae Type B (Hib)

Haemophilus influenzae is a bacteria that can infect different parts of the body to cause *Haemophilus influenzae* disease, which can include several different types of diseases [101]. Common infections caused by *H. influenzae* include [102] pneumonia, meningitis, and bacteremia, among others. Symptoms of the infection will include those symptoms commonly observed in pneumonia, meningitis, and bacteremia [102]. *H. influenzae* type b (Hib) is a specific strain of the bacteria, for which there is a vaccine [103]. The CDC recommends the Hib vaccination for children less than age 5 [103]. It is a three- to four-dose vaccine with the first dose given at age 2 months, and the remaining doses given at ages 4 months, 6 months (if given as a four-dose vaccine), and 12–15 months [103]. The Hib vaccine is also recommended for unvaccinated children over the age of 5 and adults who are at increased risk for infection and for individuals who receive a bone marrow transplant [103]. The vaccine is over 90% effective in preventing Hib disease in children [103]. Annually in the United States, there are less than 50 cases of Hib disease in young children, and most of these cases occur in those young children who are unvaccinated or not fully vaccinated [103]. Since the introduction of Hib vaccination, the annual incidence of Hib disease in young children in the United States has decreased by 99% [104].

7.3.13 Respiratory Syncytial Virus (RSV)

Respiratory syncytial virus (RSV) is a viral infection that is usually mild and causes common cold-like symptoms, including [105, 106] runny nose, decreased appetite, coughing, sneezing, fever, and wheezing. RSV is transmitted through viral droplets produced when an infected person sneezes or coughs or by touching surfaces contaminated with the virus [107]. While RSV is typically a mild infection, the infection can be severe in infants and older adults, resulting in hospitalization [105, 106]. For this reason, the CDC recommends that adults 60 years old discuss with their physicians whether receiving a single-dose RSV vaccination is indicated [108]. Additionally, it is now recommended that pregnant women receive a single dose of the RSV vaccine during weeks 32 through 36 of their pregnancy [108].

7.4 EU and UK Vaccine Recommendations

A vaccination schedule has been proposed by the European Union (EU)/European Economic Area (EEA) [109].

It is unique for the entire EU region; however, some differences still exist due to age and population/risk groups, type of vaccine (depending on different ingredients as approved by the government health departments), and the number and timing of doses' combination on vaccines (when necessary or indicated).

All of that is reasonable and justified, as different countries may represent with diverse burdens and prevalence of certain diseases, as well as current trends. Also, structure and health department policies, including different regulations and health systems, account for minor modifications as they pertain to a certain country. The overall approach in regard to vaccination remains efficient though, following appropriate timeframe intervals and ensuring adequate protection.

As of now, European Centre for Disease Prevention and Control (ECDC) is strengthening the national vaccination schedule by coordinating it with the public health authorities across the EU. The schedule is available on the following website: https://vaccine-schedule.ecdc.europa.eu/ [110].

The *childhood vaccination schedules in all EU/EEA* countries include the vaccination against measles, mumps, rubella, diphtheria, tetanus, pertussis (whooping cough), poliomyelitis, *Haemophilus influenzae* type B, and human papillomavirus (adolescent/preadolescent girls).

In addition, some EU/EEA countries offer protection through vaccination against hepatitis A, influenza, invasive disease caused by *Neisseria meningitidis*, invasive disease caused by *Streptococcus pneumoniae*, rotavirus, tuberculosis, varicella, as well as seasonal influenza (flu).

As to vaccination against hepatitis B, the World Health Organization (WHO) recommends vaccination as part of the universal childhood vaccination schedule, although some EU/EEA countries only recommend vaccination of children/adults who are at high risk for infection. There is a recommended vaccination schedule in the EU/EEA for booster doses, including contraindications as to when to avoid vaccinations (including allergies, immune system disorders, medical treatments, pregnancy) [111]. Guidelines to complete routine immunization schedule, based on the most updated recommendations on complete routine immunization, selective immunization, and additional vaccination for individuals with underlying medical conditions have been developed [112].

7.5 Contraindications for Vaccination

In general, in cases of any possible adverse effects, vaccination is contraindicated. However, in the majority of cases, contraindications may be temporary, and vaccines can be administered later in life. Screening for possible contraindications is mandatory and can be assessed through vaccination programs and in accordance with the national standard practices. Details on precaution measures are available on the following website: https://vaccination-info.europa.eu/en/vaccination/when-vaccinate/when-avoid-vaccination [113].

Certain conditions are commonly considered as contraindications. Immunocompromised individuals should not receive live vaccines, pregnant women should not live attenuated vaccines due to possible harm to fetus, individuals experiencing possible side effects to pertussis-containing ingredients should not be further considered for vaccination containing the pertussis component, and severe combined immunodeficiency disease (SCID) and medical history of intussusception are contraindications for rotavirus vaccine. Contraindications and precautions to commonly used vaccines in the United States have been proposed by the CDC and are available on the following website: https://www.cdc.gov/vaccines/hcp/acip-recs/general-recs/contraindications.pdf [114].

7.6 Conclusions

Vaccines are one of the principal public health tools to reduce morbidity and mortality of a variety of diseases. Unfortunately, these economic, safe, and effective pillars of global public health are often unavailable and/or, due to an increase in vaccine resistance, underutilized.

References

1. World Health Organization, Eastern Mediterranean Region. Health promotion and disease prevention through population-based interventions, including action to address social determinants and health inequity. Available at: https://www.emro.who.int/about-who/public-health-functions/health-promotion-disease-prevention.html Accessed 8 Nov 2023.
2. World Health Organization. Vaccines and immunization: what is vaccination? Available at: https://www.who.int/news-room/questions-and-answers/item/vaccines-and-immunization-what-is-vaccination. Accessed 8 Nov 2023.
3. U.S. Department of Health and Human Services. Vaccine ingredients. Available at: https://www.hhs.gov/immunization/basics/vaccine-ingredients/index.html. Accessed 8 Nov 2023.
4. Center for Disease Control and Prevention. Administer the vaccine(s). Available at: https://www.cdc.gov/vaccines/hcp/admin/administer-vaccines.html. Accessed 8 Nov 2023.
5. Centers for Disease Control and Prevention. Understanding how vaccines work. Available at: https://www.cdc.gov/vaccines/hcp/patient-ed/conversations/downloads/vacsafe-understand-bw-office.pdf. Accessed 8 Nov 2023.
6. U.S. Department of Health and Human Services. Vaccines protect you. Available at: https://www.hhs.gov/immunization/basics/work/prevention/index.html. Accessed 8 Nov 2023.
7. U.S. Department of Health and Human Services. Vaccine types. Available at: https://www.hhs.gov/immunization/basics/types/index.html. Accessed 8 Nov 2023.
8. Omran AR. The epidemiologic transition: a theory of the epidemiology of population change. 1971. Milbank Q. 2005;83(4):731–57.
9. Center for Disease Control and Prevention. Immunization: the basics. Available at: https://www.cdc.gov/vaccines/vac-gen/imz-basics.htm. Accessed 8 Nov 2023.
10. Center for Disease Control and Prevention. State vaccination requirements. Available at: https://www.cdc.gov/vaccines/imz-managers/laws/state-reqs.html. Accessed 8 Nov 2023.
11. U.S. Department of Health and Human Services. Vaccines protect your community. Available at: https://www.hhs.gov/immunization/basics/work/protection/index.html. Accessed 8 Nov 2023.
12. Center for Disease Control and Prevention. Vaccines by disease. Available at: https://www.cdc.gov/vaccines/vpd/vaccines-diseases.html. Accessed 8 Nov 2023.
13. Kubin L. Is there a resurgence of vaccine preventable diseases in the U.S.? J Pediatr Nurs. 2019;44:115–8. https://doi.org/10.1016/j.pedn.2018.11.011. Epub 2018 Nov 29
14. Porteous GH, Hanson NA, Sueda LA, Hoaglan CD, Dahl AB, Ohlson BB, Schmidt BE, Wang CC, Fagley RE. Resurgence of vaccine-preventable diseases in the United States: anesthetic and critical care implications. Anesth Analg. 2016;122(5):1450–73. https://doi.org/10.1213/ANE.0000000000001196.
15. Gautret P, Botelho-Nevers E, Brouqui P, Parola P. The spread of vaccine-preventable diseases by international travellers: a public-health concern. Clin Microbiol Infect. 2012;18(Suppl 5):77–84. https://doi.org/10.1111/j.1469-0691.2012.03940.x. Epub 2012 Aug 6.
16. Feldman AG, O'Leary ST, Danziger-Isakov L. The risk of resurgence in vaccine-preventable infections due to coronavirus disease 2019-related gaps in immunization. Clin Infect Dis. 2021;73:1920.
17. Ochani R, Asad A, Yasmin F, Shaikh S, Khalid H, Batra S, Sohail MR, Mahmood SF, Ochani R, Hussham Arshad M, Kumar A, Surani S. COVID-19 pandemic: from origins to outcomes. A comprehensive review of viral pathogenesis, clinical manifestations, diagnostic evaluation, and management. Infez Med. 2021;29(1):20–36.
18. World Health Organization. COVID-19 situation report—51. 2020. Available from: https://www.who.int/docs/default-source/coronaviruse/situation-reports/20200311-sitrep-51-covid-19.pdf?sfvrsn=1ba62e57_10. Accessed 11 Jul 2020.
19. Lai CC, Shih TP, Ko WC, Tang HJ, Hsueh PR. Severe acute respiratory syndrome coronavirus 2 (SARSCoV-2) and coronavirus disease-2019 (COVID-19): the epidemic and the challenges. Int J Antimicrob Agents. 2020;55(3):105924.

20. Li X, Zai J, Zhao Q, et al. Evolutionary history, potential intermediate animal host, and cross-species analyses of SARS-CoV-2. J Med Virol. 2020;92(6):602–11.
21. Doremalen NV, Morris DH, Holbrook MG, et al. Aerosol and surface stability of HcoV-19 (SARS-CoV-2) compared to SARS-CoV-1. N Engl J Med. 2020;382(16):1564–7.
22. Wiersinga WJ, Rhodes A, Cheng AC, Peacock SJ, Prescott HC. Pathophysiology, transmission, diagnosis, and treatment of coronavirus disease 2019 (COVID-19): a review. JAMA. 2020;324(8):782–93.
23. Zeng L, Xia S, Yuan W, Yan K, Xiao F, Shao J, Zhou W. Neonatal early-onset infection with SARS-CoV-2 in 33 neonates born to mothers with COVID-19 in Wuhan, China. JAMA Pediatr. 2020;174(7):722–5. https://doi.org/10.1001/jamapediatrics.2020.0878. PMID: 32215598; PMCID: PMC7099530.
24. Sunjaya AP, Jenkins C. Rationale for universal face masks in public against COVID-19. Respirology. 2020;25(7):678–9.
25. Ye ZW, Yuan S, Yuen KS, Fung SY, Chan CP, Jin DY. Zoonotic origins of human coronaviruses. Int J Biol Sci. 2020;16(10):1686–97.
26. Zhang JJ, Dong X, Cao YY, et al. Clinical characteristics of 140 patients infected with SARS-CoV-2 in Wuhan, China. Allergy. 2020;75(7):1730–41.
27. Giacomelli A, Pezzati L, Conti F, et al. Self-reported olfactory and taste disorders in patients with severe acute respiratory coronavirus 2 infection: a cross-sectional study. Clin Infect Dis. 2020;71(15):889–90.
28. Recalcati S. Cutaneous manifestations in COVID-19: a first perspective. J Eur Acad Dermatol Venereol. 2020;34(5):e212–3.
29. Mao L, Jin H, Wang M, et al. Neurologic manifestations of hospitalized patients with coronavirus disease 2019 in Wuhan, China. JAMA Neurol. 2020;77(6):683–90.
30. Klok FA, Kruip MJHA, van der Meer NJM, et al. Incidence of thrombotic complications in critically ill ICU patients with COVID-19. Thromb Res. 2020;191:145–7.
31. Aggarwal K, Agarwal A, Jaiswal N, et al. Ocular surface manifestations of coronavirus disease 2019 (COVID-19): a systematic review and meta-analysis. PLoS One. 2020;15(11):e0241661.
32. Mahase E. Covid-19: concerns grow over inflammatory syndrome emerging in children. BMJ. 2020;369:m1710.
33. Verdoni L, Mazza A, Gervasoni A, et al. An outbreak of severe Kawasaki-like disease at the Italian epicentre of the SARS-CoV-2 epidemic: an observational cohort study. Lancet. 2020;395(10239):1771–8.
34. Center for Disease Control and Prevention. Available at https://www.cdc.gov/vaccines/covid-19/info-by-product/index.html
35. Center for Disease Control and Prevention. Available at: https://www.cdc.gov/coronavirus/2019-ncov/vaccines/stay-up-to-date.html. Accessed 9 Nov 2023.
36. Center for Disease Control and Prevention. COVID-19 vaccines for people who are moderately or severely immunocompromised. Available at: https://www.cdc.gov/coronavirus/2019-ncov/vaccines/recommendations/immuno.html. Accessed 9 Nov 2023.
37. CDC. Interim clinical considerations for use of COVID-19 vaccines in the United States, 2023–2024.
38. Center for Disease Control and Prevention. ACIP evidence to recommendations (EtR) for use of an updated (monovalent XBB containing) COVID-19 vaccine under an emergency use authorization. Available at: https://www.cdc.gov/vaccines/acip/recs/grade/covid-19-2023-2024-Monovalent-etr.html. Accessed 9 Nov 2023.
39. US Food and Drug Administration. Available at: https://www.fda.gov/news-events/press-announcements/coronavirus-covid-19-update-fda-authorizes-changes-simplify-use-bivalent-mrna-covid-19-vaccines
40. Center for Disease Control and Prevention. Updated (2023–24 formula) Novavax COVID-19 vaccine. Available at: https://www.cdc.gov/vaccines/covid-19/info-by-product/novavax/downloads/novavax-standing-orders.pdf. Accessed 9 Nov 2023.

41. Center for Disease Control and Prevention. Selected adverse events reported after COVID-19 vaccination. Available at: https://www.cdc.gov/coronavirus/2019-ncov/vaccines/safety/adverse-events.html. Accessed 9 Nov 2023.
42. Center for Disease Control and Prevention. Past seasons' vaccine effectiveness estimates. Available at: https://www.cdc.gov/flu/vaccines-work/past-seasons-estimates.html. Accessed 9 Nov 2023.
43. Center for Disease Control and Prevention recommendations. Available at: https://www.cdc.gov/flu/prevent/quadrivalent.htm#:~:text=All%20flu%20vaccines%20in%20the,for%20the%202023%2D2024%20Season
44. Committee on Infectious Diseases. Recommendations for prevention and control of influenza in children, 2023–2024. Pediatrics. 2023;152(4):e2023063773.
45. Grohskopf LA, Blanton LH, Ferdinands JM, Chung JR, Broder KR, Talbot HK. Prevention and control of seasonal influenza with vaccines: recommendations of the Advisory Committee on immunization practices—United States, 2023–24 influenza season. MMWR Recomm Rep. 2023;72(RR-2):1–25. https://doi.org/10.15585/mmwr.rr7202a1.
46. Restivo V, Costantino C, Bono S, Maniglia M, Marchese V, Ventura G, Casuccio A, Tramuto F, Vitale F. Influenza vaccine effectiveness among high-risk groups: a systematic literature review and meta-analysis of case-control and cohort studies. Hum Vaccin Immunother. 2018;14(3):724–35. https://doi.org/10.1080/21645515.2017.1321722. Epub 2017 Jun 16. PMID: 28481673; PMCID: PMC5890832.
47. Center for Disease Control and Prevention. People at higher risk of flu complications. Available at: https://www.cdc.gov/flu/highrisk/index.htm. Accessed 9 Nov 2023.
48. Center for Disease Control and Prevention. Influenza vaccination: a summary for clinicians. Available at: https://www.cdc.gov/flu/professionals/vaccination/vax-summary.htm#children. Accessed 9 Nov 2023.
49. Center for Disease Control and Prevention recommendations. Available at: https://www.cdc.gov/vaccines/acip/recs/grade/influenza-older-adults.html
50. Center for Disease Control and Prevention. ACIP recommendations. Available at: https://www.cdc.gov/vaccines/acip/recommendations.html. Accessed 9 Nov 2023.
51. Gasse F. Neonatal tetanus: review of progress. Int J Gynecol Obstet. 1995;50(suppl 2):S67–72.
52. Zhang C, Hu W, Ma Y, Li L, Si Y, Zhang S. Seroepidemiology of tetanus among healthy people aged 1-59 years old in Shaanxi Province, China. Vaccines (Basel). 2022;10(11):1806. https://doi.org/10.3390/vaccines10111806. PMID: 36366315
53. Khoury A, Cahill JD. Tetanus vaccination 2020 and collateral protections against pertussis and diphtheria. R I Med J (2013). 2020;103(6):38–40. PMID: 32752564
54. Bednarczyk RA, Brandt HM. Descriptive epidemiology of age at HPV vaccination: analysis using the 2020 NIS-Teen. Hum Vaccin Immunother. 2023;19(1):2204784. https://doi.org/10.1080/21645515.2023.2204784. PMID: 37138466; PMCID: PMC10161935
55. Broder KR, Cortese MM, Iskander JK, Kretsinger K, Slade BA, Brown KH, Mijalski CM, Tiwari T, Weston EJ, Cohn AC, Srivastava PU, Moran JS, Schwartz B, Murphy TV, Advisory Committee on Immunization Practices (ACIP). Preventing tetanus, diphtheria, and pertussis among adolescents: use of tetanus toxoid, reduced diphtheria toxoid and acellular pertussis vaccines recommendations of the Advisory Committee on Immunization Practices (ACIP). MMWR Recomm Rep. 2006;55(RR-3):1–34. PMID: 16557217.
56. Havers FP, Moro PL, Hunter P, Hariri S, Bernstein H. Use of tetanus toxoid, reduced diphtheria toxoid, and acellular pertussis vaccines: updated recommendations of the Advisory Committee on Immunization Practices—United States, 2019. MMWR Morb Mortal Wkly Rep. 2020;69:77–83. https://doi.org/10.15585/mmwr.mm6903a5.
57. Broder KR, Cortese MM, Iskander JK, et al. Preventing tetanus, diphtheria, and pertussis among adolescents: use of tetanus toxoid, reduced diphtheria toxoid and acellular pertussis vaccines recommendations of the Advisory Committee on Immunization Practices (ACIP). MMWR Recomm Rep. 2006;55(RR-3)
58. Kretsinger K, Broder KR, Cortese MM, Advisory Committee on Immunization Practices; Healthcare Infection Control Practices Advisory Committee, et al. Preventing tetanus,

diphtheria, and pertussis among adults: use of tetanus toxoid, reduced diphtheria toxoid and acellular pertussis vaccine recommendations of the Advisory Committee on Immunization Practices (ACIP) and recommendation of ACIP, supported by the Healthcare Infection Control Practices Advisory Committee (HICPAC), for use of Tdap among health-care personnel. MMWR Recomm Rep. 2006;55(RR-17):1–37.

59. Liang JL, Tiwari T, Moro P, et al. Prevention of pertussis, tetanus, and diphtheria with vaccines in the United States: recommendations of the Advisory Committee on Immunization Practices (ACIP). MMWR Recomm Rep. 2018;67(RR-2):1–44.
60. CDC. Updated recommendations for use of tetanus toxoid, reduced diphtheria toxoid, and acellular pertussis vaccine (Tdap) in pregnant women—Advisory Committee on Immunization Practices (ACIP), 2012. MMWR Morb Mortal Wkly Rep. 2013;62:131–5.
61. Center for Disease Control and Prevention. DtaP (diphtheria, tetanus, pertussis) VIS. Available at: https://www.cdc.gov/vaccines/hcp/vis/vis-statements/dtap.html#dtap-vaccine. Accessed 11 Nov 2023.
62. Di Pietrantonj C, Rivetti A, Marchione P, Debalini MG, Demicheli V. Vaccines for measles, mumps, rubella, and varicella in children. Cochrane Database Syst Rev. 2020;4(4):CD004407. https://doi.org/10.1002/14651858.CD004407.pub4. Update in: Cochrane Database Syst Rev. 2021; 11:CD004407. PMID: 32309885; PMCID: PMC7169657.
63. World Health Organization. Global measles and rubella strategic plan: 2012–2020. Geneva: World Health Organization; 2012. [cited 2020 Aug 19]
64. Keja K, Chan C, Hayden G, et al. Expanded programme on immunization. World Health Stat Q. 1988;41(2):59–63.
65. Rasheed MAU, Hickman CJ, McGrew M, et al. Decreased humoral immunity to mumps in young adults immunized with MMR vaccine in childhood. Proc Natl Acad Sci U S A. 2019;116(38):19071–6. World Health Organization. Mumps virus vaccines. Wkly Epidemiol Rec 2007;82(7):51–60
66. Center for Disease Control and Prevention. Measles, mumps, and rubella (MMR) vaccination: what everyone should know. Available at: https://www.cdc.gov/vaccines/vpd/mmr/public/index.html. Accessed 11 Nov 2023.
67. Marin M, Marlow M, Moore KL, Patel M. Recommendation of the Advisory Committee on Immunization Practices for use of a third dose of mumps virus–containing vaccine in persons at increased risk for mumps during an outbreak. MMWR Morb Mortal Wkly Rep. 2018;67:33–8. https://doi.org/10.15585/mmwr.mm6701a7.
68. Center for Disease Control and Prevention. Routine measles, mumps, and rubella vaccination. Available at: https://www.cdc.gov/vaccines/vpd/mmr/hcp/recommendations.html. Accessed 11 Nov 2023.
69. Patil A, Goldust M, Wollina U. *Herpes zoster*: a review of clinical manifestations and management. Viruses. 2022;14(2):192. https://doi.org/10.3390/v14020192. PMID: 35215786; PMCID: PMC8876683
70. Marin M, Leung J, Lopez AS, Shepersky L, Schmid DS, Gershon AA. Communicability of varicella before rash onset: a literature review. Epidemiol Infect. 2021;149:1–18. https://doi.org/10.1017/S0950268821001102.
71. Kett JC. Perinatal varicella. Pediatr Rev. 2013;34:49–51. https://doi.org/10.1542/pir.34.1.49.
72. Rafferty E, Reifferscheid L, Russell ML, Booth S, Svenson LW, MacDonald SE. The impact of varicella vaccination on paediatric *herpes zoster* epidemiology: a Canadian population-based retrospective cohort study. Eur J Clin Microbiol Infect Dis. 2021;40:2363–70. https://doi.org/10.1007/s10096-021-04298-z.
73. Center for Disease Control and Prevention. Chickenpox/varicella vaccination. Available at: https://www.cdc.gov/vaccines/vpd/varicella/index.html. Accessed 11 Nov 2023.
74. CDC-recommendations. FDA approval of an extended period for administering VariZIG for postexposure prophylaxis of varicella. MMWR Morb Mortal Wkly Rep. 2012;61(12):212.
75. Center for Disease Control and Prevention. Administering the vaccine. Available at: https://www.cdc.gov/vaccines/vpd/varicella/hcp/administering-vaccine.html. Accessed 11 Nov 2023.

76. Center for Disease Control and Prevention. Varicella vaccine recommendations. Available at: https://www.cdc.gov/vaccines/vpd/varicella/hcp/recommendations.html#specific-groups. Accessed 11 Nov 2023.
77. Nair PA, Patel BC. StatPearls [internet]. Treasure Island: StatPearls; 2021. *Herpes zoster*
78. Center for Disease Control and Prevention. Shingles vaccination. Available at: https://www.cdc.gov/vaccines/vpd/shingles/public/shingrix/index.html. Accessed 11 Nov 2023.
79. Cunningham AL, Lal H, Kovac M, Chlibek R, Hwang SJ, Díez-Domingo J, Godeaux O, Levin MJ, McElhaney JE, Puig-Barberà J, Vanden Abeele C, Vesikari T, Watanabe D, Zahaf T, Ahonen A, Athan E, Barba-Gomez JF, Campora L, de Looze F, Downey HJ, Ghesquiere W, Gorfinkel I, Korhonen T, Leung E, McNeil SA, Oostvogels L, Rombo L, Smetana J, Weckx L, Yeo W, Heineman TC, ZOE-70 Study Group. Efficacy of the herpes zoster subunit vaccine in adults 70 years of age or older. N Engl J Med. 2016;375(11):1019–32. https://doi.org/10.1056/NEJMoa1603800.
80. Dooling KL, Guo A, Patel M, et al. Recommendations of the Advisory Committee on Immunization Practices for use of herpes zoster vaccines. MMWR Morb Mortal Wkly Rep. 2018;67:103–8. https://doi.org/10.15585/mmwr.mm6703a5.
81. Center for Disease Control and Prevention. Clinical considerations for use of recombinant zoster vaccine (RZV, Shingrix) in immunocompromised adults aged ≥19 years. Available at: https://www.cdc.gov/shingles/vaccination/immunocompromised-adults.html. Accessed 11 Nov 2023.
82. Center for Disease Control and Prevention. HPV and cancer. Available at: https://www.cdc.gov/cancer/hpv/. Accessed 11 Nov 2023.
83. Center for Disease Control and Prevention. Genital HPV infection—basic fact sheet. Available at: https://www.cdc.gov/std/hpv/stdfact-hpv.htm#:~:text=You%20can%20get%20HPV%20by,have%20no%20signs%20or%20symptoms. Accessed 11 Nov 2023.
84. Center for Disease Control and Prevention. Reasons to get HPV vaccine. Available at: https://www.cdc.gov/hpv/parents/vaccine/six-reasons.html. Accessed 11 Nov 2023.
85. Center for Disease Control and Prevention. How many cancers are linked with HPV each year? Available at: https://www.cdc.gov/cancer/hpv/statistics/cases.htm. Accessed 11 Nov 2023.
86. Center for Disease Control and Prevention. HPV vaccine. Available at: https://www.cdc.gov/hpv/parents/vaccine-for-hpv.html. Accessed 11 Nov 2023.
87. Center for Disease Control and Prevention. Hepatitis A. Available at: https://www.cdc.gov/hepatitis/hav/index.htm. Accessed 11 Nov 2023.
88. Center for Disease Control and Prevention. Hepatitis A vaccination. Available at: https://www.cdc.gov/vaccines/vpd/hepa/index.html. Accessed 11 Nov 2023.
89. Center for Disease Control and Prevention. Hepatitis A questions and answers for the public. Available at: https://www.cdc.gov/hepatitis/hav/afaq.htm. Accessed 11 Nov 2023.
90. Center for Disease Control and Prevention. Hepatitis A surveillance 2021. Available at: https://www.cdc.gov/hepatitis/statistics/2021surveillance/hepatitis-a.htm. Accessed 11 Nov 2023.
91. Nelson NP, Weng MK, Hofmeister MG, et al. Prevention of hepatitis A virus infection in the United States: recommendations of the Advisory Committee on Immunization Practices, 2020. MMWR Recomm Rep. 2020;69(RR-5):1–38.
92. Center for Disease Control and Prevention. Hepatitis B information. Frequently asked questions for the public. Available at: https://www.cdc.gov/hepatitis/hbv/bfaq.htm. Accessed 12 Nov 2023.
93. Center for Disease Control and Prevention. Pneumococcal disease. Available at: https://www.cdc.gov/pneumococcal/index.html. Accessed 12 Nov 2023.
94. Center for Disease Control and Prevention. Pneumococcal disease: types of infection. Available at: https://www.cdc.gov/pneumococcal/about/infection-types.html. Accessed 12 Nov 2023.
95. Center for Disease Control and Prevention. Pneumococcal disease: risk factors and how it spreads. Available at: https://www.cdc.gov/pneumococcal/about/risk-transmission.html. Accessed 12 Nov 2023.

96. Center for Disease Control and Prevention. Pneumococcal disease: symptoms and complications. Available at: https://www.cdc.gov/pneumococcal/about/symptoms-complications.html
97. Center for Disease Control and Prevention. Pneumococcal disease: prevention. Available at: https://www.cdc.gov/pneumococcal/about/prevention.html. Accessed 12 Nov 2023.
98. Center for Disease Control and Prevention. Meningococcal vaccination. Available at: https://www.cdc.gov/vaccines/vpd/mening/index.html. Accessed 12 Nov 2023.
99. Center for Disease Control and Prevention. Meningococcal disease: signs and symptoms. Available at: https://www.cdc.gov/meningococcal/about/symptoms.html. Accessed 12 Nov 2023.
100. Center for Disease Control and Prevention. Haemophilus influenzae disease (Including Hib). Available at: https://www.cdc.gov/hi-disease/index.html. Accessed 12 Nov 2023.
101. Center for Disease Control and Prevention. Types of Haemophilus influenzae infections. Available at: https://www.cdc.gov/hi-disease/about/types-infection.html. Accessed 12 Nov 2023.
102. Center for Disease Control and Prevention. Hib vaccination: what everyone should know. Available at: https://www.cdc.gov/vaccines/vpd/hib/public/index.html. Accessed 12 Nov 2023.
103. Center for Disease Control and Prevention. Haemophilus influenzae disease (Including Hib): surveillance. Available at: https://www.cdc.gov/hi-disease/surveillance.html. Accessed 12 Nov 2023.
104. Center for Disease Control and Prevention. Respiratory syncytial virus infection. Available at: https://www.cdc.gov/rsv/index.html. Accessed 12 Nov 2023.
105. Center for Disease Control and Prevention. Respiratory syncytial virus infection: symptoms and care. Available at: https://www.cdc.gov/rsv/about/symptoms.html. Accessed 12 Nov 2023.
106. Center for Disease Control and Prevention. RSV transmission. Available at: https://www.cdc.gov/rsv/about/transmission.html. Accessed 12 Nov 2023.
107. Center for Disease Control and Prevention. Respiratory syncytial virus (RSV) immunizations. Available at: https://www.cdc.gov/vaccines/vpd/rsv/index.html. Accessed 12 Nov 2023.
108. European Centre for Disease Prevention and Control. Vaccine scheduler. Available at: https://vaccine-schedule.ecdc.europa.eu/. Accessed 12 Nov 2023.
109. European Center for Disease Prevention and Control recommendations. Available at: https://www.ecdc.europa.eu/en/immunisation-vaccines/EU-vaccination-schedules
110. European Center for Disease Prevention and Control recommendations. Available at: https://vaccine-schedule.ecdc.europa.eu/
111. Gov.UK. Additional vaccines for individuals with underlying medical conditions recommendations. Available at: https://www.gov.uk/government/publications/the-complete-routine-immunisation-schedule/the-complete-routine-immunisation-schedule-from-february-2022#additional-vaccines-for-individuals-with-underlying-medical-conditions. Accessed 12 Nov 2023.
112. European Center for Disease Prevention and Control recommendations. Available at: https://www.cdc.gov/vaccines/hcp/acip-recs/general-recs/contraindications.pdf. Accessed 12 Nov 2023.
113. European Center for Disease Prevention and Control recommendations. Available at: https://vaccination-info.europa.eu/en/vaccination/when-vaccinate/when-avoid-vaccination
114. Center for Disease Control and Prevention recommendations. Available at: https://www.cdc.gov/vaccines/hcp/acip-recs/general-recs/contraindications.pdf

Safe Handling of Sharps and Safe Injection Practices

8

Nisha Ganesh and Sarah Rollor

8.1 Overview of Needlestick and Sharps Injuries and the Hazards to the Healthcare Worker Worldwide

Sharps is a term that describes any device that has sharp points or edges that can puncture the skin or cut other tissue [1]. The following items are common in a healthcare setting:

- Needles
- Scalpels
- Lancets
- Razor blades
- Scissors
- Metal wires
- Retractors
- Clamps
- Pins
- Staples
- Cutters
- Glass items [2]

N. Ganesh (✉)
Department of Comprehensive Dentistry, The University of Maryland School of Dentistry, Baltimore, MD, USA
e-mail: nganesh@umaryland.edu

S. Rollor
Division of General Dentistry, Department of Comprehensive Dentistry, The University of Maryland School of Dentistry, Baltimore, MD, USA
e-mail: srollor1@umaryland.edu

L. DePaola et al. (eds.), *Infection Control in the Dental Office in the Era of COVID-19*, https://doi.org/10.1007/978-3-031-64611-9_8

In dentistry, common sharps are anesthetic needles, suture needles, burs, scalpels, endodontic files, orthodontic wire and bands, broken instruments, metal matrix bands, and broken anesthetic cartridges.

The most common sharps injury is percutaneous—through the skin. Needlestick injuries (NSIs) are a specific type of sharps injury. They are a notable hazard in the healthcare setting (including dental). NSIs can occur at any time when interacting with a needle—assembly of the syringe apparatus, administration of the medication or during aspiration, capping a needle, disassembly, or disposal [2]. The risk of contracting an infectious disease is the primary concern related to sharps injuries.

When sharps are contaminated with blood, the percutaneous injury is associated with transmission of more than 20 pathogens [3]. The most common are hepatitis B virus (HBV), hepatitis C virus (HBC), and human immunodeficiency virus (HIV). Although the risk is low for contracting an infectious disease from a sharps injury, it is a significant health concern for dental healthcare workers and providers worldwide. Without postexposure prophylaxis, the risk for an exposed, susceptible healthcare worker that will contract HBV is 6–30%. This risk is highest if the source individual has hepatitis B *e* antigen, as this is an increased marker of infectivity [4, 5]. The WHO reports that globally sharps injuries are estimated to cause 66,000 HBV, 16,000 HCV, and 200–5000 HIV infections among healthcare workers each year [6]. The Centers for Disease Control and Prevention (CDC) estimates 385,000 needlestick and other sharps-related injuries occur annually by hospital-based healthcare workers in the United States alone. Notably, these 1000 sharps injuries per day average do not account for other healthcare settings—long-term care, home healthcare, and private medical and dental offices [4]. A survey conducted by the Association of Occupational Health Professionals in Healthcare estimates 320,000+ US healthcare workers sustain sharps injuries in hospital and nonhospital environments [7]. In Canada, a 2005 national survey of the work and health nurses revealed that a little less than half the respondents reported a sharps injury in the workplace at some point in their career. Eleven percent of the participants stated the injury occurred in the previous year [8]. Conclusions from a systematic review and meta-analysis revealed a 1-year global pooled prevalence of 44.5% of needlestick injuries among healthcare workers. The highest prevalence occurred in Southeast Asia, at 58.2%. By job category needlestick injuries were the highest among dentists. Hypodermic needles were the most common cause of needlestick injuries at 55.1% [9].

8.2 The Safe Handling of Sharps and Proper Disposal

8.2.1 Prevention of Sharps Injuries

A 2010 publication in the BioMedicine International journal studied the incidence and cost of needlestick injuries—one of the primary sharps injuries for healthcare workers. The comprehensive report of peer-reviewed literature, gray literature, trade associations, and other stakeholders for the prevention of needlestick injuries compiled information from the United States, the United Kingdom, Germany,

Table 8.1 Program for prevention of sharps injuries

Organizational steps
Create multidisciplinary team
Conduct baseline assessment
Set priorities for action plan
Operational processes
Create culture of safety
Report injuries
Analyze data
Select evaluating devices

Source: Centers for Disease Control and Prevention [4]

France, Italy, and Spain. Table 8.1 ranks the estimated annual occurrence of needlesticks as well as injection/intravenous-related needlestick injuries [10]. The range of reported total annual number of needlestick injuries (including dentistry) was 700,000 (Germany) with the lowest incidence at 18,720 (France, nursing data only). A subset of these total numbers are injection and IV-related needlestick injuries ranging from 168,000 (Germany) to 6552 (France, nursing only). The United States reports the second highest occurrence: 384,000 total needlesticks injuries, with 123,000 of those specifically attributed to needles or IV-related [10].

The data supports the need for continued efforts to develop, gain approval, and implement effective prevention measures for sharps injuries in the healthcare field, including dentistry. The CDC provides a myriad of resources focused on the topic of sharps injuries and prevention. The program plan to reduce sharps injuries is founded on the concept of continuous quality improvement, through systematic, organization-wide approach for continually improving all processes involved in the delivery of quality products and services. The plan has two arms: organizational steps for developing and implementing a sharps injury prevention program and operational processes. Organizational steps include the creation of a multidisciplinary team, conducting a baseline assessment, and setting priorities for development of an action plan. Operational processes are focused on creating a culture of safety, reporting injuries, analyzing data, and selecting and evaluating devices. The benefit to this program plan is the inherent flexibility to adapt it to large organizations or small private practices [4].

8.2.2 Culture of Safety

Creating an environment in which safety is a primary focus is commonplace in some industrial sectors. Studies in those environments have demonstrated a correlation with productivity, cost, product quality, and employee satisfaction. Furthermore, organizations with a strong safety culture steadily report fewer injuries than those with weaker safety cultures. This concept has been recently introduced in the healthcare setting, but the principles are easily adapted. A culture of safety reflects a shared commitment to ensure the safety of the work environment. To accomplish this goal, the employer and the employees must actively engage in creating and maintaining a safe workspace [4, 11].

The Occupational Safety and Health Administration (OSHA) has developed an e-learning tool to guide organizations in creating a culture of safety. To be successful, all members of the organization have responsibilities that must be met. Employers need to facilitate safety planning. They need to provide resources, appropriate safety devices, and protective equipment, including training in the handling of SEDs and the disposal of sharps. To maintain awareness and commitment, employers should create and contribute to a feedback system for communicating safe practices. This can include items such as newsletters, bulletin boards, brochures, regular meeting agenda items, and easy access to online resources. Positive reinforcement in the form of accolades and recognition for success can yield great results. A safe, reliable method for recommending quality improvement is equally important so that employees can highlight areas of improvement without fear of repercussions. Employees have an equal stake in the creation and propagation of a culture of safety. They need to take an active role in maintaining safe practices when handling sharps. Proactive management of sharps hazards is key to preventing injury. Lastly, their feedback and participation in the communication cycle are essential for a thriving culture of safety [4, 5].

8.2.3 Legislation Regarding Sharps Safety and Needlestick Prevention

In 1992, regulatory legislation that established strict standards to help protect healthcare and other workers from bloodborne pathogens became effective. Created and enforced by the Occupational Safety and Health Administration (OSHA), the standard was amended in late 2000 pursuant to the Needlestick Safety and Prevention Act. The standard stipulates safeguards to protect workers against health hazards related to bloodborne pathogens, including sharps injuries. In this way it is comprehensive in the approach to prevent exposure to bloodborne pathogens. The act calls for exposure control plans, engineering and work practice controls, hepatitis B vaccinations, hazard communication and training, and recordkeeping. The Needlestick Safety and Prevention Act revisions modified or added new terms in the definitions section of the bloodborne pathogen standard. Additional requirements were added to the Exposure Control Plan. It also required the employer to solicit input from employees in the identification, evaluation, and selection of engineering controls and work practices that prevent exposure. For some employers, it required the maintenance of a sharps injury log [5, 12].

Similar regulatory bodies in the 27 countries in the European Union are empowered by the Prevention of Sharps Injuries in the Healthcare Sector directive from EU-OSHA, to set strict standards to protect healthcare workers from injury and exposure to bloodborne pathogens. In 2009, European social partners HOPSEEM (European Hospital and Healthcare Employer's Association) and EPSU (European Federation of Public Services Unions) signed a Framework Agreement on prevention from sharps injuries in the hospital and healthcare sector. The statute outlines a process for employers that mirrors the creation of a culture of safety. The regulations recommend first conducting a sharps risk assessment. The next steps include how the exposure risk can be eliminated, if possible, and identifying alternative systems to remove of reduce to the risk of exposure [13]. In the United Kingdom, the Health and Safety Executive of the UK 2013 regulation on Sharp Instruments in Healthcare provides clear guidance for employers and employees. The National Health Services and Public Health of England are unified under the National Institute for Health Protection to provide guidance. The National [14] Public Health Agency of Canada issued a federal guideline in 2013 with an amendment in 2016 to develop policies and procedures for routine practices and additional precautions in healthcare settings. The Routine Practices and Additional Precautions for Preventing the Transmission of Infection in Healthcare Settings references the CDC Program for Prevention of Sharps [15].

8.2.4 Practical Scenarios When Sharps Injuries Can Occur in the Dental Setting

The risk for sharps injury and exposure presents itself initially during the preparation for a procedure and continues as a risk through breakdown, cleaning, disinfection, and sterilization. All workers who perform a duty in the dental operatory or cleaning and sterilization areas are at risk—including nonclinical staff responsible for cleaning and maintenance of the physical clinical space. Table 8.2 lists

Table 8.2 Scenarios when sharps injuries can occur

Chairside	Instrument processing	Other times
Preparing anesthetic syringe Giving injections When sharps are passed When needles are recapped When needles are discarded When exposed sharps are handled When using sharp hand instruments When sharps are laid down When manipulating scalpels and blades When making incisions When suturing When placing/removing burs from handpieces When contacting protruding burs on handpieces in their holder When manipulating wires, orthodontic bands, and dental appliances When gathering items after patient appointments	When sharpening instruments When removing needles, scalpel blades, broken items left in tray setups When hand-scrubbing and rinsing sharps When placing/retrieving sharp instruments from cleaning solutions When packaging sharps items for sterilization When organizing instrument tray setup When handling sterile packages of sharps	Laundry of reusable PPE Handling and cleaning dental appliances with clasps Handling sharps in the dental laboratory

Source: Centers for Disease Control and Prevention [16]

circumstances in which sharps injuries can occur. Each scenario presents an opportunity to create a safety-centered workflow to prioritize protection of the worker and the patient [4, 17, 18].

Figures 8.1, 8.2, and 8.3 show examples of common sharps injuries situations.

8.2.5 Review of Sharps Safety and Safe Injection Practices

Standard Precautions

In 1970, the CDC published guidelines titled "Isolation Techniques for Use in the Hospital," formally introducing the concept of precautions for the purpose of infection control. In 1983, catalyzed by the HIV/AIDS epidemic, the CDC Guideline for Isolation Precautions in the Hospital had more robust recommendations and guidelines for hospital workers to reference. The idea of universal precautions was born from this set of practices as the connection to needlestick injuries and the spread of HIV/AIDS to healthcare workers. This approach sparked the era of considering all patients should be treated with blood and fluid precautions as they can be

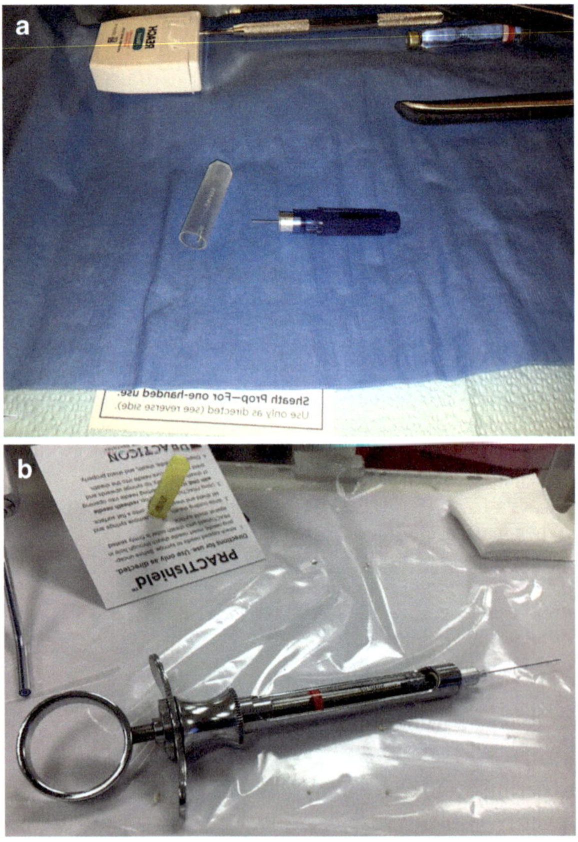

Fig. 8.1 (**a**) Needle left uncapped after removing from the syringe. (**b**) Needle uncapped after injecting anesthetic

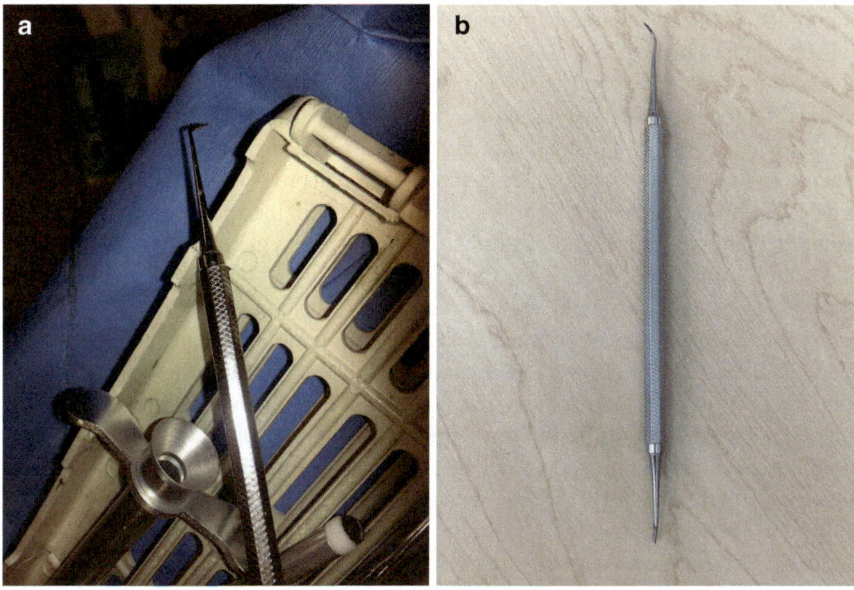

Fig. 8.2 (**a**) Jacquette scaler left in a precarious position in the instrument cassette increasing the risk for percutaneous injury. (**b**) Broken instrument used in the lab

Fig. 8.3 Bur left in handpick and bur block left open

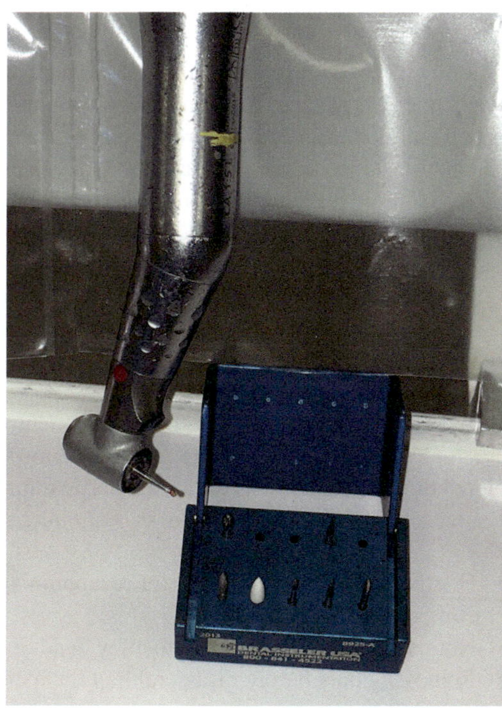

undiagnosed for an infectious disease, known as body substance isolation. In the 1990s, standard precautions emerged from the confusion of when to apply universal precautions versus body substance isolation guidelines [19]. Although initially created with a focus on the hospital setting, standard precautions have evolved to apply to all patient cares in any environment. They are based on a risk assessment and make use of common-sense practices and personal protective equipment use that protect healthcare providers from infection and prevent the spread of infection from patient to patient. Standard precautions include hand hygiene, respiratory hygiene and cough etiquette, and safe injection practices. In the dental practice, they are designed to protect the dental healthcare provider also to prevent the dental healthcare provider from spreading infections among patients. Standard precautions are used whenever and wherever healthcare is delivered, regardless of the patient's infection status. Education and training on standard precautions are critical for understanding the importance of these practices, making appropriate decisions, and complying with recommended practices. Sharps safety and safe injection practices are an essential aspect of standard precautions [16].

Specific Prevention Approaches and Best Practices in Dentistry

When addressing sharps injury prevention, there are three categories of action:

1. Eliminate the use of the sharp whenever possible.
2. Apply engineering controls.
3. Apply workflow controls.

Many of dental procedures include the incision or cutting of tissue, which necessitates the use of sharp instruments. Alternatives such as lasers or electrosurgery may be an option in certain circumstances, but the efficacy and side effects on the patient dictate the decision to use one tool versus another. Elimination of the use of sharps is rarely possible in the dental setting. However, most exposures in dentistry are preventable. Therefore, each dental practice should have policies and procedures available addressing sharps safety.

The CDC recommends that engineering controls should be the primary method to reduce the exposure to bloodborne pathogens via sharps exposure. Self-sheathing needles, needle recapping devices, safety scalpels, and needless IV ports are examples.

Work-practice controls are the complement to engineering controls when they are not available or appropriate. This behavior-based approach changes the risk of bloodborne pathogen exposure via sharps injury by changing the way the dental healthcare personnel performs tasks. Examples of work-practice controls are:

- One-handed scoop technique for recapping a needle
- Not bend or break a needle
- Not passing a syringe unsheathed by hand
- Removing burs before disassembling the handpiece from the dental unit

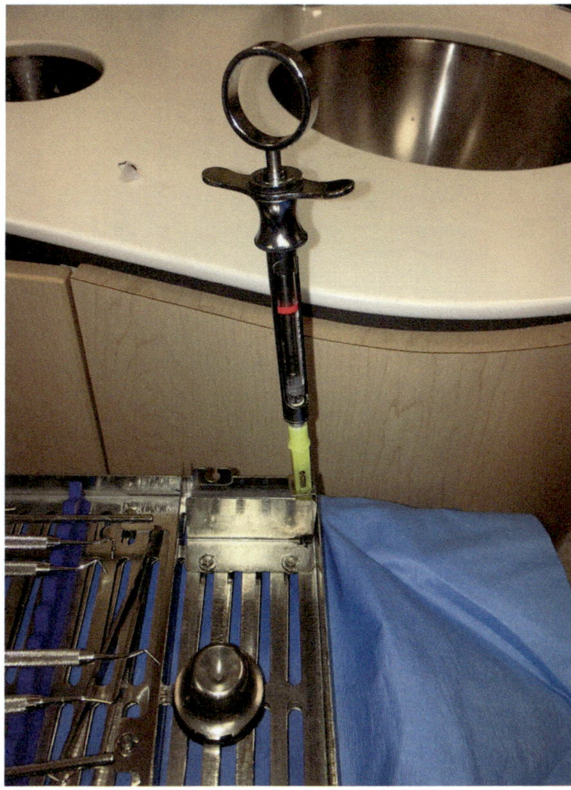

Fig. 8.4 Example of engineering control to safely cap a needle

- Using instruments instead of fingers for tissue retraction or palpation during suturing or administration of anesthesia
- Placing all disposable syringes, needles, scalpel blades, and other sharps in the appropriate puncture-resistant container

Figures 8.4 and 8.5 show examples of engineering controls to mitigate sharps injuries.

8.2.6 Proper Disposal of Sharps in Dentistry

Sharps are a form of regulated medical waste. It is differentiated by whether it has been exposed to bodily fluids. All federal agencies consider contaminated sharps to be infectious waste—capable of causing infectious disease. OSHA bloodborne pathogens standard states that immediately after use, disposable sharps are to be placed in closable, leakproof, puncture-resistant containers (i.e., sharps containers; Fig. 8.6). These containers must be labeled with a biohazard symbol and color-coded for easy identification. The CDC recommends that sharps containers are positioned as close as is practical to the work area. In the dental practice, this translates

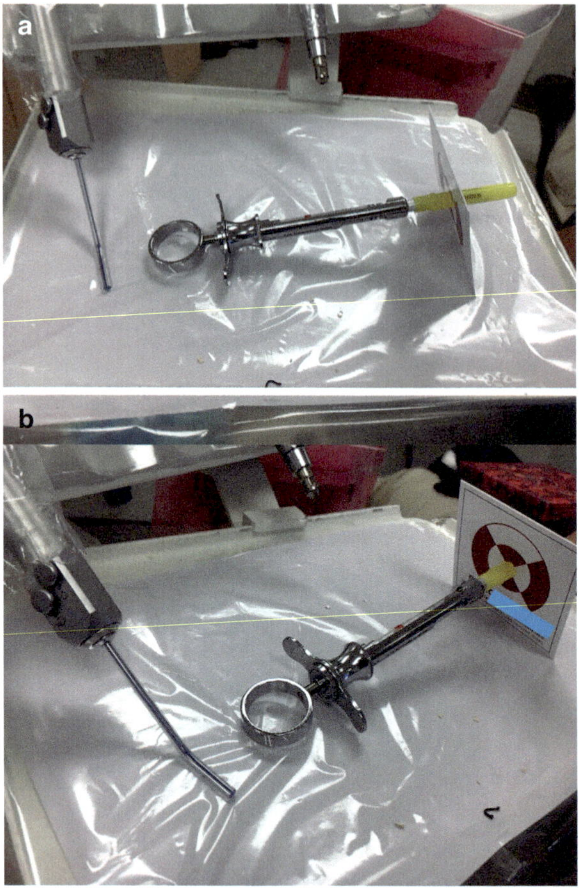

Fig. 8.5 (**a**, **b**) Example of engineering control to safely cap a needle

to having a sharps container in each operatory. Risk for injury and exposure exists until the sharp is deposited in the container. Best practices include the following:

- Use an FDA-approved container.
- Read cautionary statements on sharps containers.
- Use containers with larger bottoms to avoid tipping them over.
- Don't exceed the recommended fill line.
- Do not force sharps into containers.
- Drop syringes horizontally into containers.
- The container should be limited to sharps disposal only.
- Carefully inspect filled containers before handling.
- Securely close containers before moving them.
- Replace containers as soon as they are filled.

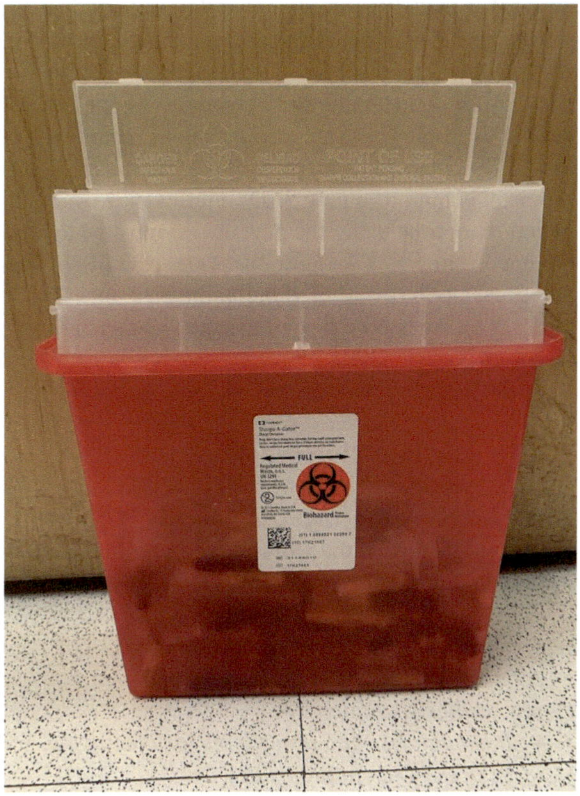

Fig. 8.6 Sharps container

8.2.7 Impact and Effectiveness of Safety Engineered Devices

In addition to safety laws, education, and injury prevention, one of the main improvements to sharps safety has been the introduction of safety engineered devices (SEDs) [20]. Safety features on these devices are designed to shield the needle or other sharp objects after use and are available for a variety of sharps including blood collection system, intravenous systems, hypodermic injection needles, suture needles, lancets, and scalpels. They utilize a variety of mechanisms such as self-retractable needles or external shielding or include reuse prevention feature. Safety devices are divided into two main categories: passive and active. Passive devices do not require the manual operation of the device, as the safety element will activate during normal use. In contrast, active devices require manual activation of the safety function. This could be the activation of a protection shield or the pressing of a button to activate the safety mechanism [21].

Many studies indicate that consistent and proper use of SEDs is effective. Research published in the journal *Infection Control and Hospital Epidemiology* in 2013 demonstrated a strong association with the increased use of SEDs and reduced injuries. Another study, however, looked at the incidence of needle stick injuries from 2014 to 2019 and found that the continued occurrence of needlestick injuries is a multifaceted issue. Data indicated that SEDs do not provide complete protection and are only effective if used and disposed of correctly and that many of these injuries may be due to failure of activation. About 1/3 of injuries were found to occur during disposal. There are also questions regarding a reasonable adjustment period that SEDs entail. This refers more to "active" SEDs compared to "passive" SEDs. When switching to a new SED, injuries may even increase during this adjustment period. Everyone using the new device must be appropriately trained and provided the opportunity to ask questions. One example of these SEDs include the Switch Safety Scalpels from Medline Industries Inc. This device has a built-in blade remover on the handle that allows the technician to safely remove the contaminated blade [20].

8.2.8 Safe Injection Practices

A study published in JADA in February 2007 identified needlestick injuries as a preventable injury in the workplace. Recommendations for dental health personnel included the following:

- *Safe work practices and recapping systems can contribute to injury prevention.*
- *All dental practices should have a comprehensive, written program for preventing needlestick injuries:*
  - *It should describe procedures for identifying, screening, and adopting safety devices (when appropriate).*
- *A mechanism to report and provide medical follow-up for percutaneous injuries should be in place.*
- *Establish a system for training staff members in safe work practices and the proper use of safety devices* [18].

As outlined by the CDC, safe injection practices are meant to prevent transmission of infectious diseases between one patient and another or between a patient and the dental healthcare worker during preparation and administration of parenteral (e.g., intravenous or intramuscular injection) medications. In dentistry, most injections are associated with administering local anesthesia, using single-use needles and cartridges containing local anesthetics. The dental cartridge syringe is cleaned and heat-sterilized between patients. Safe injection practices are a set of procedures the dental healthcare personnel should follow to perform injections in the safest possible way for the protection of patients. Additional safe practices refer to use of parenteral medications combined with fluid infusion systems, such as for patients undergoing conscious sedation [16].

The *CDC Key Recommendations for SAFE INJECTION PRACTICES in the Dental Settings* are a comprehensive guide for all dental practitioners and dental personnel to follow (Table 8.3):

Table 8.3 Key recommendations for safe injection practices in dental settings

1. Prepare injections using aseptic technique in a clean area
2. Disinfect the rubber septum on a medication vial with alcohol before piercing
3. Do not use needles or syringes for more than one patient (this includes manufactured prefilled syringes and other devices such as insulin pens)
4. Medication containers (single- and multidose vials, ampules, and bags) are entered with a new needle and new syringe, even when obtaining additional doses for the same patient
5. Use single-dose vials for parenteral medications when possible
6. Do not use single-dose (single-use) medication vials, ampules, and bags or bottles of intravenous solution for more than one patient
7. Do not combine the leftover contents of single-use vials for later use
8. The following apply if multidose vials are used:
a. Dedicate multidose vials to a single patient whenever possible
b. if multidose vials will be used for more than one patient, they should be restricted to a centralized medication area and should not enter the immediate patient treatment area (e.g., dental operatory) to prevent inadvertent contamination
c. if a multidose vial enters the immediate patient treatment area, it should be dedicated for single patient use and discarded immediately after use
d. Date multidose vials when first opened and discard within 28 days unless the manufacturer specifies a shorter or longer date for that opened vial
9. Do not use fluid infusion or administration sets (e.g., IV bags, tubing, connections) for more than one patient

Source: Centers for Disease Control and Prevention [16]

Table 8.4 International resources for sharps safety

Canada	Canadian Centre for Occupational Health and Safety	https://www.ccohs.ca/
European Union	European Agency for Health and Safety at work	https://osha.europa.eu
The United Kingdom (still part of EU)	Health and Safety Executive	http://www.hse.gov.uk

Table 8.5 Additional resources for prevention and research

Centers for Disease Control and Prevention	http://www.cdc.gov/sharpssafety
Institute for Healthcare Improvement	http://www.ihi.org/IHI/Topics/PatientSafety/
International Sharps Injury Prevention Society	http://www.isips.org/

https://www.osap.org/page/Issues_SharpsSafety

Sharps safety and safe injection practices are similar in most developed countries. In today's global economy, leaders in healthcare and research utilize each other's work to create guidelines and inform policies and new research and development. Table 8.4 lists the regulatory body and website for several key countries that recognize the significance of infection control, sharps safety, and safe injection practices.

Table 8.5 lists organizations dedicated to prevention, research, and best practices for sharps safety.

8.2.9 Sharps and Post-COVID Updates

As in many other fields, the COVID pandemic has revealed numerous vulnerabilities and challenges. It has reinforced the importance of following established and adapted standards and guidelines while also heightening awareness of sharps safety [22]. The pandemic has served as a reminder of the important role that high-quality, sterile manufacturing practices of these devices play. Consequently, the demand for these devices has risen.

During the upsurge of the pandemic in 2020, the International Safety Center maintained their watchdog efforts for the healthcare workers, issuing a consensus statement. Entitled "Moving the Sharps Safety in Healthcare Agenda Forward in the United States: 2020 Consensus Statement and Call to Action," the statement highlighted the critical role that healthcare workers play, emphasizing the importance of protecting them from workplace hazards. Amid the emergence of previously unknown pathogens, such as COVID-19, there has been increased pressure for providers to see more patients in less time, exacerbating the risk of work-related exposures. The consensus aimed to refocus attention to sharps injuries, providing updated data on rates of injuries, outlining the requirements of the OSHA Pathogens Standard, listing facility-based measures and controls, and providing policy-based recommendations. The call-to-action agenda provided an update to the system of prevention measures termed Hierarchy of Controls. The new top level capitalizes on the institutional culture of safety as the primary step. The preventive measures are identified below in order of most effective to least effective:

1. *Institutional controls*
2. *Elimination*
3. *Substitution*
4. *Engineering controls*
5. *Work practice and administrative controls*
6. *Personal protective equipment*

Specific to dentistry, the updates reinforce the "high-risk, critical environment" of the dental field. This is due to multiuse, double-ended sharp instruments utilized in the oral cavity, which is already a difficult, relatively small area to access. A significant percentage of injuries are due to anesthetic needles, as the needle cap is often removed and replaced multiple times during an appointment and a patient often requires multiple injections over the course of a single procedure. In addition to these factors, there are few sharps injury prevention (SIP) features available to dental healthcare professionals, and those that are or have not been widely accepted. The Consensus Statement reinforced the importance for dental practices to increase the use of SIP features and avoid recapping and proper handling and/or disposal of contaminated sharps [23].

References

1. Merriam-Webster. Dictionary. Sharp. [Online] https://www.merriam-webster.com/dictionary/sharps
2. Canadian Centre for Occupational Health and Safety. Needlesticks and sharps injuries. Diseases, disorders and injuries. [Online] 26 Jul 2018 [cited 2023 Oct 21]. https://www.ccohs.ca/oshanswers/diseases/needlestick_injuries.html
3. Beltrami EM, et al. Risk management of blood-borne infections in healthcare workers. Clin Microbiol Rev. 2000;13:385–407.
4. Centers for Disease Control and Prevention. Centers for Disease Control and Prevention: workbook for designing, implementing and evaluating a sharps injury prevention program. [Online] 2008. https://www.cdc.gov/sharpssafety/pdf/sharpsworkbook_2008.pdf
5. Occupational Safety and Health Administration. Bloodborne pathogens and needlestick prevention. Safety and health topics. [Online] https://www.osha.gov/bloodborne-pathogens
6. World Health Organization, editor. WHO sharps injuries: assessing the burden of disease from sharps injuries to health-care workers at national and local levels, Environmental burden of disease series. Geneva: s.n; 2005. 11:50. 924159232X
7. Industrial Safety & Hygiene News. 320,000+ sharps injuries a year among U.S. health care workers. Occupational Safety_Today's News. [Online] 13 Nov 2013. https://www.ishn.com/articles/97373-000-sharps-injuries-a-year-among-us-health-care-workers
8. Chambers A, Mustard CA, Etchens J. Trends in needlestick injury incidence following regulatory change in Ontario, Canada 2004–2012; an observational study. BMC Health Serv Res. 2015;15:17.
9. Bouya S, et al. Global prevalence and device-related causes of needle stick injuries among health care workers: a systematic review and meta-analysis. Ann Glob Health. 2020;36:35. https://doi.org/10.5334/aogh.2690.
10. Saia M, et al. Needlestick injuries: incident and cost in the United States, United Kingdom, Germany, France, Italy, and Spain. https://www.bmijournal.or. Biomed Int. 2010;1:41–9.
11. Centers for Disease Control and Prevention. Stop sticks injuries. NORA Healthcare and Social Assistance Sector Council. [Online] 26 Feb 2019. https://www.cdc.gov/nora/councils/hcsa/stopsticks/safersharpsdevices.html
12. National Institutes of Health. Legislative chronology. National Institute of Health Office of NIH History and Stetten Museum. [Online] 2010. https://history.nih.gov/display/history/Legislative+Chronology
13. European Union. Directive 2010/32/EU-prevention from sharp injuries in the hospital and healthcare sector. EU Directives [Online] 10 May 2010. https://osha.europa.eu/en/legislation/directives/council-directive-2010-32-eu-prevention-from-sharp-injuries-in-the-hospital-and-healthcare-sector
14. GOV.UK. Government creates new National Institute for Health Protection. [Online] 18 Aug 2020. https://www.gov.uk/government/news/government-creates-new-national-institute-for-health-protection
15. Public Health Agency of Canada Centre for Communicable Diseases and Infection Control. Routine practices and additional precautions for preventing the transmission of infection in healthcare settings. Publications: Diseases and conditions. [Online] November 2016. https://www.canada.ca/en/public-health/services/publications/diseases-conditions/routine-practices-precautions-healthcare-associated-infections.html%20accessed%20on%2010-21-23
16. Centers for Disease Control and Prevention. Summary of infection prevention practices in dental settings: basic expectations for safe care. DHHS. Atlanta: US Department of Health and Human Services; 2016. http://www.cdc.gov/hai/settings/outpatient/outpatient-care-guidelines.html
17. Kohn WG, et al. Guidelines for infection control in dental health care settings-2003. J Am Dent Assoc. 2004;135:33–47. https://doi.org/10.14219/jada.archive.2004.0019.

18. Cleveland JL, et al. Prevention percutaneous injuries among dental health care personnel. J Am Dent Assoc. 2007;138:169–78.
19. Siegel JD, et al. 2007 Guideline for isolation precautions: preventing transmission of infectious agents in healthcare settings. Centers for Disease Control and Prevention. s.1: https://www.cdc.gov/infectioncontrol/guidelines/isolation/; 2017. p. 1–209.
20. Dimond V. Infection prevention: sticking together on sharps safety. Healthcare Purchasing News [Online]; December 2014. https://cdn.hpnonline.com/inside/2014-12/1412-IP-Sharps.html
21. Dulon M, et al. Causes of needlestick injuries in three healthcare settings: analysis of accident notifications registered six months after the implementation of the EU Directive 2010/32/EU in Germany. J Hosp Infect. 2017;95(3):306–11. https://doi.org/10.1016/j.jhin.2016.11.015.
22. Smith E. Operating room: sticking together on sharps Safety. Healthcare Purchasing News. July 2021:14–8.
23. Sharps Injury Prevention Stakeholder Group. Moving the sharps safety in healthcare agenda forward in the United States: 2020 consensus statement and call to action. International Safety Center; 2020. p. 1–15. https://internationalsafetycenter.org/wp-content/uploads/2020/12/Moving_The_Sharps_Safety_In_Healthcare_Agenda_Forward_In_The_US.pdf

Surface Disinfection

9

Oksana Mishler and Stephanie Dennison

9.1 Introduction

A diverse population of microorganisms circulates in the healthcare environment [1]. Many of these potentially harmful bacteria and viruses contaminate surrounding surfaces and remain active while continuing to be invisible. To minimize the risk of transmission of a pathogen from an inanimate surface to a susceptible host, healthcare providers must incorporate appropriate surface cleaning and disinfecting practices and procedures into their workplace routine [1].

Dental settings are a unique subset of healthcare. Unlike many other healthcare providers, dental professionals work in close proximity with their patients, only a few inches away from the patient's nasal and oral cavity, while surrounded by numerous environmental surfaces. Such a unique work environment places both dental providers and patients at higher risk for disease transmission. While the same principles of infection prevention—*standard precautions*—apply to dental settings, there are some dentistry specific modifications that must be incorporated into infection control practices.

In essence, *any* infection could be transmitted in dental settings. However, some pathogens are more specific to dental settings than others. Considering the nature of dental procedures, blood-borne pathogens such as hepatitis B and C, human immunodeficiency virus (HIV), and upper respiratory tract viruses like influenza A and B, and COVID-19 are among the most common [2, 3]. Other pathogens that can also

O. Mishler (✉)
Department of Advanced Oral Sciences and Therapeutics, The University of Maryland School of Dentistry, Baltimore, MD, USA
e-mail: omishler@umaryland.edu

S. Dennison
Division of General Dentistry, Department of Comprehensive Dentistry, The University of Maryland School of Dentistry, Baltimore, MD, USA
e-mail: sdennison1@umaryland.edu

L. DePaola et al. (eds.), *Infection Control in the Dental Office in the Era of COVID-19*, https://doi.org/10.1007/978-3-031-64611-9_9

be transmitted in dental settings are *Mycobacterium tuberculosis*, *Staphylococcus aureus*, streptococci, measles, mumps, rubella, and human papillomavirus [3, 4].

For an infection to occur, a pathogen must reach a susceptible host. In dental settings, the most common routes of transmission are:

- *Direct contact* with blood, oral fluids, or infectious materials.
- *Indirect contact* with contaminated objects, equipment, or environmental surfaces.
- *Contact with droplets or aerosols* [5, 6].

With respect to this chapter, the focus will be on specific infection control practices that can disrupt indirect contact transmission via contaminated objects, equipment, and environmental surfaces.

9.2 Pathogens in Dental Settings

Considering that many bacteria and viruses circulate in dental settings, dental providers must be aware of the pathogens' ability to remain active. Some pathogens survive *only* inside a host, while others remain virulent on inanimate surfaces, where they await the opportunity to transfer to the next host [7]. To prevent the transmission, it is providers' responsibility to keep dental instruments, equipment, and environmental surfaces free of potentially infectious microorganisms. Pathogen persistence on inanimate surfaces varies and has been summarized by Wibmann and colleagues (Fig. 9.1) [7]. As specified for SARS-CoV-1, pathogen survival ability is influenced by several factors:

- Surface material (therefore, avoid carpeted flooring and upholstered furnishings).
- Temperature (with low temperatures associated with longer persistence).
- Humidity.
- Initial titer.

Even though some pathogens can remain potentially infectious for a long time, the risk of transmission can be significantly decreased by adherence to standard cleaning and disinfecting procedures [7].

9.3 Environmental Dental Surfaces

In dental settings, pathogens can take temporary residence on various environmental surfaces. Environmental dental surface is an umbrella term for a surface or equipment that does not come in direct contact with patients during treatment [8]. Environmental surfaces can be further categorized as *clinical contact* or

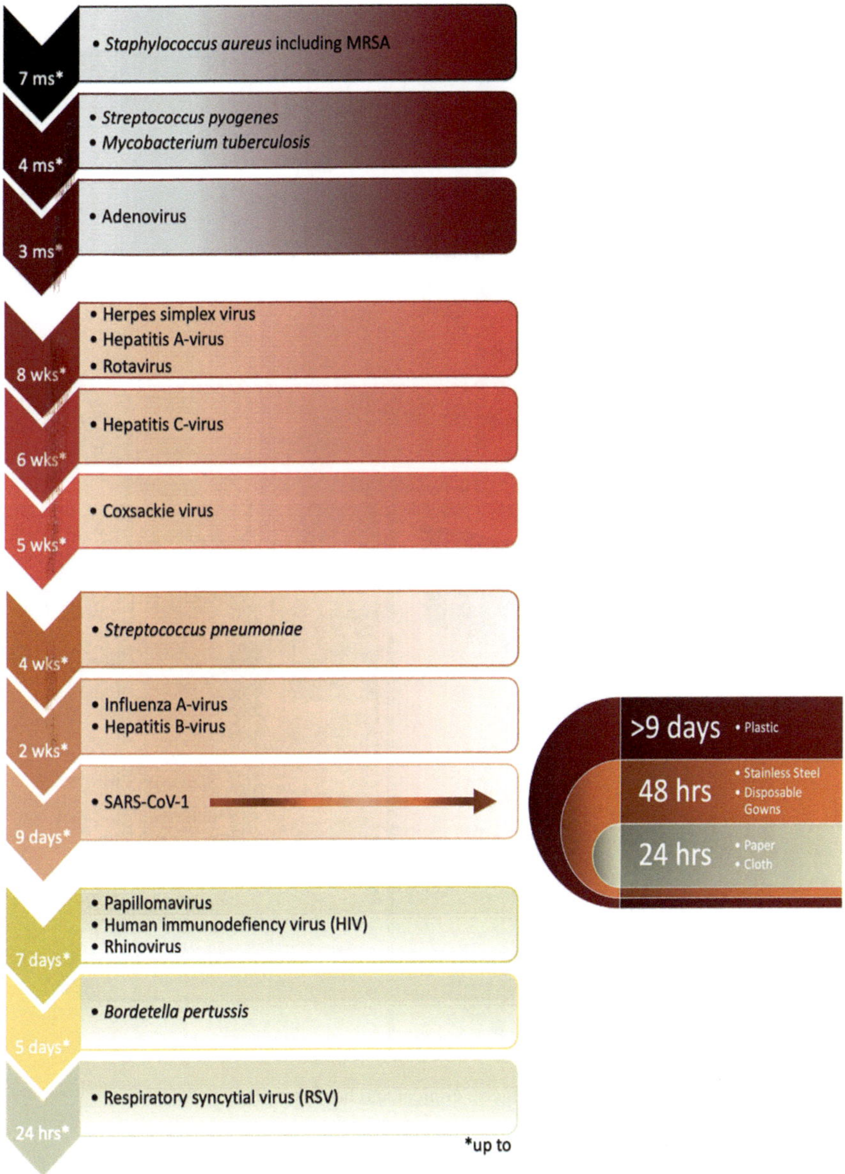

Fig. 9.1 Pathogen persistence on inanimate surfaces

housekeeping surfaces (Photo 9.1). As a general rule, the level of disease transmission defines the category of an environmental surface.

Clinical contact surfaces pose the highest risk of disease transmission as they may easily become contaminated with blood or bodily fluids during patient care, considering that clinical contact surfaces are relatively close to the patient treatment

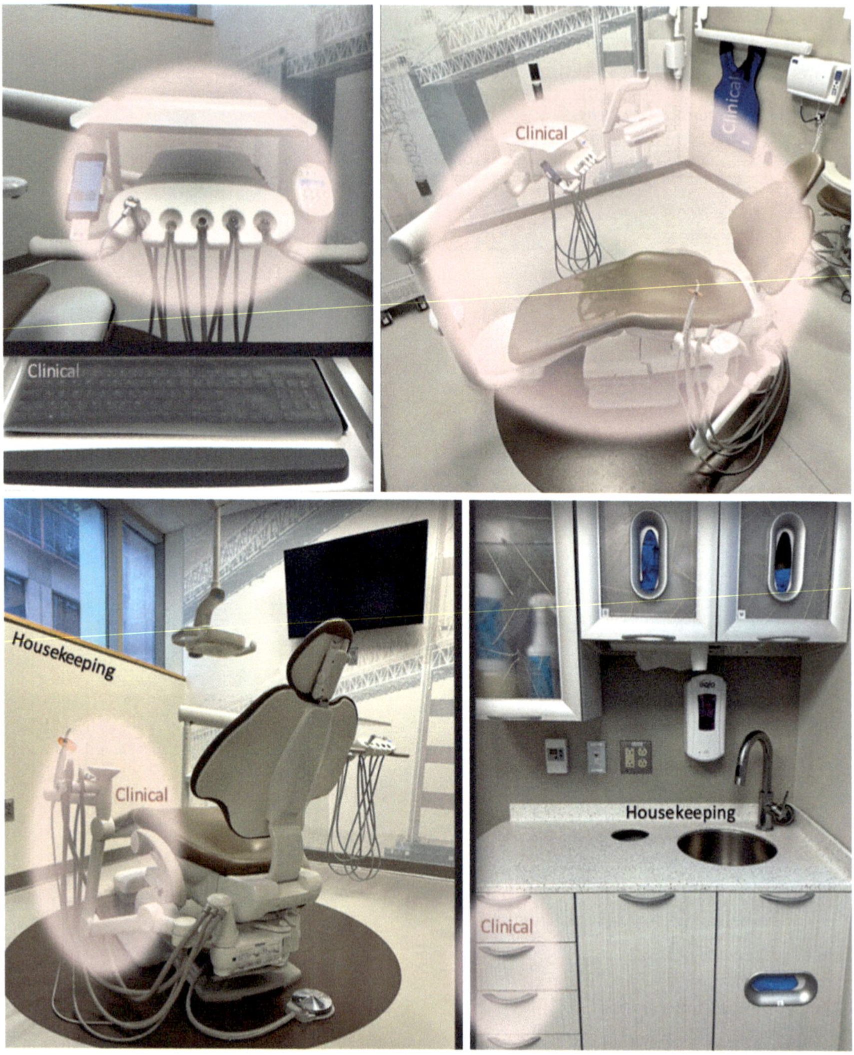

Photo 9.1 Environmental dental surfaces: clinical and housekeeping

area and can become contaminated either *directly*, via spray or splatter generated during dental procedures, or *indirectly*, through contact with the provider's gloved hands and dental instruments or devices [9]. Some examples of clinical contact surfaces in a dental operatory include:

- Dental chair
- Operator chair
- Operator overhead light
- Instrument tray

- Dental chair controls with multiple hoses
- Suction unit
- Air water syringe
- Operator foot control
- Dental radiology equipment
- Chairside computer with keyboard and mouse
- Cabinets and dental supply carts
- Patient safety glasses and reusable bib holder

All other environmental surfaces that are—typically—not directly touched during dental treatments are considered housekeeping surfaces. Housekeeping surfaces carry the lowest risk for disease transmission [9]. Some examples of housekeeping surfaces in a dental operatory are listed below:

- Floor
- Walls
- Ceiling
- Window covering
- Sink

Even though environmental surfaces and patient care items must be pathogen-free for each patient use, the recommendations are not the same for clinical versus housekeeping surfaces, or dental instruments and other items used during dental procedures. Keeping environmental dental surfaces and other patient care items pathogen-free can be achieved with cleaning, disinfection, and sterilization.

9.4 Cleaning, Disinfection, and Sterilization

Cleaning is a *physical removal* of organic materials and visible soils from objects and environmental surfaces [10]. Proper cleaning with detergents and sufficient rinsing with water is required prior to disinfection and sterilization to ensure germicidal activity of a disinfecting agent and effectiveness of a sterilization process [9]. Although cleaning removes substantial numbers of microorganisms, it does not destroy them all.

Unlike cleaning that simply removes microorganisms, disinfection can destroy pathogens. In healthcare settings, disinfection is typically achieved by liquid chemicals [10]. Based on their level of effectiveness, disinfectants can eliminate many or all pathogens. Disinfectants can be used alone or in combinations, with each product designed for a specific purpose. Unlike sterilization, disinfection does not destroy bacterial spores. However, disinfection provides a certain level of pathogen elimination:

- High level
  - Consider chemical sterilants.

  - Destroy all microorganisms and some bacterial spores [11].
  - Should never be used on environmental surfaces [12].
- Intermediate level
  - Destroy vegetative bacteria, most fungi, and viruses.
  - Have tuberculocidal claim.
  - Do not kill all bacterial spores.
  - May be used to clean and disinfect any clinical contact or housekeeping surface regardless of the presence or absence of blood [8].
- Low level
  - Inactivate vegetative bacteria, fungi, enveloped viruses, and some nonenveloped viruses.
  - Do not have tuberculocidal claim.
  - Do not kill bacterial spores [12].
  - May be used to clean and disinfect clinical contact and housekeeping surfaces that are not visibly contaminated with blood [8].

9.5 Clinical Versus Housekeeping Surfaces

When feasible, clinical contact surfaces should be barrier-protected, especially when surfaces are difficult to clean. For clinical contact surfaces that are not barrier-protected or whose barrier was breached, surface cleaning and disinfection is required between patients [8–10]. Environmental Protection Agency (EPA)-registered hospital disinfectants with *intermediate*-level pathogen elimination can be utilized to clean and disinfect clinical contact surfaces, with or without visible contamination by blood. EPA-registered hospital disinfectants with *low*-level pathogen elimination can be used to clean and disinfect clinical contact surfaces that are not visibly contaminated with blood. At the end of each day, all clinical contact surfaces must be cleaned and disinfected by an EPA-registered hospital disinfectant [8, 10, 13, 14].

Housekeeping surfaces require routine evaluation, cleaning, and disinfection. While cleaning and disinfection protocols and schedules for housekeeping surfaces vary among different healthcare realms, it is generally recommended that high-touch housekeeping surfaces such as doorknobs and light switches be cleaned and disinfected more frequently than minimal contact housekeeping surfaces such as floors and ceilings. Most housekeeping surfaces can be adequately cleaned with soap and water. Detergents and disinfectants may also be used according to the type and degree of contamination. When housekeeping surfaces in the dental setting are visibly soiled, EPA-registered hospital disinfectants of low and intermediate level are required for cleaning and disinfection. Facility-specific policies and procedures for cleaning and disinfection of housekeeping surfaces are typically determined via a risk assessment for contamination [13].

9.6 Use of Barriers

Even though dental provides aim to keep every environmental surface free of harmful pathogens, some surfaces—like a keyboard or a mouse of a chairside computer—cannot be properly cleaned or disinfected. In these instances, the surface should be covered with a disposable barrier to protect it from potential microbial contamination [8]. Considering the digital advances in dental radiology, special attention should be paid to the digital radiology sensors. To protect the sensors from potential contamination, a Food and Drug Administration (FDA)-approved barrier must cover the sensor during use. If the manufacturer instructions indicate that the sensor cannot tolerate heat sterilization, an intermediate-level disinfectant must be used to prevent contamination between patients [8].

Different types of surface barriers are used in dental settings (Photo 9.2). While materials range from clear plastic wrap to aluminum foil, the most important property of any barrier is to be impermeable [14]. Clean barriers should be placed with clean ungloved hands. Used barriers should be removed with gloved hands. Barriers must be changes after each patient use. After removing the barrier, the underneath surface should be examined for potential contamination and cleaned and disinfected as needed [14]. Surface disinfection is not required between patients for barrier-protected clinical contact surfaces whose barrier remains intact and whose surface shows no sign of contamination upon removal of the barrier. The general considerations for barrier placement during patient care are indicated below:

- Frequency of potential contact with gloved hands.
- Likelihood of contamination.
- Difficulty of cleaning the surface [14].

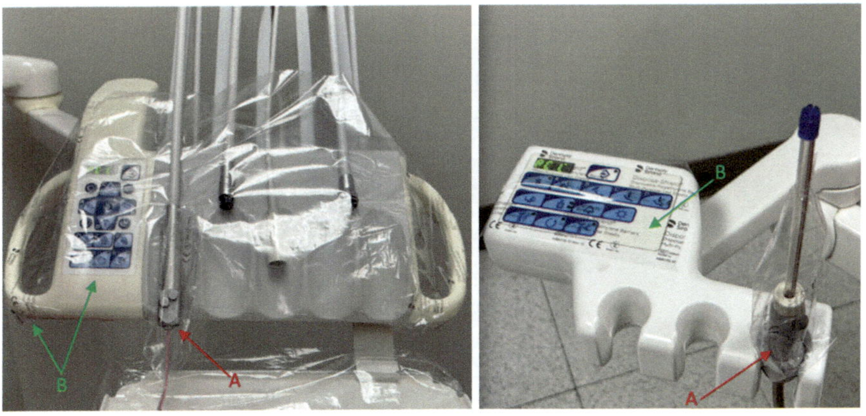

Photo 9.2 Surface barriers: (**a**) difficult to clean surfaces; (**b**) frequent contact with gloved hands

9.7 Cleaning and Disinfecting Procedures and Techniques

As previously mentioned, a thorough cleaning must precede disinfection procedures in order to prepare environmental surfaces for the next level of pathogen elimination. Water and detergent will remove visible organic and inorganic residues [14]. When mop or cloths are used for cleaning, mop heads and reusable cleaning cloths must be decontaminated—laundered or dried—regularly to prevent contamination. When spills of blood or other potentially infected materials occur, promptly clean and *then* decontaminate potentially infectious surfaces, and discard blood-contaminated items in accordance with federal regulations [14].

To ensure proper disinfection post-cleaning, the two-step procedure, spray-wipe-spray or wipe-discard-wipe, is recommended to ensure that environmental surfaces—especially, clinical contact surfaces—are free of potentially virulent pathogens [9]. When using liquid disinfectant, first "spray-and-wipe" the surface to ensure it is clean, and then proceed with another "spray" as part of the disinfection step. If using commercially available disposable disinfectant wipes, use the first wipe to clean the surface, and then use the second wipe to disinfect the surface [9] (Photo 9.3).

Even though patients are not in the treatment room when cleaning and disinfection of environmental surfaces takes place, providers performing these procedures must still wear appropriate personal protective equipment (PPE). To prevent

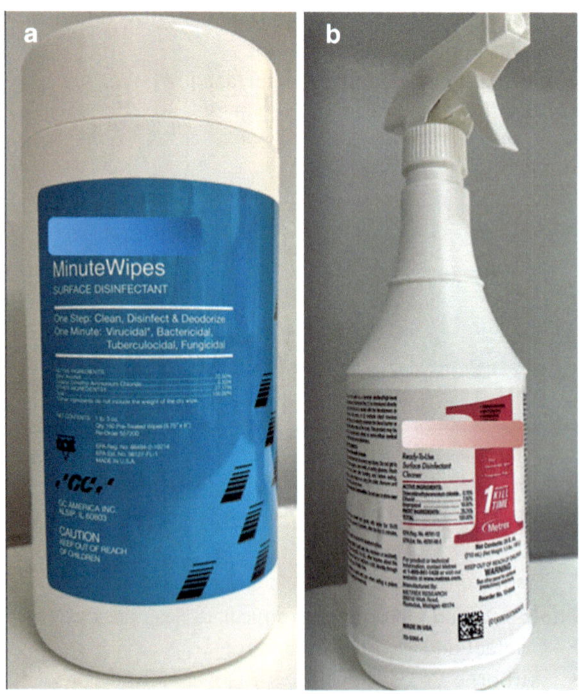

Photo 9.3 Surface disinfectants: (**a**) wipes; (**b**) spray

exposure to pathogens that could potentially linger in the room posttreatment and to ensure *personal* protection against harmful chemicals contained within cleaning and disinfecting products—at a minimum—a mask, gloves, protective clothing, and eye protection must be worn by dental providers involved in cleaning or disinfection [9]. It is important to note that chemical- and puncture-resistant utility gloves provide a higher level of protection against harmful chemicals than exam gloves. Typically, these gloves are not disposable and can be reused after cleaning and disinfection.

9.8 Chemical Disinfectants

The most common liquid chemicals used in healthcare settings are summarized in Fig. 9.2. When selecting disinfecting products, it is essential to be familiar with their bactericidal and virucidal properties for proper use and application. For patient and provider safety and product efficacy, always follow manufacturers' directions and read the labels carefully [5].

9.9 Properties of an Ideal Disinfectant

Keeping in mind the different levels of *pathogen persistence* on inanimate surfaces and considering safety of patients and healthcare providers, many factors should be taken into consideration when identifying properties of an ideal disinfectant. An ideal disinfectant should be effective against a wide spectrum of pathogens and have good cleaning properties without causing harm to the users or patients [10]. An ideal disinfectant should also be compatible with various surfaces without being corrosive or causing deterioration of the surface. Ideal disinfectant should be water-soluble, stable in concentrate and use dilution, and leave an antimicrobial film—known as a residual effect—on the treated surfaces [10]. Figure 9.3 summarizes properties of an ideal disinfectant.

Considering that microorganisms have various degrees of *resistance* to chemical germicides, an ideal disinfectant should target the most resilient pathogen [10]. As indicated in Fig. 9.4, *Mycobacterium tuberculosis* has one of the highest innate ability to resist chemical disinfectants. Therefore, an ideal disinfectant should be able to destroy *Mycobacterium tuberculosis* [10]. When selecting a disinfectant for your practice, keep in mind that a disinfectant with a tuberculocidal claim is capable of destroying less resistant microorganisms such as blood-borne pathogens inclusive of Hepatitis B and C, and HIV [10].

	Overview	Recommendations
Alcohol: • Ethyl alcohol • Isopropyl alcohol	• Water-soluble • Rapidly bactericidal rather than bacteriostatic • Optimum bactericidal concentration: 60%-90% • Bactericidal activity drops sharply below 50% concentration • Evaporates rapidly • Flammable (must be stored in a cool, well-ventilated area) • Does not destroy spores • Damages shellac mountings of lensed instruments, rubber and certain plastic tubing after prolonged and repeated use	• Tuberculocidal • Fungicidal • Virucidal • Not recommended as a sterilant or high-level disinfectant
Chlorine and Chlorine Compounds	Household Bleach (5.25%-6.15% sodium hypochlorite): • Broad spectrum antimicrobial activity • No toxic residue • Unaffected by water hardness • Fast acting • Inexpensive • Corrosive to metals (concentration >500 ppm) • Inactivated by organic matter • Discoloration of fabrics • Releases toxic chlorine gas when mixed with ammonia or acid	• Decontamination of blood spills; however, large spills must be cleaned first to compensate for inactivation in the presence of blood • Can be used as an irrigating agent in endodontic treatment, disinfectant for manikins, and dental appliances
Formaldehyde*	Formalin (37% formaldehyde by weight): • Bactericidal • Fungicidal • Virucidal • Sporicidal *Should be handled in the workplace as a potential carcinogen by OSHA	• Chemical sterilant and high-level disinfectant • Health-care use is limited due to its irritating fumes and pungent odor, and potential link to nasal and lung cancer
Glutaraldehyde	• Saturated dehydrate • Not sporicidal in aqueous solution • Becomes sporicidal once the solution is activated • Shelf-life and use-life have improved over the years • Noncorrosive to metal • Does not damage lensed instruments, rubber, or plastic	• Chemical sterilant and high-level disinfectant • Widespread use in health-care facilities • Should not be used for cleaning non-critical surfaces: too toxic! • Exposure should be monitored to ensure a safe work place!

Fig. 9.2 Chemical disinfectants. (Centers for Disease Control and Prevention)

Ortho-Phthalaldehyde (OPA)	• Superior mycobactericidal activity to glutaraldehyde • Stability over a wide pH range (pH 3-9) • Does not require activation • Does not require exposure monitoring • Excellent material compatibility	FDA-approved high-level disinfectant (since 1999)
Hydrogen Peroxide	• Bactericidal • Fungicidal • Virucidal • Sporicidal Extremely stable if stored in dark containers!	• Stable and effective disinfectant for use on inanimate surfaces* • Chemical sterilant and high-level disinfectant* *Dependent upon concentration and exposure time
Iodophors: Iodine + Solubilized Agent of Carrier	• Bactericidal • Mycobactericidal • Virucidal • Fungicidal • Sporicidal {Fungicidal, Sporicidal} Can require prolonged contact time	• Disinfectants • Antiseptics: - Not suitable for use on as hard-surface disinfectant - Should not be used on silicon catheters
Peracetic Acid	• Rapid action against *all** microorganisms • Sporicidal even at low temperatures • Lacks harmful decomposition products • Enhances removal of organic material • Leaves no residue • Corrosive effects can be reduced by additives and pH modification *Dependent upon concentration and exposure time	• Chemical sterilant
Phenolics: used by Joseph Lister in his work on antiseptic surgery	• Bactericidal • Fungicidal • Virucidal • Tuberculocidal • Absorbed by porous materials • Residual disinfectant can irritate skin	• Disinfectants: - Environmental surfaces - Non-critical devices
Quaternary Ammonium Compounds	• Bactericidal • Fungicidal • Virucidal • Microbicidal activity affected by water hardness and materials (cotton and gauze pads)	• Disinfectants: - Housekeeping surfaces - Equipment or items that contact intact skin

Fig. 9.2 (continued)

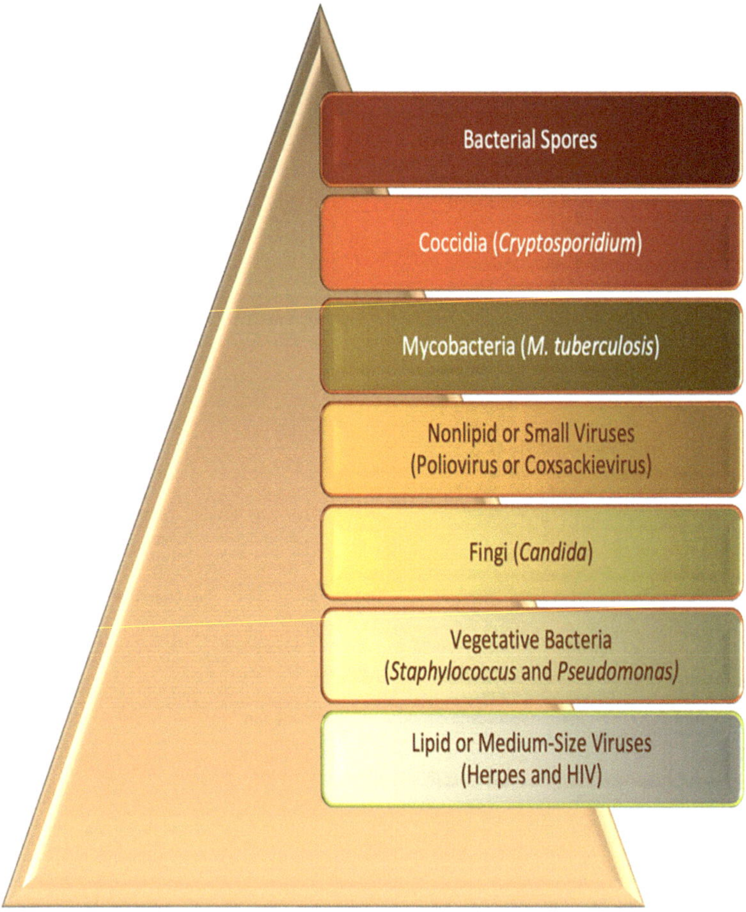

Fig. 9.3 Properties of an ideal disinfectant. (Centers for Disease Control and Prevention)

9.10 Sterilization

While cleaning removes pathogens from objects and environmental surfaces without destroying them and disinfection can eliminate most pathogens but not bacterial spores, sterilization destroys *all* forms of microbial life if performed correctly [9]. In dentistry, saturated steam under pressure has been the most common and reliable form of sterilization [15]. It is important to note that the efficacy of sterilization—similar to that of disinfection—depends on the following factors:

- Preceding cleaning.
- Type and level of microbial contamination.

Fig. 9.4 Degrees of pathogen resistance. (Centers for Disease Control and Prevention)

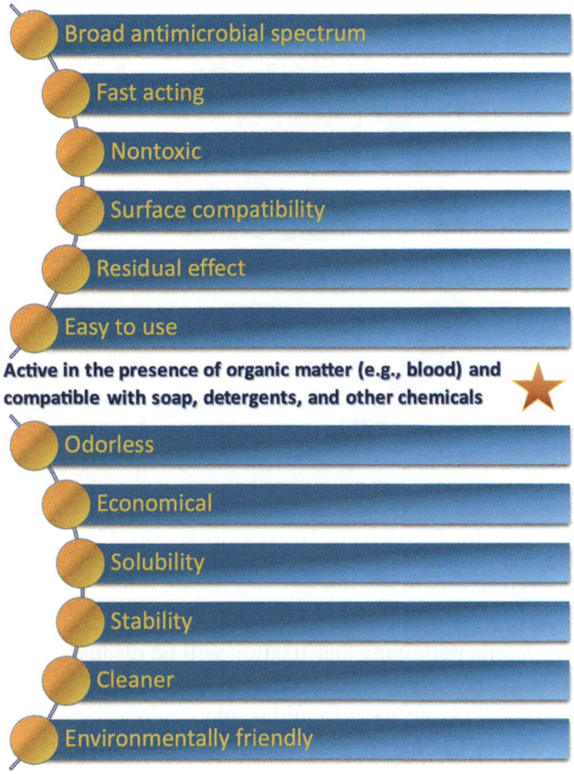

- Concentration and exposure time.
- Physical nature of an object including crevices, hinges, etc.
- Presence of biofilms.
- Temperature and pH [9].

As previously indicated, cleaning should *always* occur before sterilization and disinfection. Removal of organic and inorganic debris helps with microbial inactivation during the sterilization process. [16] Regardless of the selected cleaning process—manual or automated—dental providers and dental personnel must comply with the following recommendations when handling used instruments and devices:

- Wear appropriate PPE, including puncture-resistant, heavy-duty utility gloves.
- Use appropriate detergent or chemical solution.
- Remove residual detergent or chemicals by rinsing with water.
- Take extra precautions to eliminate splashing.
- Avoid retrieving sharp instruments by hand; use forceps instead or empty them onto a towel [16].

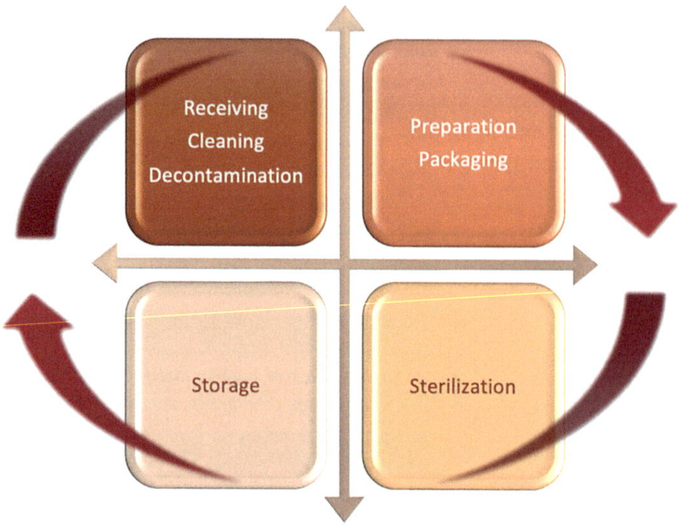

Fig. 9.5 Instrument processing area in the dental settings. (Centers for Disease Control and Prevention)

Details pertaining sterilization will be discussed in subsequent chapters. For the flow of the instrument processing, please refer to Fig. 9.5. When feasible, instrument processing areas should be physically divided. Otherwise, each section should be clearly labeled from contaminated to sterile [16].

9.11 Disinfection and Sterilization Guideline and Regulatory Framework

When considering disinfection and sterilization of instruments and other items involved in patient care, dental providers must be aware of a classification that has been in place for over 30 years. Originally invented by Earle H. Spaulding, this classification takes into consideration the degree of infection occurrence for specific patient care procedures [10]. In accordance with the classification, all patient care items can be classified as critical, semi-critical, or noncritical.

- *Critical:*
  - Patient care items that *penetrate* soft and hard tissues or vasculature when being used. Because of this, critical items confer the greatest risk of infection transmission when contaminated with pathogens. Critical items that are tolerant to heat must be heat-sterilized. Those that are sensitive to heat may be sterilized by a low-temperature sterilization process or liquid chemical sterilant [8, 13, 14, 17].
  - *Examples:* surgical instruments, scalpels, periodontal scalers, and explorers.

- *Semi-critical:*
  - Patient care items that *contact* mucous membrane or non-intact skin without penetration when being used. Because of this, semi-critical items confer a lower risk of infection transmission when contaminated with pathogens as compared to critical items. Semi-critical items that are tolerant to heat must be heat-sterilized. Semi-critical items that are not tolerant to heat must be high-level disinfected using an FDA-registered chemical sterilant [8, 13, 14, 17].
  - *Examples:* cheek retractors, mouth mirrors, handpieces, and air water syringes.
- *Noncritical:*
  - Non-critical items include both patient care and clinical contact surfaces. Non-critical items contact *intact skin*, but not mucous membranes when being used. Because intact skin is an effective barrier to most pathogens, non-critical items are considered low-risk infection transmission [8, 13, 14].
  - *Examples:* dental chair, operator chair, operator overhead light, curing light, radiographic equipment, and instrument tray.

Non-critical items should be barrier-protected when possible. Those that are not barrier-protected or are visibly soiled with blood must be cleaned and disinfected between all patients using an EPA-registered, hospital-level disinfectant [8, 13, 14]. Intermediate-level disinfectants may be used on all non-critical items regardless of the presence or absence of blood, while low-level disinfectants can be utilized to disinfect non-critical items that are not visibly soiled by blood.

In the United States, every step of the disinfection and sterilization process—from distribution to proper use of disinfectants and sterilants—is governed by the federal laws and regulations [10]. Two governmental agencies that are part of the regulatory framework are the EPE and FDA. Low- and intermediate-level disinfectants are regulated by the EPA. High-level disinfectants, heat, liquid, and chemical sterilants are controlled by the FDA [9]. Although the Centers for Disease Control (CDC) provides overall guidance on selection of products based on the principles of infection prevention and control, it does not test or evaluate specific chemical germicides.

9.12 Summary and Conclusion

To prevent the spread of infection via indirect contact with contaminated objects, equipment, or environmental surfaces, dental providers must be aware of the pathogen persistence on inanimate surfaces and the means of effective pathogen elimination. Knowing the difference between cleaning, disinfection, and sterilization procedures and understanding the degree of pathogen resistance are critical in order to select the proper pathogen elimination procedure and product to prevent the transmission of harmful pathogens from an inanimate surface to a susceptible host.

References

1. Centers for Disease Control and Prevention. Reduce risk from surfaces. Healthcare-Associated Infections (HAIs); 13 Oct 2020. Retrieved from: https://www.cdc.gov/hai/prevent/environment/surfaces.html
2. Bromberg N, Brizuela M. Preventing cross-infection in the dental office. [Updated 2023 Mar 2019]. In: StatPearls [Internet]. Treasure Island: StatPearls Publishing. Retrieved from: https://www.ncbi.nlm.nih.gov/books/NBK589669/; 2023.
3. McCarthy GM. Risk of transmission of viruses in the dental office. J Can Dent Assoc. 2000;66(10):554-5–557.
4. Amato A, Caggiano M, Amato M, Moccia G, Capunzo M, De Caro F. Infection control in dental practice during the COVID-19 pandemic. Int J Environ Res Public Health. 2020;17(13):4769.
5. Sebastiani FR, Dym H, Kirpalani T. Infection control in the dental office. Dent Clin N Am. 2017;61(2):435–57.
6. Upendran A, Gupta R, Geiger Z. Dental infection control. In: StatPearls [internet]. Treasure Island: StatPearls Publishing; 2023.
7. Wibmann JE, Kirchhoff L, Bruggemann Y, Todt D, Steinmann J, Steinmann E. Persistence of pathogens on inanimate surfaces: a narrative review; 2021. Retrieved from: https://www.ncbi.nlm.nih.gov/pmc/articles/PMC7916105/
8. Centers for Disease Control and Prevention. Guidelines for infection control in dental health-care settings, 2003. MMWR Morb Mortal Wkly Rep. 2003;52(RR-17):1–68.
9. Centers for Disease Control and Prevention. Cleaning & disinfecting environmental surfaces. Oral Health; 26 Mar 2016. Retrieved from: https://www.cdc.gov/oralhealth/infectioncontrol/faqs/cleaning-disinfecting-environmental-surfaces.html
10. Centers for Disease Control and Prevention. Cleaning. Infection control; 18 Sept 2016. Retrieved from: https://www.cdc.gov/infectioncontrol/guidelines/disinfection/cleaning.html
11. Rutala WA, Weber DJ, The Healthcare Infection Control Practices Advisory Committee (HICPAC). Guideline for disinfection and sterilization in healthcare settings. Atlanta: Centers for Disease Control and Prevention; 2008.
12. Sehulster LM, Chinn RYW, Arduino MJ, Carpenter J, Donlan R, Ashford D, Besser R, Fields B, McNeil MM, Whitney C, Wong S, Juranek D, Cleveland J. Guidelines for environmental infection control in health-care facilities. Recommendations from CDC and the Healthcare Infection Control Practices Advisory Committee (HICPAC). Chicago: American Society for Healthcare Engineering/American Hospital Association; 2004.
13. Sehulster L, Chinn RY, CDC, HICPAC. Guidelines for environmental infection control in health-care facilities. Recommendations of CDC and the Healthcare Infection Control Practices Advisory Committee (HICPAC). MMWR Recomm Rep. 2003;52(RR-10):1–42.
14. Rutala WA, Weber DJ, The Healthcare Infection Control Practices Advisory Committee (HICPAC). Guideline for disinfection and sterilization in healthcare facilities, 2008. CDC; 2019.
15. Laneve E, Raddato B, Dioguardi M, Di Gioia G, Troiano G, Lo Muzio L. Sterilization in dentistry: a review of the literature. Int J Dent. 2019;2019:6507286. Retrieved from: https://pubmed.ncbi.nlm.nih.gov/30774663/
16. Centers for Disease Control and Prevention. Sterilization: cleaning. Oral Health. April 2020. Retrieved from: https://www.cdc.gov/oralhealth/infectioncontrol/faqs/cleaning.html
17. Food and Drug Administration (FDA). FDA-cleared sterilants and high-level disinfectants with general claims for processing reusable medical and dental devices. Rockville: U.S. Department of Health and Human Services, Food and Drug Administration; 2015.

Cleaning and Sterilization of Dental Instruments

10

Eve Desai and Daniel Cheng

10.1 Introduction

Dental instrument sterilization is a critical process in dental practices to prevent the spread of infection and ensure patient safety. Each office must develop standard protocols to prevent the transmission of pathogens to patients and staff members via contact with infected blood, bodily fluids, or tissues. All clinical personnel are responsible for understanding and implementing the guidelines for proper cleaning and sterilization of dental instruments. Dentists and their staff work within close contact with patients on a consistent basis and risk acquiring pathogens or spreading pathogens to their patients if proper infection control is not maintained. For example, contaminated instruments could spread viruses such as hepatitis B, which can live outside a human host for up to a week in dried blood [1].

One of the most famous case reports detailing the spread of infectious disease in the dental setting due to poor sterilization practices was detailed by the Centers for Disease Control (CDC) in 1991. The CDC reported on six patients infected with HIV in a Florida dental office that had no established infection control policy or procedures for reporting any injuries, such as needlesticks. The office lacked any consistent policy for instrument processing and breakdown which may have facilitated the transmission of HIV from the practicing dentist to patients [2]. This incident demonstrated not only the need for proper infection controls but also how a consistent plan could have prevented multiple people from contracting a chronic illness.

Manufacturers of dental products must comply with FDA regulations and must provide information about the "intended use" and "the instructions for use" (IFUs) of their products that allow the end user to operate within recommended safe

E. Desai (✉) · D. Cheng
Division of General Practice, Department of Comprehensive Dentistry, The University of Maryland School of Dentistry, Baltimore, MD, USA
e-mail: edesai@umaryland.edu; dcheng@umaryland.edu

L. DePaola et al. (eds.), *Infection Control in the Dental Office in the Era of COVID-19*, https://doi.org/10.1007/978-3-031-64611-9_10

practices. Successfully implementing a process that incorporates IFUs and clinical best practices into operational standards is required to operate safely. It is mandated that those who process instruments must provide clean and sterile instruments for each patient [3]. This section will provide a general overview of best practices and provide additional resources for professionals seeking to leverage research outside of their immediate realm of understanding. This will help to ensure they are following all infection control guidelines at the national and state level.

10.2 Definitions and Levels of Disinfection

Cleaning, disinfection, and sterilization are unique processes, and each has their own utility in safe processing of dental instruments. Cleaning removes foreign material through scrubbing with water and detergents but does not guarantee all microbial life has been killed. During disinfection, a chemical is used that eliminates most pathogens from the instrument surface but still does not always kill all microbial life, such as spores. Sterilization is the utilization of a chemical or physical method to destroy all microbial life, including bacterial spores.

The CDC categorizes items into three groups, according to how they are used in dental care. Critical items like surgical handpieces and forceps penetrate soft tissue and bone, creating the greatest risk to spread infection. These instruments need to be sterilized. Semi-critical items are those that touch mucous membranes or non-intact skin, such as explorers and retractors, and pose a decreased threat of transmission. They should be managed using high-level disinfection or heat sterilization if possible. Noncritical items, such as X-ray tubeheads, only contact intact skin and thus pose the least risk for infection spread. These items can usually be wiped down with an intermediate or low-level disinfectant [4].

10.3 Instrument Processing

A plan that provides guidance and defines instrument-specific procedures ensures sterilization and cleaning processes are effective, efficient, and cost-conscious. All dental clinics should have a designated area to process instruments, away from patient care. The instrument-processing area should have designated areas for receiving and cleaning, packaging, sterilization, and storage. This prevents contamination of clean areas and instruments. Healthcare providers are also at risk of infection through injury and contact with mucous membranes of the eyes, nose, and mouth, or contact with open skin. Therefore, operator protection is essential during instrument processing. To avoid injury from sharp instruments, dental personnel must wear heavy-duty gloves and refrain from blindly reaching into tray; use forceps or empty the tray onto a towel. Operators should protect themselves with masks, face shields, eye protection, and gowns [5]. There are six steps widely recognized steps of instrument processing.

10.3.1 Step 1: Cleaning

Prior to sterilization, instruments must be cleaned to remove biological soil, which can hinder microbial inactivation and disrupt the sterilization process. All instruments are considered contaminated until they undergo sterilization. Instruments not cleaned immediately should be soaked in a dedicated detergent, disinfectant-detergent combination, or enzymatic cleaner to prevent material drying and simplify cleaning. Manual scrubbing, while basic and cost-effective, has drawbacks: it is time-consuming and operator-dependent and may not detect all contaminants. The CDC recommends using long-handled brushes to reduce the risk of injury to dental personnel:

- Two separate sinks should be used: a sink for soiled instruments and a sink for cleaned instruments. Soiled instruments should be submerged in a detergent solution, cleaned individually, and rinsed in clean water. They should then be dried and inspected for cleanliness under proper lighting.
- Ultrasonic immersion is a less labor-intensive option. Instruments are placed in a cleaning solution, and ultrasonic action loosens and removes soil. However, this process is still operator-dependent, and hollow instruments should not be cleaned this way.
- Industrial washer-disinfector machines can clean and dry multiple instruments at once, minimizing operator errors and sharps injuries [5]. The washer uses fresh solution each cycle, reducing bacterial contamination, and is consistent with cleaning and drying cycles in terms of water temperature, detergent solution, drying temperature, and cycle times. The disadvantages of the washer-disinfector machines are larger initial cost, longer cycle times, and larger water requirements. It is better for offices to have multiple small machines for backup redundancy and staggered finish times for increased instrument turnover.

10.3.2 Step 2: Inspection

A visual inspection detects any remnants of foreign materials and other contamination prior to sterilization. Each instrument is required to meet the standards of sterilization and is to be verified at this point [6]. A visual inspection can also be used as a quick screening for repairing or retiring instruments. There are limits to the visual inspection, as some biological material (saliva) may be colorless and hard to detect.

10.3.3 Step 3: Packaging

Proper packaging of dental instruments for sterilization is critical to ensure that they remain sterile until they are used on patients. Instruments should be separated whenever possible, with hinged instruments opened and unlocked, and loaded into cassettes based upon procedures. Cassettes improve organization, save time for personnel, and increase instrument longevity [7]. Cassettes and instruments without containers should then be wrapped with packaging materials to allow sterilization agents to penetrate [5].

To maintain instruments in their original status, the use of different storage and packaging measures is required. The use of individual pouches with chemical indicators is demonstrated in Fig. 10.1 for isolated instruments. Quality assurance is vital to validate that processed instruments and equipment conform to CDC guidelines. Visual indicators serve to verify that instruments have met and maintain their sterile status. Inclusion of the chemical indicators inside of pouches ensures that the instruments maintain their sterile status until they reach chairside. If chemical indicators cannot be seen within sterile packaging, indicators must be placed on the outside packaging for verification [5].

To provide an effective barrier, two sheets of sterilization wrap are required when wrapping for instrument trays or cassettes as shown in Figs. 10.2 and 10.3. The Association for the Advancement of Medical Instrumentation recommends this particular technique for wrapping instruments as it still allows for aseptic opening [8]. All wraps are required to meet material-specific guidelines from manufacturers and

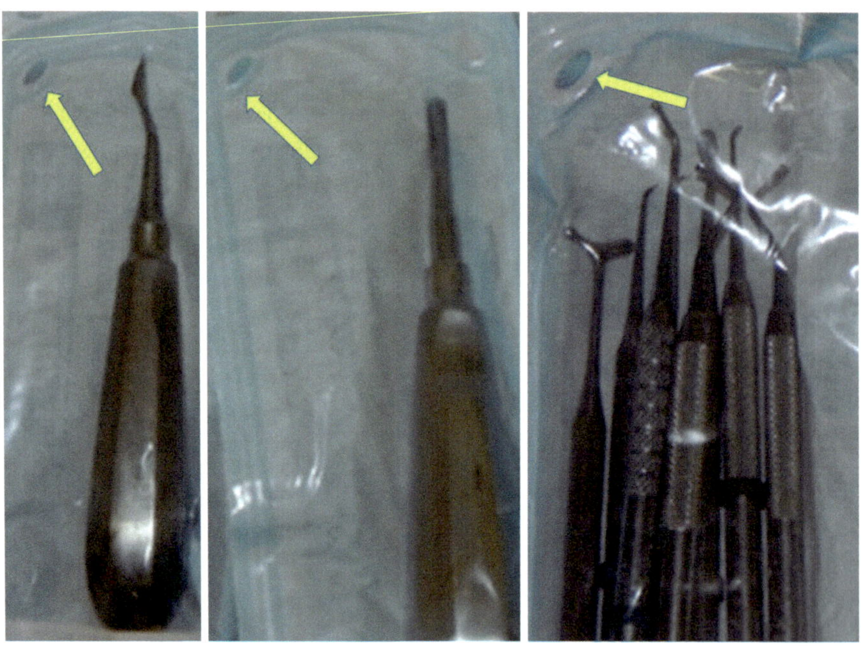

Fig. 10.1 Chemical indicators should be placed internally and externally on every instrument pack and/or wrap. The chemical indicators used in the above change from green to purple when the proper sterilization parameters have been met. In this image multiple instrument packs demonstrated that the chemical indicator(s) had not turned the proper color. This indicates that conditions for sterilization had not been met and these packs must be repackaged and reprocessed before the instruments are used for patient care. (Image Courtesy of Dr. Louis G. DePaola)

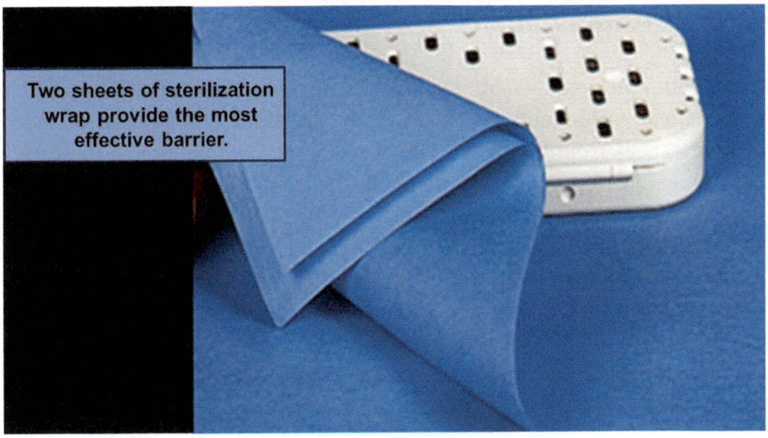

Fig. 10.2 To provide an effective barrier, two sheets of sterilization wrap are required when wrapping for instrument trays or cassettes. (Image Courtesy of Dr. Louis G. DePaola)

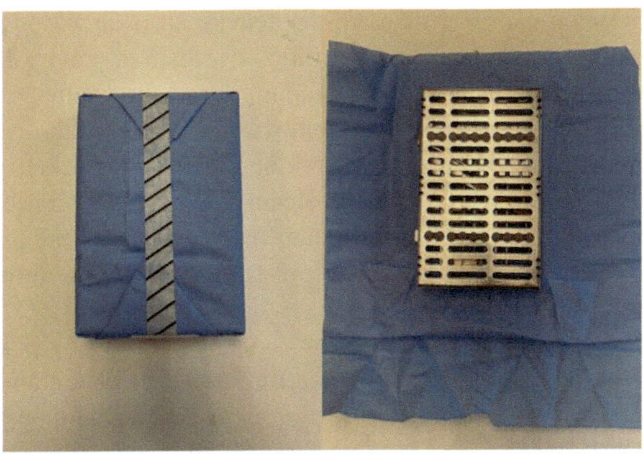

Fig. 10.3 Sterilized basic examination cassette wrapped using the ANSI/AAMI-approved double wrap technique for use in a dental clinic. This cassette neatly contains dental instruments necessary to complete a comprehensive oral evaluation or limited/problem-focused examination and prevents delicate instruments, such as probes from being damaged. Aseptic opening of these cassettes is easily done (right side), and the outer wrapping can be used to drape bracket tables and keep instruments sterile

the FDA. Securing wraps with sterile indicator tapes secures instruments and provides additional quality assurance. Similar to pouched instruments, wrap manufacturers recommend not stacking wrapped items during storage, as this can compromise sterility [9].

10.3.4 Step 4: Sterilization

The most common methods of sterilization of dental instruments are the use of steam, chemical vapor, and dry heat/rapid heat transfer. The use of sterilizers requires clearances from the FDA to ensure that the equipment and their packages are able to meet the required level of cleanliness and hygiene [10]. Sterilizers come in different sizes and processes to fit specific office needs.

Steam under pressure (autoclaving) is the process of choice whenever possible as it is considered safe, fast, and cost-effective for dental healthcare facilities. Steam sterilization is microbicidal and sporicidal and is the most dependable method of sterilization of all the methods available. It can penetrate fabrics (wraps). Each item is exposed to direct steam contact at a required temperature and pressure for a specific length of time.

The three key types of steam sterilizers include gravity displacement (gravity cycles), high-speed prevacuum, and steam flush pressure pulse (SFPP). All the above procedures are able to employ the use of air in sterilizing equipment [11]. In gravity displacement (gravity cycles), steam enters from the top and/or sides of the chamber. Since steam is lighter than air, the heavier air is displaced out of the bottom drain vent of the chamber. The penetration of steam in gravity displacement is delayed because it must displace the remaining air in the chamber. In high-speed prevacuum autoclaves, a vacuum pump removes air from the sterilization chamber before the steam enters. The steam will not be blocked by pockets of air, and the sterilization process is much quicker. In steam flush pressure pulse (SFPP) autoclaves, there are a series of alternating steam flushes and pressure pulses that push air out. This happens above atmospheric pressure to prevent reintroduction of air into the machine.

Flash sterilization is a modification of conventional packaged sterilization in which the flashed item is placed in an open tray or a special container to allow for rapid penetration of steam. Flash sterilization is an acceptable method of sterilization of critical instruments [12, 13]. This is not recommended as a routine sterilization method because of the absence of a protective wrap, possible contamination during transportation to operatories, lack of timely biologic monitors, and minimal sterilization cycle times. Some healthcare facilities have addressed these issues by moving equipment for flash sterilization close to operating rooms, increasing steam exposure time, using special biological indicators that provide results in one hour, and using protective wraps. Another disadvantage is that instruments that have been flash-sterilized are hot enough to cause clinical burns. These instruments must be air-cooled or immersed in a sterile liquid to prevent patient injury. Flash sterilization is acceptable for processing items that cannot be packaged, sterilized, and stored before use. It is also used when there is not enough time to sterilize an item by the preferred method. However, flash sterilization is not to be used as an alternative to purchasing more instrument sets or more equipment.

Each item must be exposed to steam at a required temperature and pressure for a required amount of time. Thus, the four components of steam sterilization are steam, pressure, temperature, and time. Raising pressure enables the autoclave to reach the required temperature faster. A high temperature must be maintained to kill microorganisms. The minimum required exposure time for wrapped healthcare supplies are 30 minutes at 121 °C in a gravity displacement sterilizer or 4 minutes at 132 °C in a prevacuum sterilizer. The conditioning phase of the sterilization cycle refers to the elimination of all air from the chamber. Steam must contact all surfaces to be sterilized. The various methods autoclaves use to achieve this have been detailed above. Some devices need extended time to reach all surfaces and extended cycles must be used. Sterilization will fail if steam cannot reach all surfaces of the instruments. Disadvantages of steam heat include corrosion and combustion of lubricants associated with handpieces [14]. The process is heavily dependent on all air elimination. In studies, some items, such as burs and other rotary cutting instruments, have been found to be difficult to clean and sterilize. After processing, there was evidence of soil, structural damage from steam processing, and bacterial spores. This has led some researchers to recommend all rotary cutting instruments be considered single-use instruments [15] (Figs. 10.4 and 10.5).

Other commercially available sterilization processes include chemical vapor, dry heat, ethylene oxide, vaporized hydrogen peroxide, and ozone. Chemical vapor sterilization utilizes heated alcohol in 0.23% formaldehyde within a closed pressure chamber. Instruments must be dry prior to sterilizing, but this method decreases corrosion to carbon steel instruments, such as dental burs. A major downfall for this process is that local authorities must be contacted to ensure proper handling and disposal of sterilizing solution. Dry heat sterilization is reserved for instruments that cannot tolerate moist heat, such as some burs and orthodontic appliances. There are two types of dry heat sterilizers used in the dental setting: static air and forced air. Static air types or oven-type sterilizers use convection heating through coils within the unit to expose instruments to hot air. Forced air or rapid heat-transfer sterilizers rapidly circulate heated air through the chamber [5].

Ethylene oxide or "gas" sterilization is used when heat sterilization will cause unacceptable damage to instruments and involves five stages: preconditioning and humidification, gas introduction, exposure, evacuation, and air wash. The average

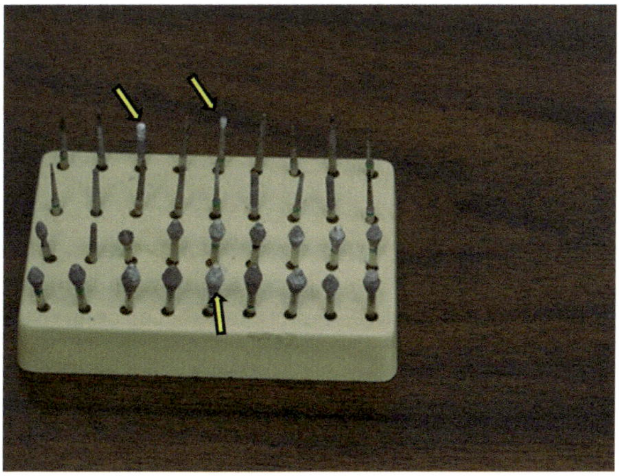

Fig. 10.4 Rotary cutting instruments such as burs should be thoroughly cleaned, packaged, and sterilized between each use. The burrs in the photo above cannot be sterilized in their current condition. (Image Courtesy of Dr. Louis G. DePaola)

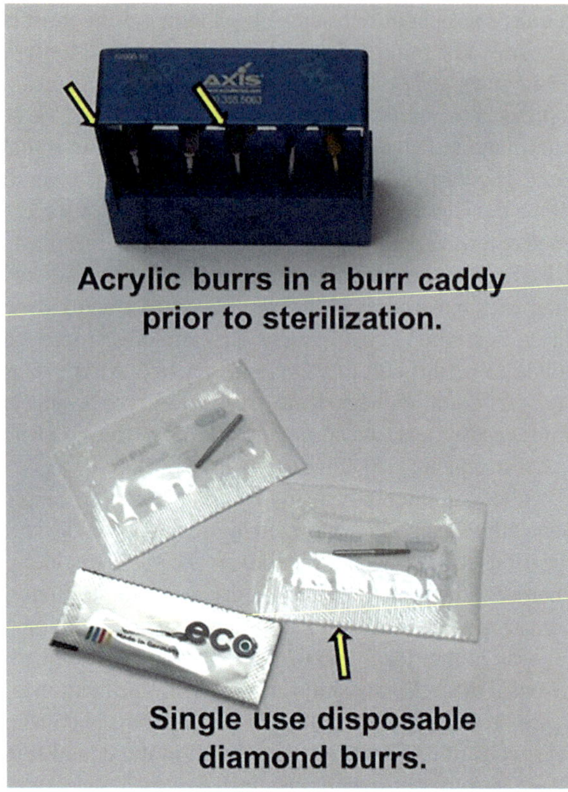

Fig. 10.5 After processing, there was evidence of soil, structural damage from steam processing, and bacterial spores. This has led to the recommendation that all rotary cutting instruments be considered single-use instruments whenever possible. More expensive acrylic and/or finishing burrs should be thoroughly cleaned placed in a burr caddy and sterilized between each use. (Image Courtesy of Dr. Louis G. DePaola)

cycle takes 2.5 hours, excluding aeration time to remove residual gas. The biggest concern with this method is that ethylene oxide is a documented carcinogen and has been linked to several occupational diseases, such as spontaneous abortion and cancer. Most local authorities require environmental controls, making this method only practically available to large-scale dental operations. Hydrogen peroxide gas plasma (vaporized) uses hydrogen peroxide solution that is injected and vaporized in a chamber, exposing surfaces for 50 minutes. An electrical field is applied within the chamber to create gas plasma, generating free radicals and killing microbes before the chamber is vented and filled with filtered air. Some current variations of the gas plasma system, such as diffusers, are not cleared for use by the FDA, restricting the availability of this method. Ozone, a low-temperature sterilization method, has recently been cleared by the FDA for sterilization of some reusable devices. Devices use medical grade oxygen, steam-quality water, and electricity, and the ozone is converted back into water vapor and oxygen before being purged from the room. The average cycle takes 4 hours and has been demonstrated to kill resistant microbes, such as *Geobacillus stearothermophilus* [16].

Although each of these processes offers advantages and disadvantages, the decision about which sterilization process the healthcare facility should choose lies with the instrument manufacturer as to what is validated in their IFU. For patient safety, the process must be compatible as to not cause damage to instruments but still ensure surface sterility.

10.3.5 Step 5: Sterile Storage

Sterilized packages should be stored in a manner that reduces the potential for contamination, i.e., clean, dry, and temperature- and traffic-controlled areas. They must be handled with care: avoid dragging, crushing, bending, compressing, or puncturing. Sterilized instruments should be stored in a location which is protected from environmental contaminants [17]. Each package should be inspected before use (Figs. 10.6 and 10.7).

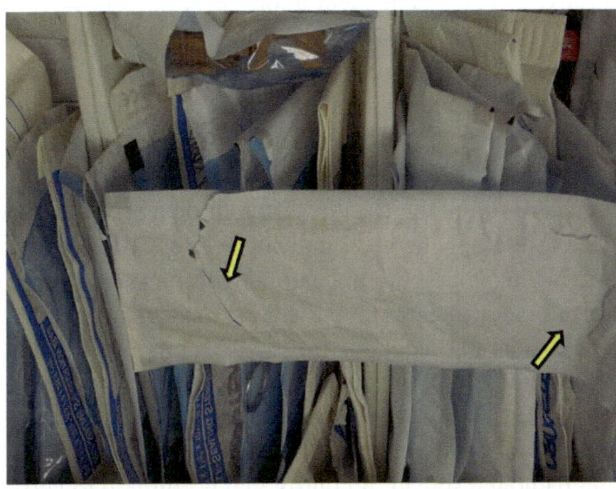

Fig. 10.6 Sterilized packages should be stored in a manner that reduces the potential for contamination and inspected for integrity before use. The instrument pack pictured above have been breached and should be repackaged and sterilized before they are used for patient care. (Image Courtesy of Dr. Louis G. DePaola)

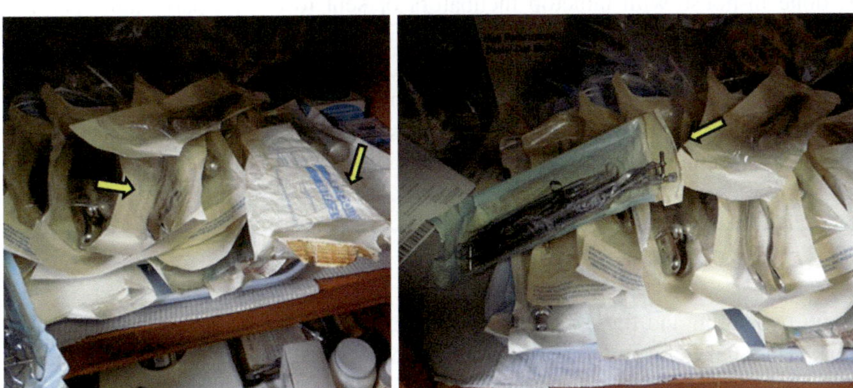

Fig. 10.7 Sterilized packages should be stored in a manner that reduces the potential for contamination and inspected for integrity before use. The instrument pack pictured above have been breached and should be repackaged and sterilized before they are used for patient care. (Image Courtesy of Dr. Louis G. DePaola)

10.3.6 Step 6: Quality Assurance

Quality assurance of processed instruments requires routine verification using three types of indicators: physical, chemical, and biological. The CDC guidelines specify the appropriate indicators for different instrument types and sterilization methods to ensure compliance.

Physical indicators are built into sterilizers to monitor time, temperature, and pressure during cycles [18]. Deviations indicate equipment malfunctions, but correct readings do not guarantee effective sterilization. Printouts are available from large-scale sterilizers but not in smaller office autoclaves [5].

Chemical indicators are placed inside or outside of the pouch. They are sensitive to either heat or chemicals used in sterilization and will change color when the particular element has been exposed long enough. Chemical indicators are divided up into five classes, dependent upon the Association for the Advancement of Medical Instrumentation (AAMI) guidelines. External chemical indicators make up Class I and Class II types. Autoclave tape placed on the outside of packages is an example of Class I indicators and demonstrates that the package has been exposed to a temperature of 121 °C for 15 minutes. It does not guarantee sterility. Class II indicators are specific tests, such as the Bowie-Dick test for dynamic air removal sterilizers, which are run in the sterilization unit on a stand-alone cycle. Classes III–V indicators are internal chemical indicators. Class III indicators are single-variable indicators, while Class IV indicators will measure two or more variables. Class V indicators, or integrating indicators, measure all variables within a sterilizer but are not considered acceptable for use with implanted medical devices [19].

Biological indicators, containing bacterial spores (e.g., *Bacillus subtilis* for dry heat and *Geobacillus stearothermophilus* for steam autoclaves) [5], are the gold standard. They should be used weekly or at each dental implant sterilization to prevent pathogen spread. A control vial is cultured to verify spore viability. Testing can be done in-house with tabletop incubators or sent to a third-party laboratory. A major concern with in-house kits is that they do not provide unbiased verification. Any biological indicator test that fails must be autoclaved at 250 °F/121 °C for 30 minutes prior to disposal. A repeat test should then be completed to determine if the first was a false positive. If the second test fails, the sterilizer must be serviced before it can return to duty [20].

10.4 Current Regulations

Input, oversight, and regulation of dental sterilization occur in multiple organizations. This makes formulating a single standard difficult. A partial list of organizations that have input into sterilization protocols are as follows:

- The American Dental Association (ADA) tests dental products and provides guidelines for use.

- The Organization for Safety, Asepsis and Prevention (OSAP) advocates for safe and infection-free delivery of oral healthcare.
- The Association for the Advancement of Medical Instrumentation (AAMI) produces standards, recommended practices, and technical information.
- The American National Standards Institute (ANSI) works with AAMI to create and publish American standards for healthcare equipment.
- The International Association of Healthcare Central Service Materiel Management (IAHCSMM) represents Central Sterile technicians by providing training and certification.
- The Association of periOperative Registered Nurses (AORN) provides recommendations for the sterilization of medical instruments.
- The Commission on Dental Accreditation (CODA) accredits dental education programs.
- The Centers for Disease Control (CDC) is responsible for controlling the introduction and spread of infectious diseases.
- The Joint Commission accredits and certifies healthcare organizations in the United States.
- The Food and Drug Administration inspections compliance and enforcement of patient safety.
- The Occupational Safety and Health Administration (OSHA) establishes workplace safety standards.
- European Centre for Disease Prevention and Control (ECDC).
- European Society of Clinical Microbiology and Infectious Diseases (ESCMID).
- UK Health Security Agency (UKSA).
- Disease Control and Prevention Center (Japan).
- National Institute of Infectious Diseases (NIID) (Japan).
- Chinese Center for Disease Control and Prevention.
- National Health Commission of the People's Republic of China.
- Santé Publique France.
- Istituto Superiore di Sanita (Italy).
- Robert Koch Institute (Germany).
- Australian Commission on Safety and Quality in Health Care.
- Australian Centre for Disease Control.
- Korea Disease Control and Prevention Agency (KDCA).

10.5 Breaches in Infection Control

The CDC is a nonregulatory, nonenforcement, agency and recommends that any infection control breach be reported to state and/or local agencies. Specific advice and procedures can also be requested or may be mandated from those agencies.

There are some guidelines for evaluating an infection control breach. First, identify the type of breach and the nature of the substance involved. For breaches involving a medical instrument, review recommended reprocessing methods, and start corrective actions as soon as possible. Determine if key steps were done in a suboptimal manner, or if they were omitted altogether. Directly observe the cleaning and sterilization procedures, with the understanding that actual practice and the observed practice may be different. Fear of retaliation may be a factor in the veracity of direct interviews. Examine disinfection processing records to evaluate whether a breach occurred during processing or a deficit exists in the cleaning and sterilization procedures. If there is an ongoing breach, stop all procedures until a new plan can be implemented. The plan should include a method to assess if the new procedures have been effective. Next, determine when the breach happened, the number of patients, and healthcare providers involved and which patients and/or providers were exposed. If available, the blood-borne pathogen infection status of patients should be determined. If transmission of blood-borne pathogens from the breach is suspected, then further epidemiological investigations should be initiated. Then, consult infection control experts, state, and local agencies, risk management, and licensing authorities. These may vary depending on the situation [14].

A qualitative assessment of the breach should be performed. It will be assigned to one of two categories. Category A indicates high-risk practice and egregious error, with high likelihood of blood exposure. Category B indicates a breach with lower likelihood of blood transmission. If the breach falls in Category A, notify and test the patients, as there is a significant risk of blood-borne pathogens. If Category B, consider these risks, in conjunction with key stakeholders, before notifying patients: the likelihood of transmission, public concern, perceived risk among patients and the community, and duty to warn vs harm of notifying patients [21].

When communicating with the patients, develop materials in consultation with key stakeholders. The key stakeholders should agree upon the method and type of communication and who is primarily responsible for communication. The key stakeholders should agree and explore postexposure testing and prophylaxis. Legal and media issues should be anticipated. Communication should use a multipronged approach with direct patient mail, Internet postings, telephone postings, and press releases.

10.6 Conclusions

Effective cleaning and sterilization of dental instruments is a critical component of infection control in the dental setting. This responsibility falls upon the dentist and auxiliary staff. Adherence to established infection control guidelines provided by the CDC helps prevent the spread of pathogens. Every office should have a written protocol for the sterilization of dental instruments and is responsible for the training of staff in this area. Efficient sterilization processes protect the patient, dentist, and the staff alike.

References

1. Bond WW, Favero MS, Petersen NJ, Gravelle CR, Ebert JW, Maynard JE. Survival of hepatitis B virus after drying and storage for one week. Lancet. 1981;1:550–1.
2. Centers for Disease Control. Update—transmission of HIV infection during an invasive dental procedure—Florida. MMWR Morb Mortal Wkly Rep. 1991;40:21–27, 33.
3. Kohn WG, Collins AS, Cleveland JL, Harte JA, Eklund KJ, Malvitz DM, Centers for Disease Control and Prevention. Guidelines for infection control in dental health-care settings—2003. MMWR Recomm Rep. 2003;52:1–61.
4. Wann O. Back to basics: infection control and prevention. Dental Economics. 2016;109(9):88.
5. Resuggan JC. The cleaning and sterilisation of bottles and other glass containers. London: United Trade Press; 1957.
6. ES HSA. Cleaning validation manual: a comprehensive guide for the pharmaceutical and biotechnology industries. Boca Raton: CRC Press; 2010.
7. Molinari JAHJ, Nelson P. Instrument cassettes: an effective infection control precaution. Inside Dentistry. 2013;9:1–7.
8. Association for the Advancement of Medical Instrumentation ANSI. 9.6- Wrapping techniques. In: ANSI/AAMI ST79:2017. Arlington: Association for the Advancement of Medical Instrumentation; 2017.
9. Rutala WAWD. Choosing a sterilization wrap for surgical packs. Infection Control Today. 2000;4:70.
10. Voss J. Cleaning and cleaning validation: a biotechnology perspective. London: Taylor and Francis; 2017.
11. Association for the Advancement of Medical Instrumentation ANSI. 10.2- Sterilization parameters. In: ANSI/AMMI ST79:2017. Arlington: Association for the Advancement of Medical Instrumentation; 2017.
12. Maki DG, Hassemer CA. Flash sterilization: carefully measured haste. Infect Control. 1987;8:307–10.
13. Rutala WA, Weber DJ. Disinfection, sterilization, and antisepsis: principles, practices, current issues, new research, and new technologies. Am J Infect Control. 2019;47S:A1–2.
14. CDC. Guideline for disinfection and sterilization in healthcare facilities, 2008. Update May 2019. p. 61–62.
15. Uchoa-Junior F, et al. Biofilm on and structural damage of rotary cutting instruments after 5 cycles of clinical use and processing. J Am Dent Assoc. 2023;154(6):495–506.
16. Lewis K. Persister cells, dormancy and infectious disease. Nat Rev Microbiol. 2007;5:48–56.
17. Andersen HK, Fiehn NE, Larsen T. Effect of steam sterilization inside the turbine chambers of dental turbines. Oral Surg Oral Med Oral Pathol Oral Radiol Endod. 1999;87:184–8.
18. Centers for Disease Control and Prevention. Guideline for disinfection and sterilization in healthcare facilities: recommendations of CDC and the Healthcare Infection Control Practices Advisory Committee (HICPAC). MMWR Morb Mortal Wkly Rep. 2008.
19. Burke FJ. Handling, cleaning and sterilization of instruments. Surbiton: Ansell Medical; 1997.
20. Brady RJ. Cleaning and sterilization processes. Bowie: Robert J. Brady Company; 1977.
21. Centers for Disease Control and Prevention. Summary of infection prevention practices in dental settings: basic expectations for safe care. Atlanta: Centers for Disease Control and Prevention, US Dept of Health and Human Services; October 2016.

Maintenance and Sterilization of Dental Handpieces

11

John McDaniel and Glenn Canares

11.1 Introduction

A dental handpiece is classified as a Class 1 medical device, which is regulated by the US Food and Drug Administration (FDA). In order for Class 1 devices to be approved by the FDA, manufacturers must submit 510(k) forms containing information demonstrating the device's safety and effectiveness compared to substantially identical devices already approved by the FDA [1]. The 510(k) is the FDA's required premarket submission form. Air- and electricity-powered handpieces with contra-angle, straight, and oscillating attachments, along with electric-driven systems, are covered by 510(k) submissions for dental rotary handpieces. Other countries have similar requirements under a variety of different regulatory agencies [1].

FDA approval requires a device to be sterilizable completely by an approved method and to demonstrate continued performance after repeated sterilizations. After sterilization parameters are clearly defined, biological monitoring is necessary to document external and internal sterility. Under the 510(k) process, new or modified dental handpieces and/or attachments must be as safe and effective as approved handpieces which makes it substantially equivalent [1]. Recently, the American Dental Association (ADA) has also developed extensive guidelines regarding dental handpieces, along with product reviews. Biological monitoring is necessary to ensure that the sterilization parameters are effective and that the dental handpieces

J. McDaniel (✉)
Bien Air USA, Inc., Irvine, CA, USA
e-mail: john.mcdaniel@bienair.com

G. Canares
Department of Pediatric Dentistry, The University of Maryland School of Dentistry, Baltimore, MD, USA
e-mail: gcanares1@umaryland.edu

L. DePaola et al. (eds.), *Infection Control in the Dental Office in the Era of COVID-19*, https://doi.org/10.1007/978-3-031-64611-9_11

and/or attachments meet safety requirements. The ADA guidelines provide a comprehensive set of standards that dental professionals can use to ensure that the products are safe and effective [2].

11.2 Dental Handpieces and Motors (American Dental Association (ada.org))

All sterilization processing departments (SPDs), dental students, faculties, hygienists, and dentists should receive continuous training to make sure they are up to date with the latest standards and comprehend the importance of adhering to the requirements. Standard operating procedures (SOPs) are recommended for all critical processes. Appropriate personal protective equipment (PPE) is required for all stages of the processes. All personnel should read and understand the SOPs before performing their duties. They should also inspect the PPE before each use to make sure it is in good condition. Finally, all personnel should be aware of the potential risks of the process and take steps to minimize risk as much as possible.

At the point of use, you should prepare the handpiece to be returned for transport and reprocessing as soon as possible after use. Do not wait until the full procedure has ended to clean the instruments. To remove gross soil from the instruments during the surgical procedure, a dental student or dental assistant should wipe the surfaces with a sterile surgical sponge moistened with sterile water to thoroughly remove visible soil. Removing gross soil from surgical instruments is necessary to reduce microorganisms on the instruments. When blood, organic matter, debris, and saline are allowed to dry on surgical instruments, they can also cause corrosion, rusting, and pitting. Not only are they highly corrosion-causing, but they can also cause corrosion, rust, and pitting when they are allowed to dry on surgical instruments for an extended period [3–6].

PPE should also be tested in order to ensure its effectiveness. All personnel should practice proper hand hygiene before and after handling handpieces. Point-of-use cleaning allows the instrument to remain free of blood and debris and inhibits biofilm or bioburden from building up on the tool. Biofilm can start to form within minutes; therefore, instruments should be wiped off or rinsed with sterile water periodically throughout the procedure. Lumened instruments should be flushed as much as practical during the procedure and immediately after the procedure. Remove any attachments such as burs, and clean the work area thoroughly. And ensure all tools are properly put away. Also, check the work area for any remaining debris. Dispose of any disposable items in a biohazard bag. Wash your hands thoroughly with soap and water. Clean and disinfect all surfaces according to your standard operating procedure (SOP) [3–6].

Considerations for viral contamination in response to COVID-19 are covered in the new CDC guidance document published on June 17, 2020. The recommendations complement the following documents. Infection Prevention and Control Recommendations for Patients with Coronavirus Disease 2019 (COVID-19) in healthcare facilities [7]. This covers changes in non-COVID-19 clinical care in healthcare systems during the COVID-19 pandemic. There is no longer a recommendation to wait 15 minutes after clinical care and patients have left the room before cleaning and disinfecting room surfaces in accordance with the Interim Infection Prevention and Control Recommendations for Patients with Suspected or Confirmed Coronavirus Disease 2019 (COVID-19) [5, 6]. A dental clinic should be notified 2 days after a dental appointment if a patient develops symptoms or is diagnosed with COVID-19, according to the CDCs or your country's equivalent health agency Healthcare Personnel with Potential Exposure Guidance.

Wipe off all debris from the surface of the handpiece, ensuring that it is clean and free of any contaminants. Check for any signs of damage; inspect any areas of concern for further damage, clean the area again if necessary, and report any found issues to the responsible personnel. Any instruments designated for return to the manufacturer for service should be thoroughly cleaned and sterilized prior to packaging, and verification of sterilization should accompany the returned instrument. An example of verification would be a handpiece placed in a sealed pouch with an indicator strip:

1. Wipe the instruments clean of gross bioburden following the procedure, and irrigate the canals when the procedure is completed.
2. Separate sharps from the rest of the waste, and place them in a puncture-resistant container.
3. Disposable blades should be removed from the reusable surgical instruments.
4. Ensure that sharp and delicate instruments are protected.
5. Make sure that multipart instruments are disassembled and the pieces are kept together.
6. Sets of instruments should be always kept together.
7. Ensure that linens, waste products, and disposable instruments are kept separately from the reusable ones.
8. Be sure to dispose of soaking solutions before transporting them.
9. Ensure that all contaminated items are stored in closed containers to prevent contamination [3–6].

Identify containers as biohazards. Disposable items, including scalpels, suture needles, sponges, and disposal containers, should be clearly marked. Personal protective equipment needs to be disposed of and replaced immediately, as well as being regularly inspected in order to detect potential problems. Also, employees need to be trained in how to use personal protective equipment properly.

The act of donning personal protective equipment (putting it on):

1. Hand hygiene must be performed.
2. If necessary, put on shoe covers.
3. Don your gown.
4. Make sure you are wearing a mask and respirator (if necessary).
5. Make sure you have eye protection on (if needed).
6. Gloves must be worn.

Taking off personal protective equipment (doffing):

1. Shoe covers (if applicable) should be removed.
2. Ensure that the gown and gloves are removed together.
3. Perform hand hygiene.
4. Remove eye protection (if applicable).
5. Remove mask/respirator (if applicable).
6. Perform hand hygiene [5, 8, 9].

Transportation of contaminated instruments and materials must be carried out in a rigid, puncture-proof, leak-proof container to the sterile processing area. Alternatively, an enclosed cart may be used to transport instruments to the decontamination area. The Occupational Safety and Health Administration (OSHA) blood-borne pathogen standard contains the requirements for transporting contaminated sharps. In addition to either transporting contaminated instruments in a rigid leak-proof container or an enclosed cart, the container or cart must contain a biohazard symbol to identify the contents as contaminated.

Removal of hardened bioburden significantly adds to the time needed to clean and decontaminate instruments; therefore, it is important to keep the instruments moist until they are cleaned. There are several methods to keep instruments moist during transport such as covering the instruments with a wet towel. Another method is to use a commercial product developed to keep instruments moist and, in the case of enzymatic sprays or gels, break down the blood and debris on the instruments prior to cleaning. This method is beneficial because it allows the enzymes more time to break down the bioburden on the instruments, thus making the cleaning process easier and faster. Additionally, gels and sprays help to reduce the risk of cross-contamination between instruments by minimizing the contact time between instruments and air [5, 8, 9].

11.3 Inspecting Handpieces for Connected Attachments

When initially spraying the handpiece with cleaner to remove any debris, also inspect the attachments for any cracks or chips, and replace any damaged or worn parts if necessary. The enzymatic spray cleaner will remove any dirt and grime that could be in the attachments and will help prevent any further damage. The inspection of the attachments will let you know if there is any damage that needs to be addressed or if any parts need to be replaced. If new parts are required, it should be addressed immediately to ensure that the device is working properly.

Ensure all items are secured, covered, and identified as contaminated prior to transporting to decontamination. Enzymatic sprays are designed to break down organic matter such as dirt and bacteria, which can quickly spread and cause contamination. By spraying the items before transporting them, it helps to ensure that all the organic matter is removed prior to further handling.

11.4 The Decontamination Processes

Do not use a dental handpiece that cannot be heat-sterilized or does not have FDA approval and validated reprocessing instructions. Follow the manufacturer's instructions when cleaning, lubricating, and sterilizing handpieces and other intraoral devices that can be removed from air and water lines of dental units. The equipment includes reusable prophylaxis angles, nose cones, and contra-angles as well as electric, endodontic, surgical, high-speed, and low-speed handpieces, as well as all handpiece motors and attachments. Air and water lines in dental units should also be cleaned and sterilized before use.

US Food and Drug Administration (FDA) regulations should be followed for handpieces that do not require air and water lines in dentistry, such as cordless devices. To reprocess these devices (clean, lubricate, and/or sterilize), follow manufacturer instructions, and only use FDA or your country's regulatory agency-approved devices [5, 10, 11].

11.5 Reverse Osmosis (RO)

Purification use within the sterilization department is highly recommended. This type of purification uses membranes to physically separate the water from other solid particles and heavy metals.

Reverse osmosis uses a pressure-driven membrane to separate dissolved solids from water. This membrane allows water to pass through while rejecting large molecules such as salt, sugars, and proteins. The concentrated stream of rejected molecules can then be used for other purposes such as industrial processes, cooling tower blowdowns, and dewatering holding ponds. Reverse osmosis is an effective and economical way of purifying water and removing any unwanted impurities.

Some portable reverse osmosis (RO) systems offer varying flow rates and onboard filtration, making it a convenient option for removing dissolved solids and total organic carbon (TOC). Numerous systems are commercially available, and clinicians should test their local water source to determine which, if any, of these devices are indicated. These systems may also be equipped with an adjustable flow rate that allows you to customize the flow output to your specific needs. Other features such as onboard filtration help to further purify the water and reduce the amount of TOC.

Depending on the water quality, RO systems can be set up for single-pass or double-pass operation. For instance, if the source water contains high dissolved solid content, a double-pass RO system may be more effective in reducing the concentration of these solids. Most of these systems are also easy to operate and maintain, making them an ideal choice for both residential and commercial applications. Furthermore, they have a low environmental impact, making it a sustainable solution [12].

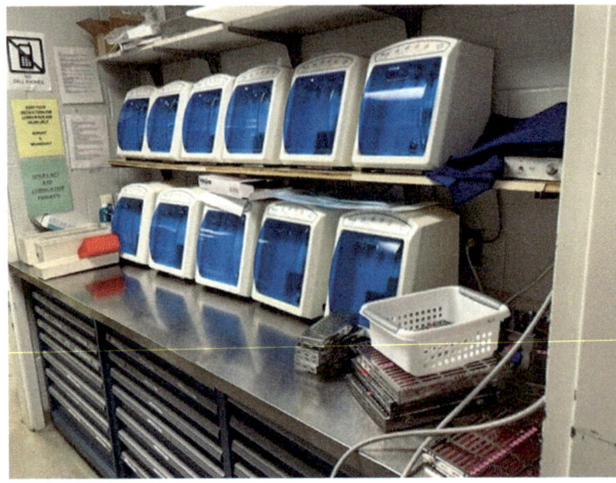

Fig. 11.1 Bien Air handpiece Lubricare units: picture. (Courtesy of UMSOD and Bien Air USA™)

11.6 Lubrication

Lubricating certain handpieces may be critical for daily use. Automatic lubrication equipment is designed to maintain turbines, handpieces, and contra-angles. An example is Bien Air Lubricare unit which makes maintaining devices easy, fast, and economical when combined with the company's Spraynet and Lubrifluid products, each are tailored to a specific phase of the maintenance cycle (Figs. 11.1 and 11.2). The Spraynet system dissolves impurities both inside and outside instruments, while Lubrifluid effectively lubricates them. Maintenance systems like Lubricare with the appropriate supplementary products are essential to ensure instruments are functioning at optimal performance and to ensure a long-life cycle. In short, lubrication and maintenance of devices form an effective combination for comprehensive, efficient, and cost-effective maintenance [13].

11.7 Packaging

One of the most important aspects of handpiece care is proper wrapping and storage of dental instruments. AMI ST 79 recommends maintaining packaging materials at room temperature for at least 2 hours between 20 °C and 23 °C [68 °F to 73 °F], with a relative humidity of 20% to 60%. To ensure compliance with manufacturer recommendations, it is essential to develop packaging policies and procedures to ensure that defects and extraneous matter are checked on a regular basis. A regular inspection for defects is recommended for all packaging materials, whether they are woven or nonwoven. In acute care settings, double wrapping is recommended for terminal sterilization, and some dental products may also benefit from double wrapping because of their strength and barrier properties. Particularly if you use only one wrapper, it is especially important to select packaging that provides excellent barrier

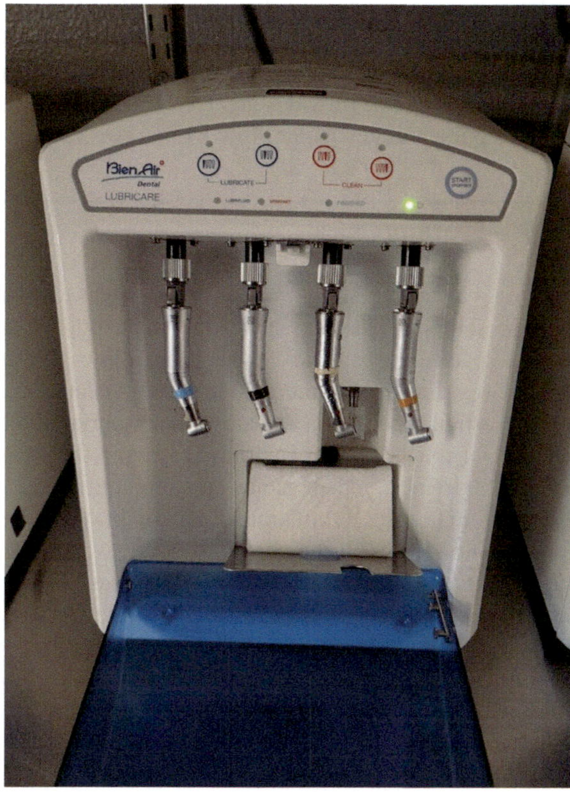

Fig. 11.2 Lubricare unit and handpieces. (Courtesy of UMSOD and Bien Air USA™)

protection. The highest level of barrier protection should be chosen when choosing packaging.

Using double barrier layers has several advantages, including:

- *Decreases opportunity for bacterial contamination:* Adding two more layers to a microorganism's path forces them to travel along a longer and more tortuous path. Bacteria have a longer distance to travel when they have to go through two layers. The addition of two layers helps prevent infectious diseases from spreading.
- *Backup protection:* If one layer has been snagged and torn, a layer may still remain intact. Additionally, it is unlikely that two breaches within the same layer will align perfectly, which means microorganisms will be able to enter unhindered if one is within one layer and the other within another. Microorganisms are unable to pass through each layer because they are made up of fibers tightly woven together. In addition, each layer is overlapped by approximately 20%, which further hinders microorganism movement. By compressing the fibers in the overlapped area, the microorganisms are unable to pass through the fibers, providing additional protection. Furthermore, the overlapping layer also provides a barrier to microorganism migration from one layer to another.

- *Protection from physical damage:* Overlapping two sheets provides additional cushioning and loft to the packaged item. The additional layer of cushioning helps to reduce the impact and vibration of the product when transported, while the additional loft provides greater surface area for air to circulate, which helps to keep the product cooler [4–6, 14].

11.8 Storage

The best way to keep supplies clean and sterile is to remove them from their original exterior shipping packages and store them outside of a clean and sterile area. External packaging cannot be cleaned and allows dust and bacteria to accumulate in the grooves. Ensure that the products are protected from damage, including puncture, crushing, bending, stacking inappropriately, being accidentally kicked, bumped, or touched when entering or leaving the storage area; dust, vermin, temperature extremes, and moisture contamination; and direct exposure to sunlight, airflow from heating, ventilation, or air conditioning. For instance, cardboard boxes are often lined with plastic or waxed paper, which can repel moisture and prevent the box from collapsing when stacked. The use of portable fans, humidifiers, and heaters in clean storage areas is not recommended. Before using, check for tears, dampness, dried water marks, excessive dust or dirt, and expiration date. If a package is wet or damp, comes in direct contact with the floor, or has passed its expiration date, it cannot be used. Whenever sterile items are uncertain about their sterility, they are discarded. Reusable items are reprocessed. These items are not meant to be used in clean storage areas because they can easily contaminate the sterile items. The dust and dirt from the fan, humidifier, or heater can spread to the sterile items, and the moisture can cause the items to become damp or wet. This can cause the sterility of the items to be compromised, and they need to be discarded or reprocessed [4–6, 14].

11.9 Handpiece Sterilization Asset Management

Before placing packaged instruments in the sterilizer, they should be labeled with the following information:

- The sterilizer used
- Cycle number or load number
- Date of sterilization
- Date of expiration, if applicable

Dental instruments and supplies should not be stored under sinks or any area where they may get wet. They should be stored in covered or closed cabinets. Before opening and using sterilized instruments, it is crucial to inspect them to ensure the packaging has not been damaged during storage (i.e., wet, torn, or punctured).

This is important because if the packaging is damaged, it can allow bacteria and other contaminants to enter the instrument and contaminate it. This can then lead to an increased risk of infection for the patient if the instrument is used.

The length of time a sterilized instrument can be stored based on its date or event varies. In some facilities, sterilized packages are dated, and designated shelf-life practices have been instituted. In other locations, event-based practices have been implemented. Whether manual or automated asset management establishes defined processes for ensuring that current operating standards are being adhered to and are trackable [4–6, 14].

11.10 Reviewing of Cleaning and Maintenance of Dental Handpieces in Dental Office

In dental offices, cleaning and maintaining dental handpieces is very important for maintaining the performance of the handpieces. The most common method of cleaning and maintaining dental handpieces is through the use of steam sterilization (Figs. 11.3 and 11.4), most commonly a tabletop sterilizer. To properly sterilize dental handpieces, the tabletop sterilizer should be operated according to the manufacturer's instructions. The sterilizer should also be regularly inspected to ensure that it is working correctly. Additionally, handpieces should be regularly lubricated to ensure they are running properly. The tabletop sterilizer works by exposing the handpieces to high pressure and steam, which kills any bacteria or viruses on the handpieces. Regular inspection is necessary to ensure that no parts of the sterilizer

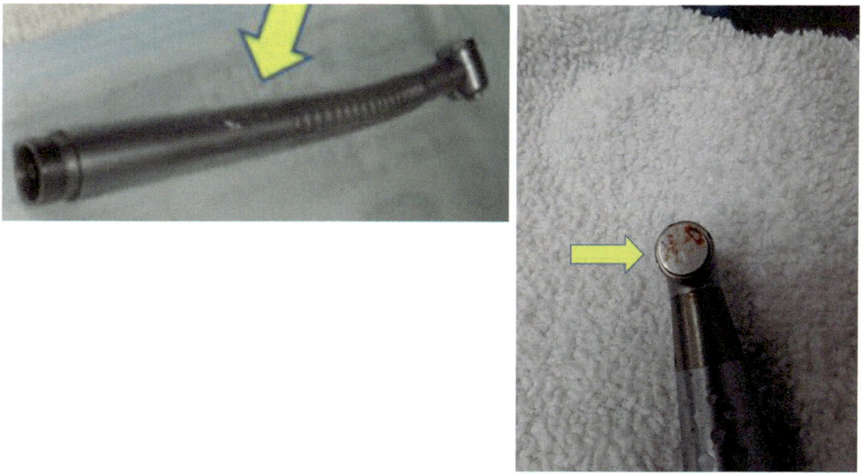

Fig. 11.3 Handpieces shown have not been properly cleaned. All handpieces should be cleaned of all debris, lubricated according to the manufacturers DFU, packaged, and heat-sterilized between every patient. (Image: Courtesy of Dr. Louis G. DePaola, University of Maryland School of Dentistry)

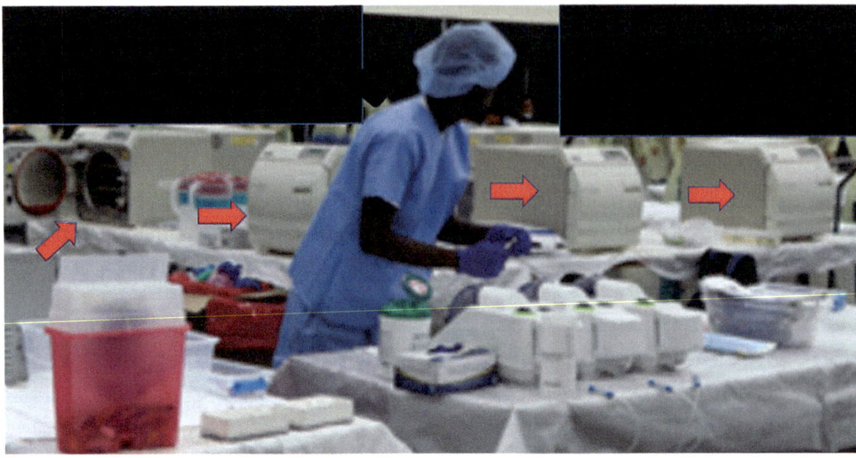

Fig. 11.4 Gravity steam sterilizers at large chartable dental event during which almost a thousand disenfranchised people were treated. All instruments inclusive of dental handpieces were sterilized between each patient. (Image: Courtesy of Dr. Louis G. DePaola—University of Maryland School of Dentistry)

are malfunctioning, which could lead to the handpieces not being properly sterilized. For example, the sterilizer should be inspected daily for any signs of leakage, and any loose parts should be tightened. In addition, regular lubrication, if required by the manufacturer, ensures that the system is running smoothly and that they are not overheating. In summary, regular inspection and lubrication (if necessary) of the sterilizer are essential to ensure that the handpieces are effectively sterilized:

- Cleaning your tabletop sterilizer on a daily, weekly, and monthly basis should be conducted in accordance with the instructions provided by the manufacturer.
- A tabletop sterilizer should only be used with distilled water to ensure successful sterilization, which can be assured by preserving the original water quality prior to sterilization.
- Sterilizer must be loaded in accordance with its manufacturer's instructions. In the absence of a rack, you can align the pouches properly on the sterilizer tray. Most sterilizers come with pouch racks and cassette racks. Follow the instructions for loading the racks to make sure they are loaded properly. Also, orient the load in accordance with the manufacturer's instructions.
- If a load contains wet loads or wet instruments at the end of the cycle, then this can be an indication that there is a problem with the sterilization process. Either the drying process has been interrupted during the drying cycle or the manufacturer's recommendations regarding the drying time have not been followed. If the drying cycle has been interrupted, the moisture will remain in the handpiece and can cause corrosion and damage to the internal components.

The Spaulding Classification system offers three levels of classification, critical, semi-critical, and non-critical that support the safe use of instruments and devices. Handpieces are considered medical devices that have contact with sterile body tissues or fluids and are considered critical items. This includes surgical instruments, and these instruments, or devices, if contaminated, can cause infection or damage to the tissue they contact. Therefore, it is important to ensure that they are sterile before being used. Any instrument in the critical category should be sterilized. Steam sterilization is the most frequently used type of heat sterilization in dentistry. Steam sterilization works by exposing instruments to high temperatures and pressures, killing all microorganisms present on the instruments.

However, check the manufacturer's directions for the instrument and sterilizer to ensure the correct type of sterilization is used and the correct sterilization parameters are followed. Not all instruments are suited for the same type of sterilization. It is important to ensure that all instruments are autoclaved at a temperature that meets the manufacturer's instructions. All instruments should be inspected before use to ensure they are sterile. Additionally, it is important to monitor and document the autoclave cycle to ensure the instrument is sterilized correctly. Finally, all instruments should be inspected before use to ensure they are sterile. By following these steps, healthcare professionals can ensure they are using the proper sterilization technique to ensure patient safety [4–6, 14].

11.11 Conclusions

11.11.1 Implementing a Process for Training and Preparing Personnel

In order to process handpieces safely for reuse, dental teams must follow infection control guidelines as well as safe use of cleaning products. Understanding the manufacturer's cleaning, maintenance, and sterilization instructions, as well as how to use cleaning products in a safe manner, is essential. Handpieces should not be cleaned, maintained, or sterilized by untrained employees without following the manufacturer's instructions. The Centers for Disease Control and Prevention recommends that dental staff receive continuous training in infection control and pathogen prevention. In addition, the Centers for Disease Control recommends that dental personnel be trained in infection control if their responsibilities or tasks exceed the standards of the federal Office of Safety and Health Administration (OSHA) concerning blood-borne pathogens. This is important to ensure that dental personnel are aware of the most up-to-date safety protocols for working with infectious diseases and bodily fluids. Additionally, it helps to reduce the risk of transmission of infectious diseases among dental personnel, patients, and other workers. By staying up-to-date on the latest safety protocols, dental personnel can reduce the risk of spreading infectious diseases to their patients and other workers. Additionally, being aware of the latest safety protocols can help dental personnel avoid potential legal or financial risks associated with not properly handling infectious diseases. Altogether, staying informed on the latest safety protocols can help dental personnel better protect patients, staff, and themselves from infectious diseases.

References

1. United States Food and Drug Administration (FDA). Premarket notification 510(k); 3 Oct 2022. https://www.fda.gov/medical-devices/premarket-submissions-selecting-and-preparing-correct-submission/premarket-notification-510k. Accessed 11 Nov 2023.
2. American Dental Association. Dental products: standards, technical specifications and technical reports; Dental handpieces and motors ANSI/ADA standard No. 35 executive summary. https://www.ada.org/resources/practice/dental-standards/dental-standards-executive-summaries/dental-instruments/dental-handpieces-and-motors. Accessed 11 Nov 2023.
3. Seavey R. Decontamination begins in the OR outpatient surgery; 27 Apr 2015. https://www.aorn.org/outpatient-surgery/article/2015-May-decontamination-begins-in-the or#:~:text=Any%20biohazard%20%E2%80%94%20in%20this%20case,solutions%20to%20contact%20all%20surfaces. Accessed 11 Nov 2023.
4. Centers for Disease Control and Prevention (CDC). Guidelines for infection control in dental health-care settings, 2003. https://www.cdc.gov/mmwr/preview/mmwrhtml/rr5217a1.htm. Accessed 11 Nov 2023.
5. Centers for Disease Control and Prevention (CDC). Summary of infection prevention practices in dental settings: basic expectations for safe care; 2016. https://www.cdc.gov/oralhealth/infectioncontrol/pdf/safe-care2.pdf. Accessed 11 Nov 2023.
6. Centers for Disease Control and Prevention (CDC). Infection prevention checklist for dental settings: basic expectations for safe care; 28 Mar 2016. https://www.cdc.gov/oralhealth/infectioncontrol/pdf/safe-care2.pdf
7. Centers for Disease control and Prevention. Guidance for dental settings, interim infection prevention and control guidance for dental settings during the COVID-19. Response, Updated 17 Jun 2020. https://www.cdc.gov/oralhealth/infectioncontrol/summary-infection-prevention-practices/. Accessed 11 Nov 2023.
8. Infection control results. Point-of-use instrument cleaning and transport. https://www.infectioncontrolresults.com/point-of-use-cleaning. Accessed 11 Nov 2023.
9. AAHA. Sequence for donning and doffing personal protective equipment (PPE). https://www.aaha.org/aaha-guidelines/infection-control-configuration/protocols/personal-protective-equipment/, https://www.infectioncontrolresults.com/point-of-use-cleaning. Accessed 11 Nov 2023.
10. CDC statement on reprocessing dental handpieces. CDC. 11 Apr 2011. Retrieved September 23, 2023, from https://www.cdc.gov/oralhealth/infectioncontrol/statement-on-reprocessing-dental-handpieces.htm. Accessed 11 Nov 2023.
11. OSHA review. CDC clarifies handpiece reprocessing procedures—infection control March 28, 2018. https://oshareview.com/2018/03/cdc-clarifies-handpiece-reprocessing-procedures-infection-control/. Accessed 11 Nov 2023.
12. Diversified industrial services. Reverse osmosis (RO). https://www.mpwservices.com/reverse-osmosis/?gclid=Cj0KCQjw1aOpBhCOARIsACXYv-frYxhEgxj1h5M-FJgmgzGCwn-Kanrv0umgrY1EgcX9SFYbDQMBGpwaAnqxEALw_wcB. Accessed 11 Nov 2023.
13. BianAir. Lubricare 2. https://dental.bienair.com/en_us/products/maintenance/device/lubricare-2.html#technical_data. Accessed 11 Nov 2023.
14. Halyard. Packaging dental instruments for sterilization. https://www.halyardhealth.com/articles/dental/packaging-dental-instruments-for-sterilization. Accessed 11 Nov 2023.

Dental Unit Waterlines

12

Dana R. Weikel and Christine Livesay

12.1 Introduction

Dental units supply electricity, air, suction, light, and water to devices needed for dental treatment. Contained in each dental unit is narrow-bore tubing made from either plastic, polymer, or silicone rubber, which runs water from a reservoir to the handpieces, scalers, and air/water syringe [1]. Within this tubing, or dental unit waterline (DUWL), microorganisms can colonize and form biofilms—communities of microorganisms that attach easily to surfaces and coexist in a moist or wet environment, posing a potential threat to those who encounter this water source (Fig. 12.1a). If left untreated, biofilms can lead to waterborne infection in

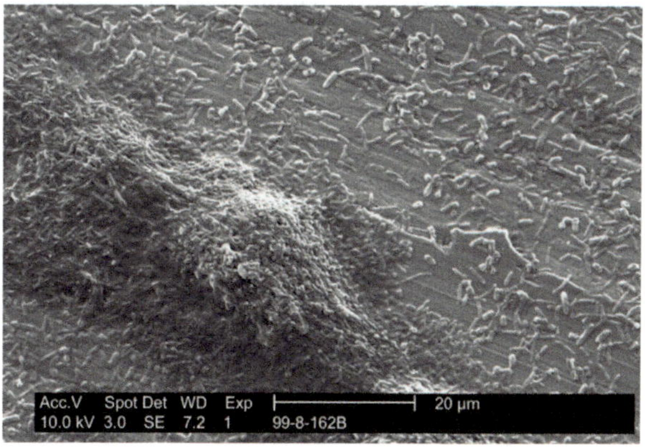

Fig. 12.1a Scanning electron microscopic (SEM) image depicts biofilm from potable water; revealed is the presence of numerous aquatic bacteria. Waterborne organisms cause healthcare-associated infections and bacteremia in immunocompromised patients. (Image source: Courtesy of CDC Image Library: https://phil.cdc.gov/Details.aspx?pid=2263)

D. R. Weikel (✉) · C. Livesay
Department of Oncology and Diagnostic Sciences, The University of Maryland School of Dentistry, Baltimore, MD, USA
e-mail: dweikel1@umaryland.edu; CLivesay@umaryland.edu

L. DePaola et al. (eds.), *Infection Control in the Dental Office in the Era of COVID-19*, https://doi.org/10.1007/978-3-031-64611-9_12

patients and therefore require regular treatment and monitoring to ensure patient and environmental safety.

12.2 Biofilms

Microbes such as bacteria, fungi, algae, and yeasts have adapted to coexist in various settings. They accomplish this by forming biofilms or heterogeneous communities of microorganisms interacting commensally within an extrapolysaccharide matrix. These species may adhere to surfaces in moist environments, living tissues, indwelling medical devices, and water systems by excreting a slimy, glue-like substance to form the matrix that contains the biofilm. Not all biofilms are detrimental; for example, wastewater may be treated by biofilms as the microbes break down harmful organic material, effectively filtering the wastewater as it passes through [2]. However, there are also instances of biofilms negatively impacting their host or the environment.

In orthopedic surgeries such as total joint replacement as well as arthroplasty and internal fixation, the risk of biofilm formation on and around prosthetic materials presents a challenge to clinicians and microbiologists as antibiotic resistance continues to rise [3]. Another pathogenic biofilm that is well described in the literature is the *Pseudomonas aeruginosa* biofilm infection found in the sputum and mucus of cystic fibrosis patients, which is also able to resist antimicrobial treatment mechanisms [4]. *Clostridium difficile* is yet another pathogen responsible for increasing morbidity and mortality, which may be attributed to biofilm formation, and is often resistant to treatment modalities leading to infection relapse [5]. Due to their complex interspecies and cross-kingdom compositions, coupled with the physical protective barrier of the matrix within which they are embedded, biofilms have been the focus of study across biomedical, pharmacological, and microbiological investigations for decades.

Microcolonies of one or multiple species of microbe(s) initiate the formation of the biofilm within the extrapolysaccharide matrix, and these adhere preferentially to plastic surfaces [6, 7]. Once formed, biofilms are able to propagate by detaching either individual or groups of cells that may adhere to another surface or biofilm downstream of the original location (Fig. 12.1b) [9]. The diversity of microorganisms interacting within a single biofilm has been well documented, and the overlap of gene expression comparing the proteome and transcriptome among Group A *Streptococcus*, for example, was diminished in samples taken from biofilms, suggesting regulation of protein expression by means other than transcription [10]. Functionally, a variety of virulence factors may be employed by microbial biofilms to maintain their own survival, such as glucan and fructan polysaccharides found in the matrix of dental plaque biofilms, which are important in the development of dental caries [11].

Biofilms are ubiquitous and form on almost any substrate surface. The plastic tubing found in DUWLs is an ideal surface facilitating biofilm growth when coupled with the perpetually moist environment and low water pressure through the

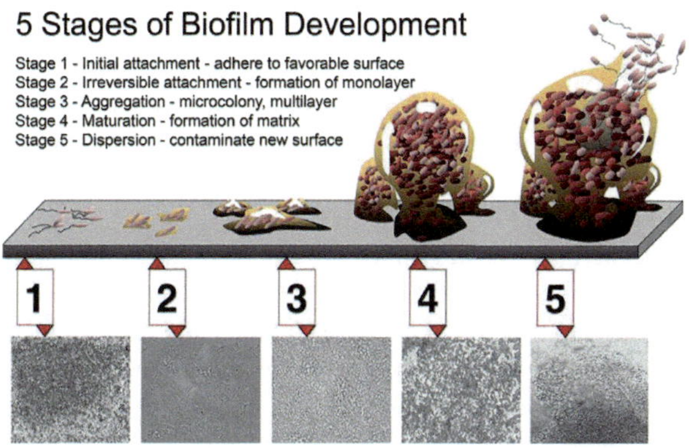

Fig. 12.1b Biofilm maturation Stage 1, initial attachment; Stage 2, irreversible attachment, cell-to-cell adhesion; Stage 3, aggregation, microcolony formation and proliferation; Stage 4, maturation—colonies' mature bacteria secrete protective matrix; Stage 5, dispersion, disperse cells to contaminate new surfaces. (Image source: Adapted from Monroe [8])

small lumen size (0.5–2 mm). During business hours, water flows intermittently throughout the day for cooling, rinsing, or irrigating during treatment. However, after hours when not in use, the water stagnates. Microbes attach more rapidly to hydrophobic, nonpolar surfaces with increased surface roughness, preferring plastic or Teflon surfaces over glass or metals [12]. These conditions facilitate the proliferation of microorganisms and the subsequent formation of biofilm on the interior surface of the waterline tubing. The microorganism growth and colonization on the inner surface of the waterline tubing in the DUWLs are nonpathogenic aerobic and heterotrophic environmental bacteria. However, occasionally opportunistic disease-causing microorganisms, including *Legionella*, *Pseudomonas aeruginosa*, and nontuberculous *mycobacteria* (NTM) can form, especially if left untreated in the dental unit waterlines [13].

12.3 Outbreaks

Biofilm-associated infections are a significant cause of morbidity and mortality in all healthcare settings. These infections are also a major concern for dental providers due to the potential for increased danger of spreading biofilm-mediated infections to patients. A confirmed case of *Legionella pneumophila* strain-associated infection of an 82-year-old woman was reported in *The Lancet.* She presented with fever and respiratory distress and was admitted to the ICU of an Italian hospital in Forli, Italy. This 82-year-old woman developed fulminant and irreversible septic shock despite the immediate administration of systemic antibiotic treatment and died 2 days following admission. A urinary antigen test and chest radiograph confirmed she suffered from Legionnaire's disease. Legionellae are gram-negative bacteria found in freshwater environments that cause respiratory disease in humans who inhale aerosolized water or aspirate water containing the bacteria. After a rigorous search to find the source of the contamination, her water system cultured no bacteria; this led the investigation then to the patient's dental office, the only place she had visited within the previous 10 days. The *Legionella pneumophila* strain found in her urinary antigen test matched the strain found in the dental water line. Cultures obtained from the dental office waterlines contained 6.0×10^4 CFU/L of *Legionella pneumophila* [14].

Nontuberculous *mycobacteria* (NTM) are opportunistic pathogens that regularly inhabit soil and drinking water systems. *Mycobacterium abscessus* is the most rapidly growing pathogen and the cause of many lung diseases and healthcare-associated infections. *Mycobacterium abscessus* has been found to be resistant to most antibiotics, thus making the bacteria exceedingly difficult to treat [15].

Over the years, there have been several documented cases of odontogenic NTM infections directly associated with DUWLs. Peralta and colleagues reported that the Georgia Department of Public Health was notified by a Georgia hospital reporting of a cluster of pediatric *Mycobacterium abscessus* odontogenic infections in September of 2015 [16]. The Center for Disease Control (CDC) reported 24 cases of odontogenic NTM in children receiving pulpotomy treatment in a Pediatric Dental Clinic in Georgia. It was later found that five of the six dental water units showed multiple species of NTM and microbial counts higher than the level recommended by CDC [17]. One of the largest reported outbreaks of *Mycobacterium abscessus* infections occurred in a pediatric dental clinic in Orange County, California, as reported by Singh and colleagues in 2016 [18]. Of 1082 patients at risk following pulpotomy procedures, a total of 71 pediatric patients were identified as part of this outbreak, 22 confirmed, and 49 probables [18]. According to the CDC, the children affected by the outbreaks in California and Georgia were as young as 4 to 8 years of age and developed severe infections with clinical diagnoses such as cervical lymphadenitis and mandibular or maxillary osteomyelitis.

Despite surgical procedures and intravenous antibiotics, complications from their infections caused permanent tooth loss, hearing loss, facial nerve palsy, and incision fibrosis. In October 2022, the CDC issued a health alert in response to another suspected cluster of children infected with NTM following procedures at a pediatric dental clinic. The DUWLs were tested and reported higher microbial counts than the level recommended by CDC [17]. This health alert contains recommendations for monitoring water quality and treating DUWLS to prevent such outbreaks from happening in dental practices nationwide.

12.4 Management of DUWLs

In 1993, it was advised by the CDC that dental waterlines be flushed at the beginning of the clinic day to reduce the microbial load in the dental unit water. However, the most recent studies have proved this practice has been shown to reduce the levels of planktonic bacteria in the water but has not been shown to affect biofilm in the waterlines [19]. Microorganisms existing as biofilm can be minimized by the application of chemical biocides, but strongly attached biofilms are difficult to eradicate [20].

There are several treatment options available for limiting bacterial growth within DUWLs, and the manufacturer of the dental unit should be consulted to determine an appropriate method for management. The most utilized waterline treatment methods are independent reservoirs, chemical treatment options, and filtration systems.

12.5 Independent Reservoirs

Independent water reservoirs are self-contained water systems for single-chair or entire-practice waterlines and are used for water isolation purposes (Fig. 12.2). It separates the dental unit from the municipal water supply and provides conditioned or treated water to the dental unit by removing or inactivating microorganisms [21]. However, use of the independent reservoir alone does not reliably ensure that the water supplied to the dental unit meets safety standards. Chemical treatment methods must be added to the use of independent reservoirs, as drying waterlines and reservoirs overnight does not sufficiently reduce bacterial loads [22].

12.5.1 Chemical Treatment

One method of chemical DUWL treatment is a daily maintenance tablet or daily liquids (Fig. 12.3). The tablet/liquid is added to an independent reservoir each time the reservoir is refilled. Its active ingredients remain effective for 14–28 days, and a

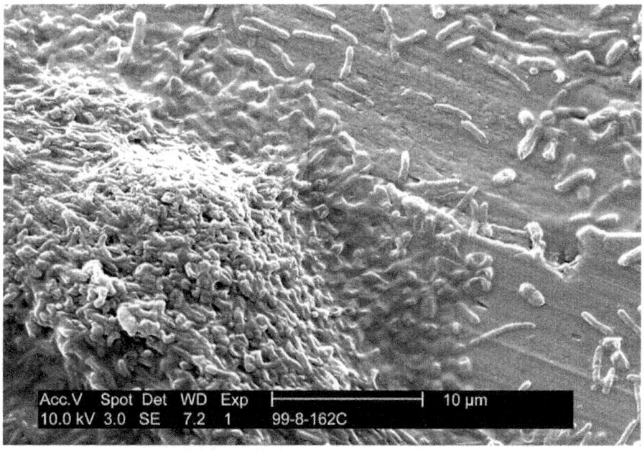

Fig. 12.2 Scanning electron microscopic (SEM) image revealed *L. pneumophila* bacteria as well as other unidentified bacteria existing on potable water biofilms. *Legionellae* are bacteria that can be found in contaminated DUWLs that cause respiratory disease in humans who inhale aerosolized water or aspirate water containing the bacteria. (Image source: Courtesy of CDC Image Library—https://phil.cdc.gov/Details.aspx?pid=6892)

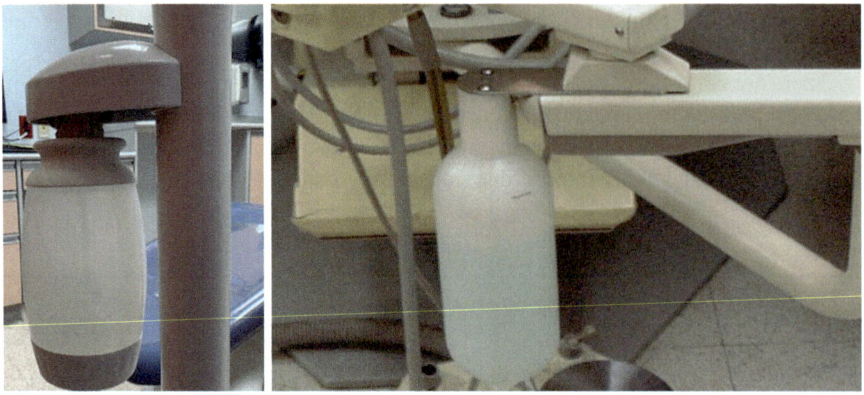

Fig. 12.3 Independent reservoir (bottle system) as it relates to the entire dental chair unit. A chemical treatment method should be combined with independent reservoirs for efficacious decontamination. (Image credit: D. Weikel & L. DePaola)

low-dose antimicrobial agent is slowly released. United states environmental protection agency (EPA)-registered shock treatments include a liquid form and a tablet. Shock treatments are effective in destroying bacteria and breaking down biofilm. However, this treatment should only be used when the unit is shut down. With continuous chemical treatment, shocking should only be performed quarterly or less depending on the monitoring test results [23]. Options available include [24–27]:

- 0.02% hydrogen peroxide (with or without 0.25% hydrogen peroxide shocks weekly).
- 0.12% ethanol and 12% ethanol overnight.
- 1:50 original Listerine overnight.
- 2% sodium perborate.
- 2% EDTA for 5 minutes in the morning.
- Chlorine dioxide cleaners [28].
- Commercial disinfectants (e.g., Oxygenal 6©, Calbenium©, Sterispray©) may be used prophylactically.

12.5.2 Filtration

Filtration systems are an adjunctive measure that can be taken to reduce microbial content when paired with chemical treatment methods and independent reservoirs—they should not be used alone [29]. One example of filtration includes 0.2 μm filters used upstream of the handpiece or air/water syringe that can help to reduce bacterial load of the water supply used in dental treatment [14, 30].

12.5.3 Other Treatment Protocols

As research evolves our understanding of biofilm behavior and bacterial resistance, DUWL treatment modalities are updated and expanded upon. For instance, iodine cartridges have demonstrated disruption of biofilms within waterlines [25, 31]. D-Amino acids were also shown to be an effective agent in biofilm dispersion [32]. The use of silver, known for its antimicrobial properties, has also been investigated as a potential solution to DUWL decontamination; however, a 2022 systematic review concluded that there is currently insufficient evidence for its efficacy specifically in DUWL treatment [33]. When selecting the appropriate treatment method, follow the instructions for use, and consider what best fits the practice's desired workflow. Regardless of the product option, it is important to verify the product compatibility to the manufacturer's instructions. All members of the dental team should be familiarized with safety standards and DUWL treatment and monitoring protocols.

12.6 Recommended Testing and Monitoring

Regardless of the dental unit system, monitoring is critical to assess how well the product itself and treatment management protocols are functioning effectively. Routine monitoring of colony-forming units per milliliter (CFU/mL) ensures compliance with agency recommendations and results in higher-quality water used during dental treatment [34]. Though several studies have compared water quality testing modalities in the DUWL setting, the R2A spread plate method remains the gold standard for monitoring bacterial growth [35, 36]. In-office and outsourced testing systems are available options, as well as the SimPlate method that has historically been considered acceptable, though this method was still shown not to be as effective in detecting bacterial growth as the R2A plate method [36].

12.7 Safety and Standard Levels

- Water must meet EPA regulatory requirements for drinking water to be used in routine dental treatment (i.e., < 500 CFU/mL heterotrophic water bacteria per the CDC, or < 200 CFU/mL per the ADA; 100–200 CFU/mL per UK guidelines [37]).
- For irrigation of open surgical sites, reduction or shaping of bone, or as a coolant during surgical procedures, sterile water or sterile saline should be used.
- Adhere to equipment maintenance according to the dental unit manufacturer's instructions.
- Follow dental unit or water treatment product manufacturer's recommendations for monitoring water quality.
- Anti-retraction valves should be installed and maintained.
- Daily flushing of the DUWLs for minutes at the start of the day, and flush for 20–30 seconds between patients [38].

12.8 Summary

Colonization of microorganisms poses an increased risk of transmission of infection to patients due to contaminated DUWLs. However, the DUWL is necessary to render safe and efficient dental treatment. Therefore, the units must be maintained according to environmental and infection control agency guidelines. This maintenance includes treating the tubing of the DUWLs to prevent biofilm accumulation and monitoring to verify adherence to safety standards.

References

1. Dental Unit Waterlines. United States Food and Drug Administration (FDA). https://www.fda.gov/medical-devices/dental-devices/dental-unit-waterlines#:~:text=The%20waterlines%20of%20a%20dental,oral%20cavity%20during%20dental%20procedures. Accessed 15 Oct 2023.
2. Cuningham AB, et al. Biofilms: the hypertextbook. Ch1: Introduction to biofilms. Eds. 2001–2010. https://www.cs.montana.edu/webworks/projects/stevesbook/contents/chapters/chapter001/section005/green/page001.html#:~:text=Water%20and%20wastewater%20treatment&text=Treating%20Waste%20Water%20with%20a,in%20dead%20plants%20and%20animals. Accessed 22 Oct 2023.
3. McConoughey SJ, Howlin R, Granger JF, Manring MM, Calhoun JH, Shirtliff M, Kathju S, Stoodley P. Biofilms in periprosthetic orthopedic infections. Future Microbiol. 2014;9(8):987–1007. https://doi.org/10.2217/fmb.14.64. Erratum in: Future Microbiol. 2014;9(10):1234. PMID: 25302955; PMCID: PMC4407677.
4. Høiby N, Bjarnsholt T, Moser C, Jensen PØ, Kolpen M, Qvist T, Aanaes K, Pressler T, Skov M, Ciofu O. Diagnosis of biofilm infections in cystic fibrosis patients. APMIS. 2017;125(4):339–43. https://doi.org/10.1111/apm.12689.
5. Maldarelli GA, Piepenbrink KH, Scott AJ, Freiberg JA, Song Y, Achermann Y, Ernst RK, Shirtliff ME, Sundberg EJ, Donnenberg MS, von Rosenvinge EC. Type IV pili promote early biofilm formation by Clostridium difficile. Pathog Dis. 2016;74(6):ftw061. https://doi.org/10.1093/femspd/ftw061. Epub 2016 Jun 30. PMID: 27369898; PMCID: PMC5985507.
6. Costerton JW. Introduction to biofilm. Int J Antimicrob Agents. 1999;11(3-4):217–221; discussion 237–219.
7. Fletcher M, Loeb GI. Influence of substratum characteristics on the attachment of a marine pseudomonad to solid surfaces. Appl Environ Microbiol. 1979;37(1):67–72.
8. Monroe D. Looking for chinks in the armor of bacterial biofilms. PLoS Biol. 2007;5(11):e307. https://doi.org/10.1371/journal.pbio.0050307.
9. Vasudevan R. Biofilms: microbial cities of scientific significance. J Microbiol Exp. 2014;1(3):00014. https://doi.org/10.15406/jmen.2014.01.00014.
10. Freiberg JA, Le Breton Y, Tran BQ, Scott AJ, Harro JM, Ernst RK, Goo YA, Mongodin EF, Goodlett DR, McIver KS, Shirtliff ME. Global analysis and comparison of the transcriptomes and proteomes of Group A *Streptococcus* biofilms. mSystems. 2016;1(6):e00149–16. https://doi.org/10.1128/mSystems.00149-16. PMID: 27933318; PMCID: PMC5141267.
11. Jakubovics NS, Goodman SD, Mashburn-Warren L, Stafford GP, Cieplik F. The dental plaque biofilm matrix. Periodontol 2000. 2021;86(1):32–56. https://doi.org/10.1111/prd.12361. Epub 2021 Mar 10. PMID: 33690911; PMCID: PMC9413593.
12. Donlan R. Biofilms: microbial life on surfaces. Emerg Infect Dis. 2002;8(9):881–90. https://doi.org/10.3201/eid0809.020063.

13. Akbar J, Behbehni J, Karched M. Biofilm growth and microbial contamination of dental unit waterlines at Kuwait University dental center. Front Oral Health. 2023;3:1071018. https://doi.org/10.3389/froh.2022.1071018.
14. Spagnolo A, Sartini M, Italy G. Microbial contamination of dental unit waterlines and potential infection: a narrative review. Pathogens. 2020;9(8):651. https://doi.org/10.3390/pathogens9080651.
15. Winthrop K, Roy E. Chapter 5: Mycobacteria and immunosuppression. In: Handbook of systemic autoimmune diseases, vol. 16; 2020. p. 83–107. https://doi.org/10.1016/B978-0-444-64217-2.00005-1.
16. Peralta G, Tobin-D'Angelo M, Parham A, Edison L, Lorentzson L, Smith C, Drenzek C. Notes from the field: *Mycobacterium abscessus* infections among patients of a pediatric dentistry practice—Georgia, 2015. MMWR Morb Mortal Wkly Rep. 2016;65(13):355–6. https://doi.org/10.15585/mmwr.mm6513a5.
17. Centers for Disease Control and Prevention. Outbreaks of nontuberculous mycobacteria infections highlight importance of maintaining and monitoring dental waterlines. Emergency Preparedness and Response; October 2022. https://emergency.cdc.gov/han/2022/han00478.asp
18. Singh J, O'Donnell K, Nieves D, Adler-Shohet F, et al. Invasive Mycobacterium abscessus outbreak at a pediactric dental clinic. Open Forum Infect Dis. 2021;8(6):ofab165. https://doi.org/10.1093/ofid/ofab165.
19. Rice E, Rich W, Johnson C, Lye D. The role of flushing dental water lines for the removal of microbial contaminants. Public Health Rep. 2006;121(3):270–4. https://doi.org/10.1177/003335490612100308.
20. Yin W, Xu W, Wang Y, Zhang Y, Chou S, Galperin M, He J. Ways to control harmful biofilms: prevention, inhibition, and eradication. Crit Rev Microbiol. 2021;47(1):57–78. https://doi.org/10.1080/1040841X.2020.1842325.
21. Dental unit water quality. https://www.cdc.gov/oralhealth/infectioncontrol/faqs/dental-unit-water-quality.html. Accessed 29 Oct 2023.
22. Fiehn NE, Larsen T. The effect of drying dental unit waterline biofilms on the bacterial load of dental unit water. Int Dent J. 2002;52(4):251–4.
23. Complete guide to treating dental unit waterlines. ProEdge Denta Water Labs. Complete guide to treating dental unit waterlines by ProEdge (proedgedental.com); August 2022. Accessed 20 Oct 2023.
24. Pawar A, Garg S, Mehta S, Dang R. Breaking the chain of infection: dental unit water quality control. J Clin Diagn Res. 2016;10(7):ZC80.
25. Lin S-M, Svoboda KKH, Giletto A, Seibert J, Puttaiah R. Effects of hydrogen peroxide on dental unit biofilms and treatment water contamination. Eur J Dent. 2011;5(1):47–59.
26. Costa D, Girardot M, Bertaux J, Verdon J, Imbert C. Efficacy of dental unit waterlines disinfectants on a polymicrobial biofilm. Water Res. 2016;91:38–44.
27. Wu M, Shi Z, Yu X, Xu Y, Jin X, Zhang L, Fu B. Disinfection methods of dental unit waterlines contamination: a systematic review. J Med Microbiol. 2022;71(6) https://doi.org/10.1099/jmm.0.001540.
28. Wirthlin MR, Marshall GW Jr, Rowland RW. Formation and decontamination of biofilms in dental unit waterlines. J Periodontol. 2003;74(11):1595–609.
29. Murdoch-Kinch CA, Andrews NL, Atwan S, Jude R, Gleason MJ, Molinari JA. Comparison of dental water quality management procedures. J Am Dent Assoc. 1997;128(9):1235–91.
30. Mayo JA, Brown CE. Effect of in-line bacteriological filters on numbers of heterotrophic bacteria in water emitted from non-autoclavable dental air-water syringes. Am J Dent. 1999;12(5):256–60.
31. Petchphayaprai C, Chotipan C, Sa-Ngiampak P, Thotsaporn K, Ampornaramveth RS. Effectiveness of iodine for continuous decontamination of dental unit waterline. BDJ Open. 2023;9(1):34. https://doi.org/10.1038/s41405-023-00160-w. PMID: 37481614; PMCID: PMC10363156.

32. Ampornaramveth RS, Akeatichod N, Lertnukkhid J, Songsang N. Application of D-amino acids as biofilm dispersing agent in dental unit waterlines. Int J Dent. 2018;2018:9413925.
33. Hong F, Chen P, Yu X, Chen Q. The application of silver to decontaminate dental unit waterlines-a systematic review. Biol Trace Elem Res. 2022;200(12):4988–5002. https://doi.org/10.1007/s12011-022-03105-w. Epub 2022 Jan 8. PMID: 34997534; PMCID: PMC8741583.
34. Ji XY, Fei CN, Zhang Y, Zhang W, Liu J, Dong J. Evaluation of bacterial contamination of dental unit waterlines and use of a newly designed measurement device to assess retraction of a dental chair unit. Int Dent J. 2016;66(4):208–14. https://doi.org/10.1111/idj.12225. Epub 2016 Mar 21. PMID: 27000421; PMCID: PMC9376651.
35. Porteous N, Sun Y, Dang S, Schoolfield J. A comparison of 2 laboratory methods to test dental unit waterline water quality. Diagn Microbiol Infect Dis. 2013;77(3):206–8. https://doi.org/10.1016/j.diagmicrobio.2013.07.010. Epub 2013 Sep 17. PMID: 24054735; PMCID: PMC3842227.
36. Porteous N, Sun Y, Schoolfield J. Evaluation of 3 dental unit waterline contamination testing methods. Gen Dent. 2015;63(1):41–7. PMID: 25574718; PMCID: PMC4450747.
37. Yates L. Biofilm and dental unit waterline management. Dent Nurs. 2021. https://www.dental-nursing.co.uk/features/biofilm-and-dental-unit-waterline-management. Accessed 10 Nov 2023.
38. Kohn WG, Collins AS, Cleveland JL, Harte JA, Eklund KJ, Malvitz DM. Guidelines for infection control in dental health-care settings-2003. MMWR Recomm Rep. 2003;52(RR-17):1–61.

Infection Control for Oral Surgical and Dental Implant Procedures

13

Behzad Mostoufi and Harlan J. Shiau

13.1 Introduction

Surgical procedures of the oral cavity, including extractions, periodontal surgery, and implant placements, are performed daily in outpatient dental settings. Most of these procedures have in common the incision, excision, or reflection of soft tissue that exposes a normally sterile region of the oral cavity. The oral cavity is home to the oral microbiome, consisting of over 700 species of bacteria, in addition to other fungi, viruses, and protozoa; the oral microbiome resides in unique niches including the oral mucosa, dentition, and gingival sulcus/pocket [1].

Dental infection control is a scientifically grounded approach that involves employing practical measures designed to prevent harm caused by infection to patients, the healthcare provider, and staff. In the context of oral surgical and implantology procedures, the dentist must establish a protocol that prevents or limits the spread of infection in dental practice.

B. Mostoufi (✉)
Department of Oral & Maxillofacial Surgery, The University of Maryland School of Dentistry, Baltimore, MD, USA
e-mail: BMostoufi@umaryland.edu

H. J. Shiau
Department of Advanced Oral Sciences and Therapeutics, The University of Maryland School of Dentistry, Baltimore, MD, USA
e-mail: Hshiau@umaryland.edu

L. DePaola et al. (eds.), *Infection Control in the Dental Office in the Era of COVID-19*, https://doi.org/10.1007/978-3-031-64611-9_13

13.2 Basis for Enhanced Infection Control Considerations for Oral Surgical Procedures

Dental procedures are performed in "clean" settings, by routine use of personal protective equipment and protocols that endeavor to disinfect surfaces and sterilize instruments. These *standard precautions* are considered the minimum best practices for all ambulatory care settings, inclusive of dentistry. Specifically, *standard precautions* include establishing appropriate rules and workflows that address hand hygiene, use of personal protective equipment, proper respiratory hygiene, sharps safety, handling of sterile instruments, and management of environmental surfaces [2]. Together with transmission-based precautions (e.g., COVID-19 Infection Prevention and Control Guidance), *standard precautions* offer a systematic and effective means for the dental healthcare provider to protect their patients, co-workers, and themselves. Many of these topics have been addressed thoroughly in this book, in previous chapters.

This chapter explores an enhanced level of infection control for oral surgical procedures. The rationale behind this concept is the heightened potential for both local and systemic infections pertaining to surgical procedures, as microorganisms may gain entry to the vascular system or even infiltrate normally sterile regions within the oral cavity [3, 4]. Epithelium is a physical barrier and is even considered a component of the human immune system [5]. For example, in a clinical crown elongation procedure, a mucoperiosteal flap is elevated to visualize and modify the relative spatial positioning of the restorative margin and bone. In this act of surgery, an incision severs the junctional epithelium which normally serves as the barrier between the oral cavity and respective oral microbiome with previously unexposed underlying tissues. The Centers for Disease Control, Division of Oral Health specifically mentions *three areas* within standard precautions to consider for oral surgical procedures: hand-washing practices, personal protective equipment, and irrigation set-up.

13.3 Hand Hygiene

- Proper hand hygiene practices represent a standard precaution that prevents cross-contamination in the dental healthcare setting, which is challenging due to the proximity of patient and provider. Maintaining this practice decreases the risk of bacterial and viral transmission from patient to patient. In addition, proper hand washing also reduces the risk of healthcare-associated infections [6]. With dental procedures involving instruments and objects that are in contact with the oral cavity that is a source of pathogens, hand hygiene practices can help protect transmission to both patients and staff. Specific to oral surgical procedures, hand-washing practices should utilize a fast-acting antimicrobial agent, with a broad spectrum of activity and a substantive effect [7].

13.4 Gloves

- Sterile gloves are a fundamental component of maintaining aseptic techniques during surgical procedures and the use of sterile surgical gloves is recommended [7]. Sterile gloves reduce the transfer of microorganisms from the hands of surgical dental healthcare personnel to patients, while also safeguarding against potential contamination of the provider by the patient's blood and bodily fluids. In the United States, sterile gloves are more thoroughly regulated by the Food and Drug Administration and therefore potentially provide an increased level of protection for the provider if exposure to blood is likely to occur. Despite the recommendation from a regulatory agency, there has been some disagreement among clinicians as to the relative necessity of individually packaged sterile gloves, as opposed to bulk non-sterile clean gloves; controlled clinical trials have repeatedly reported no significant difference in postoperative infection rates in dental and other ambulatory settings, when comparing sterile versus non-sterile glove usage [8–11].

13.5 Sterile Irrigation

- During oral surgical procedures sterile bulb syringes, and sterilizable tubing for delivery of sterile irrigating solutions should be utilized. Most implant motor/handpieces and power instrumentation systems bypass the dental unit to deliver sterile water/solutions (Fig. 13.1). Dental waterline safety is of utmost importance, [12] considering potential for aerosol generation during dental procedures to spread infection.

13.6 Sterile or Clean: What Is the Effective Infection Control Standard for the Oral Surgical Environment?

Surgical procedures of the oral cavity require enhanced infection control measures applied to the dental operatory environment. There have been studies conducted on infection control practices in dental and other ambulatory care settings comparing clean and sterile equipment and room set-ups [13–15]. These studies typically assess the effectiveness of the different infection control protocols on the risk of cross-contamination and patient safety. Outcome measures such as infection rate or complication rate are generally not different [13].

A clean and sterile dental set-up differ in terms of their select control measures; it is important to understand that the choice ultimately is tied to the risk of the dental procedure. Dental instruments for both approaches, which are critical (curette, extraction forceps, elevators, etc.) or semi-critical objects (mouth mirror, amalgam carrier, metal impression trays), are subject to steam or heat sterilization. The approach to other environmental surfaces and personal protective equipment, however, is where the clean and sterile approaches differ.

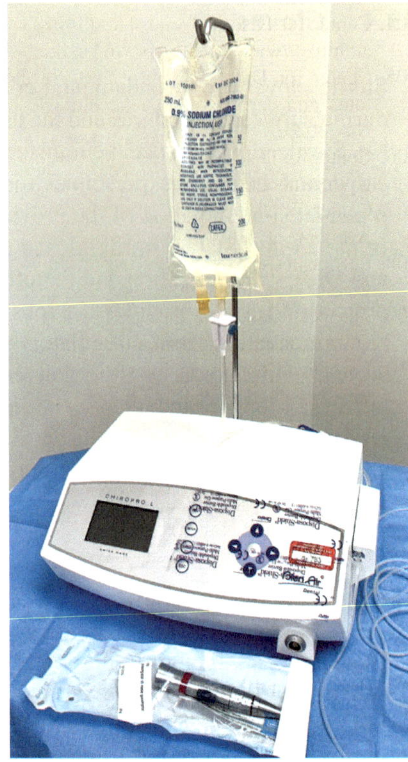

Fig. 13.1 Surgical unit with external irrigation system. Single-procedure sterile saline bags are utilized

In the typical clean dental set-up, the objective is to maintain a workspace free from visible dirt, debris, and contaminants (Fig. 13.2). Surfaces and equipment are regularly cleaned and disinfected, but not to the level of sterilization. Cleanliness in this context primarily involves the removal of surface contaminants and the reduction of microbial load to a safe level. Common measures include the use of disinfectants on noncritical items, such as dental chairs, countertops, and equipment surfaces.

In the sterile dental set-up, the infection control measures aim for complete elimination of all microorganisms, from instruments, equipment, and surfaces. Sterilization is the process used to achieve sterility, which usually involves using techniques like autoclaving (steam sterilization), dry heat, or chemical methods to eliminate all microorganisms. Sterile instruments and materials are typically used for invasive procedures where there is a direct risk of introducing infection into the bloodstream or deeper tissues. This includes items like surgical instruments, needles, and implant components. Individually dispensed sterile gloves and drapes (Fig. 13.1) are used for surgical procedures to maintain aseptic conditions. In a true sterile approach, a patient may be covered with a sterilized drape completely, with only their mouth exposed.

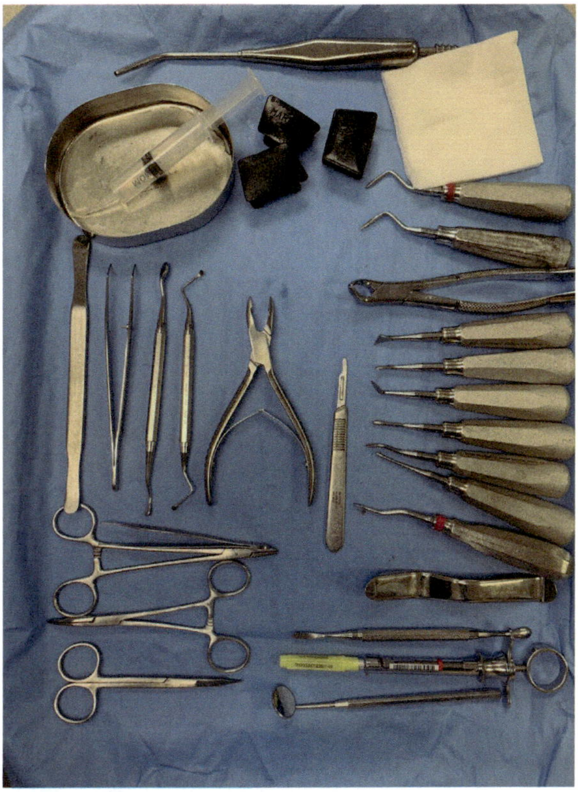

Fig. 13.2 Example of oral surgical set-up. Note the use of a sterile drape to contain or create a field for sterilized surgical instruments which are considered mostly critical objects. Order or organization of instruments is also crucial for dental infection control. Knowing where instruments are located and having all necessary equipment in close access avoids compromising established sterile and clean zones intra-surgically

Clean and sterile represent the range of infection control set-ups; *in reality, a practitioner will adopt a mix of infection control measures that place them in a hybrid category*. The dental practitioner involved with oral surgical procedures should use a risk reduction paradigm (Fig. 13.3) to determine what is the appropriate set-up protocol to implement for the specific oral surgical procedure.

Conceptually, standard precautions is the starting point for dental infection control. With additional risk, layers of surgical controls should be implemented by the practitioner for protection of patient and healthcare worker. The risk profile of each clinical scenario might consider factors such as extent of access (compare a full-arch mucoperiosteal flap for multiple implant placement versus a flapless single tooth extraction), duration of access (compare a quadrant of osseous periodontal surgery versus guided tissue regeneration at one site/defect), and open vs. closed (consider full-thickness access with deep releasing incision versus a minimally invasive surgical technique).

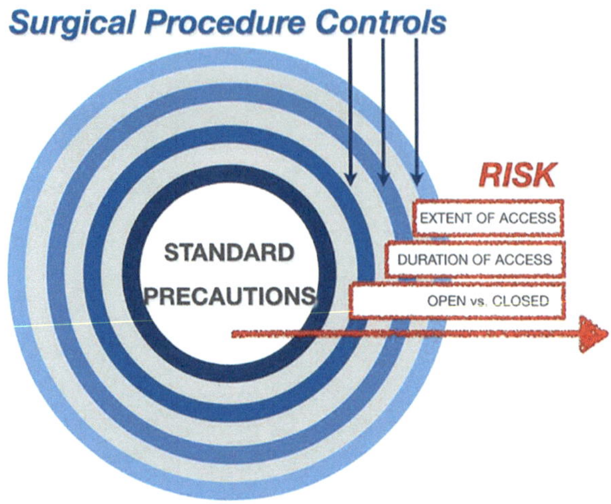

Fig. 13.3 *Implementing additional surgical controls over foundational standard precautions based on risk.* Standard precautions for dental infection control are foundational and applied to all dental procedures, whether diagnostic or therapeutic in nature. Additional surgical controls, for example, as described by the CDC, are layers of protection (blue rings) against accumulating risk (red arrow). The risk profile of each clinical scenario might consider factors such as extent of access, duration of access, and open/closed status of surgery

13.7 Managing Surgical Instruments and Equipment for Surgical Procedures of the Oral Cavity

Effective infection control for surgical instruments, implant drills, and other equipment is paramount in maintaining a sterile and safe healthcare environment. The meticulous handling and sterilization of critical and semi-critical instruments prevent transmission of microorganisms and minimize postoperative infection. Clinicians should implement rigorous protocols to ensure that instruments are thoroughly cleaned, disinfected, and sterilized according to the manufacturer's recommendation and CDC and ADA guidelines [16]. Routine inspection and maintenance of instruments are essential to identify any signs of wear or damage that could compromise the efficacy of the instruments or contribute to the risk of contamination. Finally, proper storage and packaging are equally vital to maintain the sterility of instruments until they are ready for use.

By prioritizing sterility and adhering to stringent infection control practices in handling surgical instruments, clinicians can potentially manage and minimize bacterial transmission into the surgical wound. This not only ensures the safety of both patients and dental practitioners but also adheres to the highest standards of care in surgical settings, promoting a hygienic healthcare environment.

The attention to the dental chair water line and rigorous disinfection protocols within dental settings is paramount, as untreated dental unit water can harbor potentially harmful microorganisms such as *Legionella*, *Pseudomonas aeruginosa*, and nontuberculous mycobacteria [17]. These pathogens pose a significant health risk to both dental practitioners and patients if not effectively managed. Legionella, for instance, is notorious for causing Legionnaires' disease, a severe form of pneumonia [18], while *Pseudomonas aeruginosa* can lead to opportunistic infections [19]. Nontuberculous mycobacteria, on the other hand, can cause a range of infections, particularly in individuals with compromised immune systems [20]. Regular monitoring, maintenance, and disinfection of dental unit waterlines are essential to safeguard the well-being of both patients and oral healthcare providers, emphasizing the critical role that infection control plays in the dental environment. The ADA suggests that clinicians consult with dental unit manufacturers for recommendations on cleaning and treating the water lines, regardless of internal or external water source used. Filtration, chemicals, or a combination of these methods may be required [21]. Regular training and education of dental staff on infection control protocols are also important factors to minimize complications. Dental practitioners should stay updated on the latest advancements in sterilization techniques and follow guidelines provided by regulatory bodies.

13.8 Managing Biomaterials and Implanted Devices for Surgical Procedure in the Oral Cavity

Biomaterials that are used in oral surgical, periodontal, and implantology procedures are often processed by the manufacturer to be sterile. For example, particulate bone allograft, resorbable/non-resorbable membranes, dental implant fixtures, and related components are presumed to be sterile. These biomaterials are usually packaged in layers or compartments, such that the delivery of the material can be placed into a sterile field with minimal physical handling and/or contact. Therefore, a clinician needs to develop a proper material handling *chain of command* concept to preserve the efforts that manufacturers have made to produce sterile materials. As an example, sterile drapes used for table coverings are the proper receiving point for inner envelopes/containers of processed biomaterials and implant-containing inner vials, rather than a merely chemically disinfected table.

13.9 Infection Control Considerations for Oral Surgery Procedures

Oral surgical procedures are clean contaminated surgery. The oral cavity harbors hundreds of bacterial species [22], and surgical interventions in this region may expose patients to a greater likelihood of microbial contamination. However, studies have demonstrated that despite factors such as saliva, dental plaque, and the multitude of microorganisms in the oral cavity that can contribute to the increased susceptibility of oral surgical sites to infections, infection rate remains low [23].

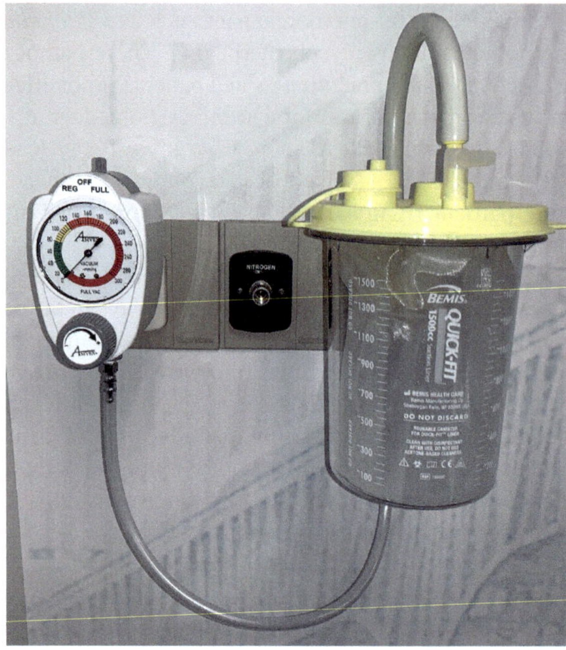

Fig. 13.4 Fluid management. A wall unit-type disposable canister and tube for suction. This is a single-use system which can deliver a hygienic, safe, and efficient method of disposal of liquid medical waste

Regardless, meticulous attention to infection control measures and stringent aseptic protocols is imperative during oral surgeries to mitigate the elevated risk of surgical site infections. This underscores the importance of healthcare practitioners employing comprehensive infection prevention strategies to ensure patient safety and favorable surgical outcomes in the realm of oral surgery [24].

In dental operatories, the choice between wall suction and dental chair suction systems for surgeries is balancing convenience and effectiveness. Wall suction with a disposable canister unit connected to individual treatment rooms is an excellent option for office-based oral surgical procedures (Fig. 13.4). This system provides robust suction power and efficient waste disposal. On the other hand, dental chair suction that integrates the suction unit directly into the dental chair offers localized and easily accessible suction during procedures. The choice often hinges on factors such as space constraints, workflow preferences, and the specific needs of the dental practice. Disinfection protocols are critical for both systems, involving regular cleaning of tubing, canisters, and filters. Diligent adherence to disinfection procedures is essential to prevent the risk of cross-contamination regardless of which systems are utilized (Fig. 13.5).

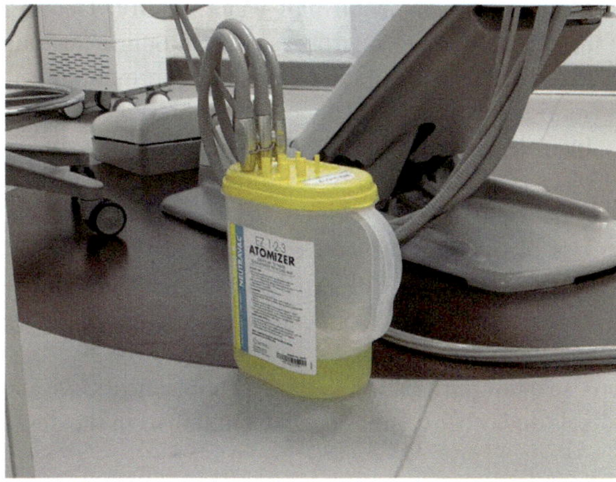

Fig. 13.5 Dental evacuation system cleaning apparatus. When lines are connected the device aspirates cleaning solutions through vacuum lines

13.10 Infection Control Considerations for Periodontal Surgery

In considering the safety of every patient, surgeon, and auxiliary personnel, proper infection control measures are essential when aerosol-generating opportunities occur with periodontal surgery. Rotary handpieces and piezoelectric instrumentation present opportunities to generate aerosol. These aerosols are minuscule droplets and/or particles that may contain bacteria, viruses, and other microorganisms from the patient's mouth [25]. The risk of inhaling aerosols can lead to a variety of health problems, including respiratory infections, such as the common cold, influenza, and pneumonia, allergic reactions, asthma attacks, Legionnaire's disease, tuberculosis, and COVID-19. Dental staff are at particularly high risk of exposure to aerosols during periodontal surgery as they work in close proximity to patients and localized work zones of aerosol generation. The aforementioned concerns are deduced from studies that mostly establish a relationship between aerosol-generating procedures and bacterial contamination-type assays that measure colony-forming units. As of 2020, there have been no direct investigations that evaluate disease transmission via aerosols in a dental setting and no direct evidence about viral contamination in aerosols [26]. Regardless, the pragmatic clinical best practices still must assume transmission risk from aerosol-generating procedures.

Assumed aerosol risk during periodontal surgery and other dental surgeries, especially utilizing a handpiece, can be reduced by the following steps:

- Use of high-volume evacuation (HVE): HVE systems are very effective at removing aerosols from the air. The HVE tip should be placed as close to the operating site as possible, typically within 1–2 cm.
- Use of preprocedural mouthrinses: Preprocedural mouthrinses such as chlorhexidine gluconate can help to reduce the concentration of microorganisms in the oral cavity and reduce the amount of aerosol generated during dental procedures.

- Maintenance of dental unit water quality: Dental unit water lines can harbor bacteria and other microorganisms. Routine flushing of the water lines can help to reduce the risk of contamination. Normal Saline is generally advised for oral surgical procedures. This can be achieved through internal or external systems. Internal systems are built in to dental chair systems that may permit attachment of a Saline source or external irrigation system as previously mentioned (Fig. 13.1).
- Use of personal protective equipment (PPE): Oral healthcare providers should wear appropriate PPE, such as surgical masks, eye protection, and gloves, to protect themselves from exposure to aerosols. A face shield is an additional PPE that can mitigate risk.
- Use of air purification systems: Air purification systems can help to remove aerosols and other contaminants from the air in the dental operatory.

This will minimize the risk for contamination during periodontal surgery.

In conclusion, the importance of adhering to proper infection control measures in oral surgical procedures cannot be overstated. In implementing strict protocols, dental healthcare professionals can safeguard the well-being of both patients and staff, thereby ensuring a safe and hygienic environment. These measures not only prevent the spread of infectious diseases but also contribute to the overall success of the surgical procedure by minimizing complications. It is imperative that all oral healthcare providers remain committed to maintaining the highest standards of infection control, as this upholds patient trust and safeguards public health. The diligence in adhering to these practices protects those in the dental office and extends to the broader community, emphasizing the significance of infection control as an essential aspect of all oral surgical dental care.

References

1. Deo PN, Deshmukh R. Oral microbiome: unveiling the fundamentals. J Oral Maxillofac Pathol. 2019;23(1):122–8. https://doi.org/10.4103/jomfp.JOMFP_304_18. PMID: 31110428; PMCID: PMC6503789.
2. Moralejo D, El Dib R, Prata RA, Barretti P, Corrêa I. Improving adherence to standard precautions for the control of health care-associated infections. Cochrane Database Syst Rev. 2018;2(2):CD010768. https://doi.org/10.1002/14651858.CD010768.pub2. PMID: 29481693; PMCID: PMC6491237.
3. Horliana AC, Chambrone L, Foz AM, Artese HP, Rabelo Mde S, Pannuti CM, Romito GA. Dissemination of periodontal pathogens in the bloodstream after periodontal procedures: a systematic review. PLoS One. 2014;9(5):e98271. https://doi.org/10.1371/journal.pone.0098271. PMID: 24870125; PMCID: PMC4037200.
4. Centers for Disease Control. Infection prevention & control in dental settings. Atlanta [updated 2022 Aug 31; cited 2023 Nov 15]. Available from: https://www.cdc.gov/oralhealth/infection-control/index.html
5. Yamamoto M, Aizawa R. Maintaining a protective state for human periodontal tissue. Periodontol 2000. 2021;86(1):142–56. https://doi.org/10.1111/prd.12367. Epub 2021 Mar 10.
6. Ataee RA, Ataee MH, Mehrabi Tavana A, Salesi M. Bacteriological aspects of hand washing: a key for health promotion and infections control. Int J Prev Med. 2017;8:16. https://doi.org/10.4103/2008-7802.201923. PMID: 28382192; PMCID: PMC5364736.

7. Centers for Disease Control. Oral surgical procedures. Atlanta [updated 2016 Mar 25; cited 2023 Nov 15]. Available from: https://www.cdc.gov/oralhealth/infectioncontrol/faqs/oral-surgical-procedures.html
8. Brewer JD, Gonzalez AB, Baum CL, Arpey CJ, Roenigk RK, Otley CC, Erwin PJ. Comparison of sterile vs nonsterile gloves in cutaneous surgery and common outpatient dental procedures: a systematic review and meta-analysis. JAMA Dermatol. 2016;152(9):1008–14. https://doi.org/10.1001/jamadermatol.2016.1965.
9. Jolly S, Court-Kowalski S, Lu V, Roberts M, Olakkengil S, Coates PTH, Bhattacharjya S. Sterile versus clean urinary catheterisation is not associated with post-transplantation infection. Int J Urol Nurs. 2023;17(1):56–61. https://doi.org/10.1111/ijun.12333. ISSN: 1749-7701.
10. Chiu WK, Cheung LK, Chan HC, Chow LK. A comparison of post-operative complications following wisdom tooth surgery performed with sterile or clean gloves. Int J Oral Maxillofac Surg. 2006;35(2):174–9. https://doi.org/10.1016/j.ijom.2005.07.003. Epub 2005 Sept 8.
11. Adeyemo WL, Ogunlewe MO, Ladeinde AL, Bamgbose BO. Are sterile gloves necessary in nonsurgical dental extractions? J Oral Maxillofac Surg. 2005;63(7):936–40. https://doi.org/10.1016/j.joms.2005.03.008.
12. Meiller TF, Depaola LG, Kelley JI, Baqui AA, Turng BF, Falkler WA. Dental unit waterlines: biofilms, disinfection and recurrence. J Am Dent Assoc. 1999;130(1):65–72. https://doi.org/10.14219/jada.archive.1999.0030.
13. Scharf DR, Tarnow DP. Success rates of osseointegration for implants placed under sterile versus clean conditions. J Periodontol. 1993;64(10):954–6. https://doi.org/10.1902/jop.1993.64.10.954.
14. Charrier L, Serafini P, Chiono V, Rebora M, Rabacchi G, Zotti CM. Clean and sterile delivery: two different approaches to infection control. J Eval Clin Pract. 2010;16(4):771–5. https://doi.org/10.1111/j.1365-2753.2009.01191.x. Epub 2010 Jun 10.
15. Wang D, Shinder R. Comparison of postoperative infection rates after office-based oculoplastic procedures using sterile and clean gloves. Ophthalmic Plast Reconstr Surg. 2023;39(2):146–9. https://doi.org/10.1097/IOP.0000000000002266. Epub 2022 Sept 9.
16. American Dental Association. Department of Scientific Information, Evidence Synthesis & Translation Research. ADA Science & Research Institute, LLC. Infection control and sterilization. Chicago [updated 2022 Oct 5; cited 2023 Nov 15]. Available from: https://www.ada.org/en/resources/research/science-and-research-institute/oral-health-topics/infection-control-and-sterilization
17. Optenhövel M, Mellmann A, Kuczius T. Occurrence and prevalence of Legionella species in dental chair units in Germany with a focus on risk factors. Eur J Clin Microbiol Infect Dis. 2023;42(10):1235–44. https://doi.org/10.1007/s10096-023-04659-w. Epub 2023 Sept 12. PMID: 37698817; PMCID: PMC10511595.
18. Fields BS, Benson RF, Besser RE. Legionella and Legionnaires' disease: 25 years of investigation. Clin Microbiol Rev. 2002;15(3):506–26. https://doi.org/10.1128/CMR.15.3.506-526.2002. PMID: 12097254; PMCID: PMC118082.
19. Riquelme SA, Prince A. *Pseudomonas aeruginosa* consumption of airway metabolites promotes lung infection. Pathogens. 2021;10:957. https://doi.org/10.3390/pathogens10080957.
20. Marshall JE, Mercaldo RA, Lipner EM, Prevots DR. Incidence of nontuberculous mycobacteria infections among persons with cystic fibrosis in the United States (2010–2019). BMC Infect Dis. 2023;23(1):489. https://doi.org/10.1186/s12879-023-08468-6. PMID: 37488500; PMCID: PMC10364346.
21. Department of Scientific Information, Evidence Synthesis & Translation Research, ADA Science & Research Institute, LLC. Dental unit waterlines. https://www.ada.org/en/resources/research/science-and-research-institute/oral-health-topics/dental-unit-waterlines
22. Kilian M, Chapple I, Hannig M, et al. The oral microbiome—an update for oral healthcare professionals. Br Dent J. 2016;221:657–66. https://doi.org/10.1038/sj.bdj.2016.865.
23. Yi EKY, et al. Prevalence of postoperative infection after tooth extraction: a retrospective study. Int J Dent. 2021;2021:6664311. https://doi.org/10.1155/2021/6664311.

24. Centers for Disease Control and Prevention. Summary of infection prevention practices in dental settings: basic expectations for safe care. Atlanta: Centers for Disease Control and Prevention, US Dept of Health and Human Services; 2016.
25. Choi JJE, Chen J, Choi YJ, Moffat SM, Duncan WJ, Waddell JN, Jermy M. Dental high-speed handpiece and ultrasonic scaler aerosol generation levels and the effect of suction and air supply. Infect Control Hosp Epidemiol. 2023;44(6):926–33. https://doi.org/10.1017/ice.2022.196. Epub 2022 Aug 8. PMID: 35938186; PMCID: PMC10262170.
26. Kumbargere Nagraj S, Eachempati P, Paisi M, Nasser M, Sivaramakrishnan G, Verbeek JH. Interventions to reduce contaminated aerosols produced during dental procedures for preventing infectious diseases. Cochrane Database Syst Rev. 2020;10(10):CD013686. https://doi.org/10.1002/14651858.CD013686.pub2. PMID: 33047816; PMCID: PMC8164845.

Infection Control When Administering N_2O and IV Sedation: Including Disinfection of Anesthesia Devices and Use of IV Infusion Solutions and Medications

14

Marvin Leventer and Glenn Canares

14.1 Introduction

The primary route of transmission of SARS-CoV-2, the causative agent of COVID-19, is through respiratory droplets. While dental procedures with forced air, water spray, and turbine handpieces are causative in mobilizing viral particles, airway manipulation is also a causative factor in transmission. Administration of sedation and general anesthesia for dental procedures increases the risk of transmission. As an example, if a patient is encouraged to take deep breaths to increase their oxygenation or levels of inhalation anesthetics, mobilization is enhanced. Moreover, if a sedated patient needs to clear their airway by coughing, there is even more pressure to mobilize viral particles. While the goal of conscious and moderate sedation is for the patient to maintain their own airway without obstructing, we know that circumstances and levels of anesthesia change during an anesthetic or sedation, and it is not guaranteed there will be no coughing or need for positive pressure ventilation. It is in this regard that many organizations in anesthesia including the American Society of Dentist Anesthesiologists, American Society of Anesthesiologists, Society for Ambulatory Anesthesia, and the Anesthesia Patient Safety Foundation have created guidelines for safe anesthesia care in regard to the pandemic. The University of Maryland School of Dentistry created guidelines based on a combination and compromise of the medical guidelines which are geared toward hospitals, operating rooms, dental offices and surgery centers. These guidelines, as presented

M. Leventer (✉)
Department of Oral Surgery, The University of Maryland School of Dentistry, Baltimore, MD, USA
e-mail: MLeventer@umaryland.edu

G. Canares
Department of Pediatric Dentistry, The University of Maryland School of Dentistry, Baltimore, MD, USA
e-mail: gcanares1@umaryland.edu

L. DePaola et al. (eds.), *Infection Control in the Dental Office in the Era of COVID-19*, https://doi.org/10.1007/978-3-031-64611-9_14

in this chapter, can serve as a format, and each organization and office are encouraged to create a set of guidelines which work for them. While not meant to be comprehensive of all the data, it is enough to create a workable document. Also, each country may have different qualifications, regulations, and/or requirements that clinicians should be aware of before initiating sedation procedures.

14.2 Preoperative Concerns

Facility construction of Heating, Ventilation, and Air Conditioning (HVAC) and air filtration varies widely depending on size, needs, accreditation standards, availability of resources, and a country's regulatory processes. A hospital operating room with a negative pressure gradient is far different than a home or a dental office. Dental care and anesthesia care can be provided in both safely. Since the COVID-19 pandemic construction of new spaces or modification of spaces for dental anesthesia may be impacted, air exchange requirements for operating rooms in volumes exchanged per hour or air exchanged per hour (ACH) is 15–20 in the United States. This can vary from country to country. Compare that to the standard home kitchen at 7–8 ACH [1]. Air exchange requirements for a typical dental office are 6 ACH. The consideration for increased ACH in an operating room is generally from an infection control standpoint to decrease surgical site infections [2]. During a dental procedure, bacterial contamination may not be as detrimental to healing as an open surgical procedure, requiring sterility for example. Increased mobilization of airway bacteria and viruses may be more relevant in consideration of infecting healthcare workers. The necessary time to wait in between cases to adequately rid the room of infecting viral and bacterial particles is determined by ACH and aerosol potential of the procedure [3]. Closed-door rooms for any anesthesia delivery are preferred [4]. External high efficiency particulate air (HEPA) filtration in a dental operatory is suggested depending on ACH and aerosol potential. Scavenging suction power requirements for nitrous oxide should be within manufacturer's guidelines. Traditional dental suctions are designed for dental materials, saliva, and blood. They are commonly used as well for anesthetic gas scavenging but are not designed for that. A secondary dry suction for scavenging anesthetic gases is preferred if available.

Patients should be screened for infectious disease(s), especially diseases affecting the upper airways. Any compromise of the ability to have optimal air exchange presents a risk in these instances, and sedation should be avoided. Patients presenting with respiratory infections should be rescheduled until the infection has been resolved. Screening questions are the same as most standard guidelines, but this can vary from region to region and country to country due to the prevalence of circulating infections, especially influenza and COVID-19. The preoperative testing guidelines for nitrous oxide are minimal. However, use of accepted surgical center guidelines for IV moderate sedation and general anesthesia is indicated due to increased possibility of airway manipulation. In the midst of the COVID pandemic, when COVID rates are elevated to high-risk transmission; preop COVID tests within a 3-day window may be indicated.

14.3 Intraoperative General Procedure Guidelines

Considerations for length and scope of the dental procedure are taken into account when choosing an anesthesia technique. Decreased aerosol with rubber dam and airway suction barrier devices such as the isolate or endotracheal intubation are warranted by behavior, health, airway status, and procedure. Strong consideration is given for general anesthesia in the hospital for complicated long procedures where maximum aerosol is expected for full-mouth rehabilitation cases on children or patients with special needs. People in the treatment room should be limited to those essential for patient care and procedural support with minimal exchange of staff. This includes the anesthesia provider, nurse, and operator. Additional roving or circulating staff members are to remain outside. Airway management should be reserved for the most experienced anesthetist if possible [5]. Procedure and recovery should be the same room with a closed door to prevent aerosols from spreading to other office areas. Caregivers and escorts should wait in their cars instead of the office for the duration of the procedure until needed for discharge.

14.4 Intraoperative Guidelines on Choice of Anesthesia Technique

The most simple and noninvasive sedation technique will have the least morbidity and least likely to cause additional aerosolized droplets due to airway instrumentation. In choosing a sedative technique, nitrous oxide potentially has less impact on airway droplet mobilization than IV moderate sedation which is less than deep sedation and general anesthesia (DS/GA).

14.5 Considerations for Nitrous Oxide Administration for Anxiolysis and Minimal Sedation

The most important principle of the nitrous oxide machine is that there is no backflow of patient gases into the machine because of a one-way valve on the bag T attached to the hoses to deliver gas (Fig. 14.1). In units that are correctly maintained, this valving is preserved, and the inside of the inhalation sedation unit will not become contaminated by human breath. As per the manufacturer, the use of a bacterial/viral filter is not necessary [6]. The scavenger assembly over the nose mask functions to remove exhaled aerosol of breathing gases from the patient's nose. Disposable nose masks are preferred over reusable autoclavable masks.

There are differences in the air circulation between a nitrous oxide machine and a general anesthesia (GA) machine and the methods of contamination of a breathing circuit. In a GA machine, the breathing circuit is a circle breathing system where exhaled gas is recycled through the system with a soda lime canister to remove

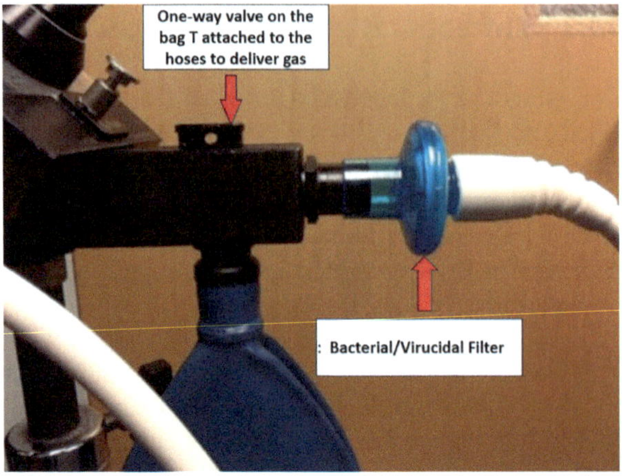

Fig. 14.1 Bag, filter, and breathing tube. One-way valve is at gas outflow before blue filter is essential to prevent backflow of patient gases into the machine

exhaled carbon dioxide. The alkalinity of the soda lime is bactericidal to *Staphylococcus aureus* and *Pseudomonas aeruginosa* but not for *Mycobacterium tuberculosis* [7]. Factors to increase the likelihood of transmission from one patient to the next depend on the number of organisms, virulence of the organism, fresh gas flows, tidal volume, frequency of use of the machine, and the time between cases. Of additional concern is that SARS-CoV-2 is able to survive outside the body for approximately 72 hours on plastic or metal surfaces [8]. In a general anesthesia machine, the recommendation of a viral, bacterial filter as per the Centers for Disease Control and Prevention (CDC) in 2009 is ambiguous except in the transmission of *M. Tuberculosis* [9]. Use of a high-quality viral filter rated to remove at least 99.7 percent of airborne particles of 0.3 microns or greater between the bag tee and the gas delivery hoses alleviates this contamination (Fig. 14.2) [5]. A clear plastic cover such as a clear trash bag, chair cover, or X-ray head cover may be placed over the nitrous oxide machine and should be used to decrease cross contamination (Fig. 14.3). Use of the breathing bag is a user preference. When nitrous oxide delivery systems such as the Porter Silhouette system are used, there is no breathing bag as per the manufacturer, and the access where the breathing bag was can be plugged with a special adaptor so as not to waste gas (Fig. 14.2). If a breathing bag is chosen, a durable non-latex bag is protected from internal contamination by the non-return valving of the flowmeter outlet. If required, it can be externally cleaned with a mild soap detergent. The breathing bag will only last for several autoclave cycles, and the temperature should not exceed 137 degrees Celsius. Lower temperatures will extend product life. It is not necessary to change the reservoir bag between patients or use disposable bags. However, a disposable bag is meant to be discarded after each use as in a dedicated anesthesia machine for general anesthesia. Gas sterilization with ethylene oxide may be used for most plastic devices that will not stand up to repeated autoclave cycles. When finished with the procedure, discard the disposable viral filter and the disposable nitrous oxide nasal mask (Figs. 14.4 and 14.5).

Disinfection of the machine is with appropriate bactericidal and virucidal wipes. Never spray onto the flowmeter itself and then wipe. Also of note, flowmeters must

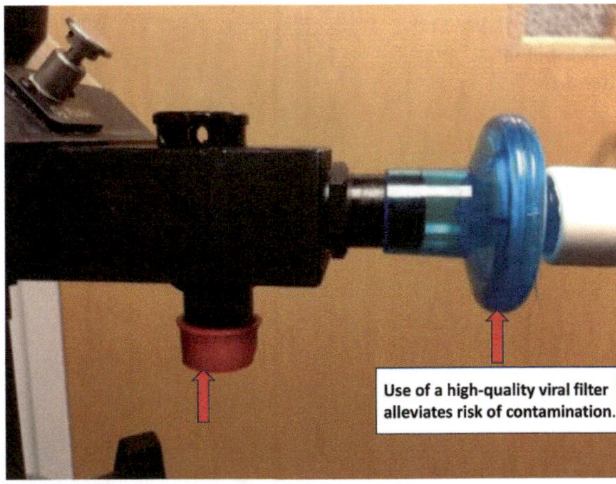

Fig. 14.2 Viral filter and red cap in place of breathing bag

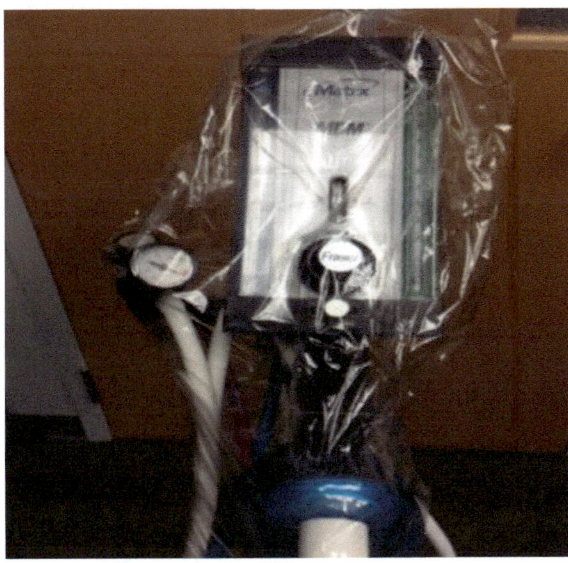

Fig. 14.3 Plastic cover over nitrous oxide machine

never be immersed in liquid. If this happens contact the distributer. The flowmeter will only become contaminated by aerosol spray [10]. The Porter Brown System has rubber and plastic parts and as recommended by the manufacturer should be placed in an ultrasonic with water and an enzymatic cleaner with soap and water and then sterilized in a steam autoclave at a low-temperature cycle of 121 degrees centigrade [10] (Fig. 14.6).

The Matrx system rubber goods follow a similar protocol for cleaning, at an autoclave temperature of 120–134 degrees Celsius. Of note, this system is said to be effective for the blue autoclavable nasal hoods as well as the white Dynomite single patient-use nasal hoods. The components are all latex-free. We urge you to contact the manufacturer on reuse of the disposable nasal hoods as this is not our practice.

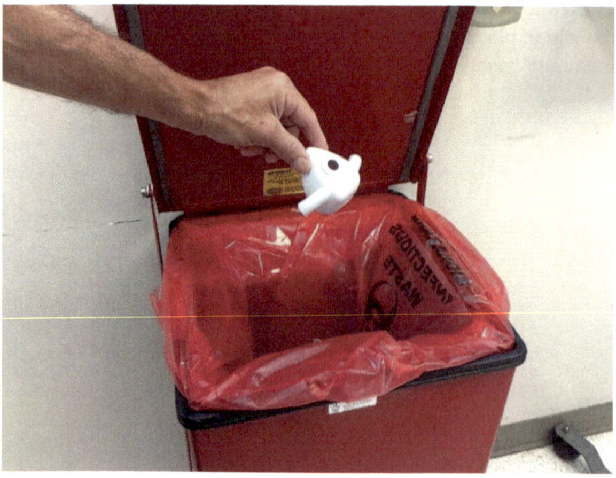

Fig. 14.4 Dispose of disposable nasal hood after use

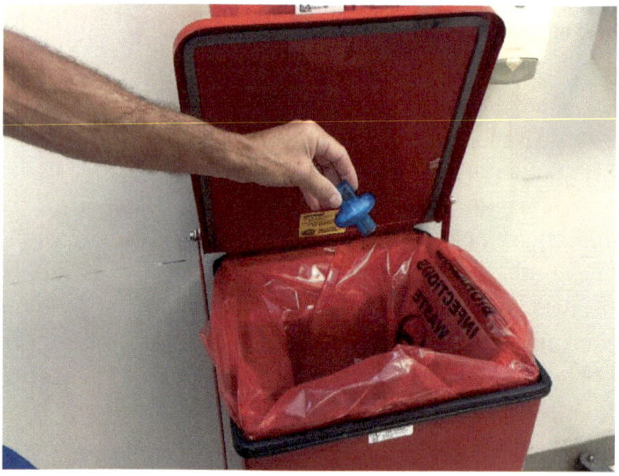

Fig. 14.5 Dispose of filter after use

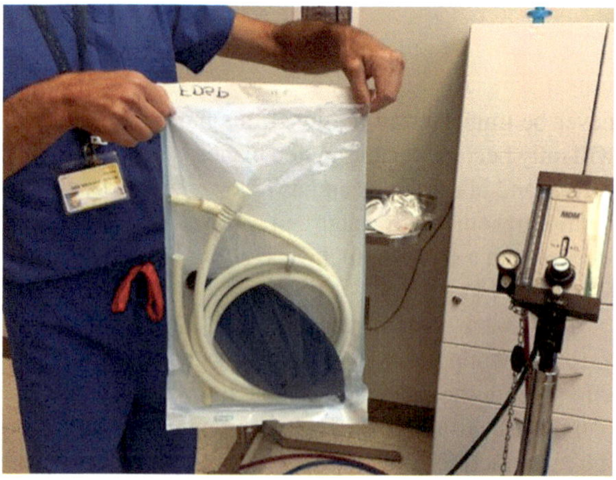

Fig. 14.6 Breathing hoses and bag in autoclave bag for sterilization

Disinfection of the Accutron Scavenger System is precleaned similar to the Matrx and Porter systems and then sterilized for a minimum of 24 minutes and 134 degrees Celsius with a dry time of 30 min. Additional recommendations for gas sterilization of rubber products may be obtained from the manufacturer or Anesthesia Associates Inc. "Guidelines for Product Cleaning and Sterilization" [11].

14.6 Considerations for IV Moderate Sedation

Advantages of this technique over general anesthesia are that airway manipulation and instrumentation are less likely to occur as the patient is awake, breathing is maintained, and the chance of obstruction of the airway requiring intervention is significantly less. Nevertheless, emergency airway supplies should be readily available in the anesthesia cart for protection from aerosol. The likelihood of immediately needing these supplies such as a nasal pharyngeal airway, oral airway, bag-valve mask, and laryngoscope with an endotracheal tube (ETT) is reasonably low during oral moderate or conscious sedation.

Many providers deliver supplemental oxygen via a nasal cannula. Keep flow to as low as possible to avoid aerosolization of the nasal mucosa. One to two liters per minute flow of 100 percent oxygen is adequate for most otherwise healthy individuals to maintain adequate oxygen saturation in the high 90s.

Use of intravenous catheters, fluid lines, and fluid bags is not treated any differently than standard protocol. It has been shown that bacterial transmission from the anesthesia work area and anesthesia machines, intravenous medications, syringe needles, intravenous lines, and ports for injection all have the potential for bacterial transmission [12]. Standard protocol would include swabbing with isopropyl alcohol all sites that will come in contact with a hypodermic needle or catheter. Standard monitoring for IV moderate sedation includes noninvasive automatic blood pressure readings, EKG interpretation, pulse oximeter, end-tidal carbon dioxide, and a pretracheal stethoscope. The physical monitor can be covered with clear plastic if it remains visible to the provider. The cables may be covered with a disposable plastic sheath if at risk for accumulation of droplets. Areas that are in contact or proximity to the patient should be disinfected with appropriate solutions as previously mentioned. The end-tidal carbon dioxide monitor poses a risk of transfer of aerosol back to the sensor at the monitor as the mechanism for gas analysis involves a small vacuum pump of expired gas. Choices of infection management include using a pretracheal stethoscope in place of an ETCO2 monitor, using an inline filter for CO2 similar to that used in an IV line or using a disposable water trap or one with a built-in filter. Regardless, always change the inline ETCO2 tubing between patients.

When considering anesthesia recordkeeping, paper generally has no infected material after 3 hours [13]. Electronic records are ideal, with integrated system to monitors or on an iPad. One may take a photo or scan paper record and upload to the electronic record.

General anesthesia and deep sedation techniques are usually warranted for those who cannot cooperate for a dental procedure such as small children or patients with special needs, or as dictated by the invasiveness of the procedure. Deep sedation and general anesthesia (DS/GA) are more likely to include airway obstruction, instrumentation of the airway with a nasal airway, oral airway, or endotracheal tube (ETT) and require positive pressure ventilation. There are therefore many more considerations for protection from aerosolized droplets from the nasal airway, oral airway, and lungs. There is also a higher likelihood of coughing, crying, vomiting, sneezing, deep suctioning, or airway obstruction requiring positive pressure ventilation with a bag valve mask (BVM) or anesthesia machine. It is important to note that the BVM and anesthesia machine should be outfitted with a viral filter as previously mentioned, attached between the mask and disposable anesthesia circuits.

Consider using the same operating area for a preop exam and recovery and treatment.

If the patient will allow an IV line to administer medications, that is ideal. If the patient will not allow an IV line due to behavior, consider an intramuscular (IM) injection for initiation of DS/GA over a mask induction which may increase exhalation of viral particles. Postoperatively consider using a simple face mask with oxygen delivery to protect against aerosolized droplets from coughing or crying. An endotracheal tube provides the most secure airway and least amount of aerosolization from the lungs during the procedure [14]. General anesthesia is mostly provided in hospitals but is increasingly available in dental offices by a dentist anesthesiologist or physician anesthesiologist. The unique risks of spreading aerosolized particles are due to the previously mentioned criteria as well as the insertion of the ETT and the extremely close proximity of the anesthesiologist to accomplish this task. Consider a N95 or powered air-purifying respirators (PAPR) for patients that are at high risk for COVID. Passively preoxygenate the patient prior to inducing general anesthesia with a non-rebreather face mask at 10 liters per minute for an adult, and try to avoid positive pressure ventilation [14]. One may also use a spontaneous breathing technique with an anesthesia full face mask. When using a laryngoscope, use double gloves, and remove one pair after intubation prior to touching the patient. Consider video laryngoscopes which allow an increased distance of the anesthesiologist from the airway. Considerations of monitoring, IV fluids, recordkeeping, and specific guidelines for an ETCO2 monitor or gas analyzer are the same as previously mentioned under IV moderate sedation.

Always use disposables where possible, including laryngoscope blades, tubing, masks, bags, and filters. Always use single versus multidose vials. Discard all opened syringes at end of case even if not used.

14.7 Conclusions

Many patients are unable to tolerate routine dental care without the use of sedation or general anesthesia. Airway maintenance is essential to deliver sedation safely requiring clinicians administering sedation/general anesthesia to have close contact with the patient's respiratory tract, often for extended periods of time. Thus, it is paramount that recommended infection control guidelines for cleaning and disinfection of devices, masks, tubing, etc. used in delivery of sedation/general anesthesia, as reviewed in this chapter, be implemented and practiced for every patient contact. This maximizes the safety of both the patients and clinicians during the delivery of these services. Emerging respiratory infections such as COVID-19 and influenza have brought the importance of infection control in this arena to the forefront, and these or newly emerging infections will persist for the foreseeable future.

References

1. The American Society of Heating, Refrigerating and Air-Conditioning Engineers (ASHRAE). Ventilation for acceptable indoor air quality, ANSI/ASHRAE Addendum ad to ANSI/ASHRAE Standard 62-2001. 3 Jul 2003. https://www.ashrae.org/File%20Library/Technical%20Resources/Standards%20and%20Guidelines/Standards%20Addenda/62-2001/62-2001_Addendum-n.pdf
2. Vonci N, et al. Association between air changes and airborne microbial contamination in operating rooms. J Infect Public Health. 2019;12(6):827–30. https://doi.org/10.1016/j.jiph.2019.05.010. Epub 2019 May 30. PMID: 31155407
3. Centers for Disease Control and Prevention. Guidelines for environmental infection control in health-care facilities; 2003. Page last reviewed: 22 Jul 2019. https://www.cdc.gov/infectioncontrol/guidelines/environmental/appendix/air.html https://www.asahq.org/about-asa/newsroom/news-releases/2020/04/joint-statement-on-elective-surgery-after-covid-19-pandemic
4. American Society of Anesthesiologists. Joint statement: roadmap for resuming elective surgery after COVID-19 pandemic. 17 Apr 2020. https://www.asahq.org/about-asa/newsroom/news-releases/2020/04/joint-statement-on-elective-surgery-after-covid-19-pandemic
5. Peng WH, Ho PL, Hota SS. Outbreak of a new coronavirus: what anaesthetists should know. Br J Anaesth. 2020;124(5):497e501. https://doi.org/10.1016/j.bja.2020.02.008.
6. RA Medical Services Ltd. Infection control guide to care of inhalation sedation, issue 4, Rev: 01/2020. www.ramedical.com. https://ramedical.com/infection-control-guide-care-inhalation-sedation/
7. Kreuger PK, et al. Cross-contamination via anesthesia equipment? Circulation 84,122. Spring 2009;24(1) https://www.apsf.org/article/cross-contamination-via-anesthesia-equipment/
8. Anesthesia Patient Safety Foundation Newsletter, June 2020.
9. Centers for Disease Control and Prevention. Guidelines for preventing the transmission of Mycobacterium tuberculosis in health care settings, 2005. MMWR Recomm Rep. 2005;54(RR17):1–147.
10. National Patient Safety Agency. The revised healthcare cleaning manual. NRLS-0949-Healthcare-clea-ng-manual-2009-06-v1. www.npsa.nhs.uk/cleaning
11. Anesthesia Associates, Inc. Guidelines for product cleaning and sterilization. San Marcos: DFU, Anesthesia Associates, Inc. https://mainlinemedical.com/wp-content/uploads/2020/07/3-0168-60-Cleaning-and-Sterilization.pdf
12. Loftus RW, Koff MD, Birnbach DJ. The dynamics and implications of bacterial transmission events arising from the anesthesia work area. Anesth Analg. 2015;120(4):853–60. https://doi.org/10.1213/ANE.0000000000000505.
13. American Society of Dentist Anesthesiologists. Interim guidance for dentist anesthesiologists practicing in the office-based setting during the COVID-19 pandemic. Last updated 5 May 2020. https://www.asda.org/wp-content/uploads/2020/05/1_Guidance-ASDA-5.7.20_0.pdf
14. American Society of Dentist Anesthesiologists. Addendum to interim guidance during the COVID-19 return to patient care, 8 May 2020. https://www.asda.org/wp-content/uploads/2020/05/2_Return-to-Patient-Care-5.8.20.pdf

Summary of Infection Control in the Dental Office in the Era of COVID-19

15

Louis G. DePaola, Robert Windsor, and Nisha Ganesh

15.1 Introduction

In the last 50 years, numerous infectious diseases challenged the delivery of oral healthcare. In the 1980s–1990s, the emergence of HIV/AIDS mandated significant changes in infection control practices to ensure safe treatment of patients in the dental office. In 2003, the respiratory infection severe acute respiratory syndrome (SARS) caused by a novel coronavirus rapidly circumnavigated the globe. Fortunately, through effective public health initiatives and infection control protocols, this pandemic was stunted, resulting in hundreds of deaths, instead of thousands. However, SARS clearly illustrated the potential for respiratory pathogens to both spread very rapidly in the modern world and cause considerable morbidity and mortality. In 2009, another respiratory infection caused by influenza A H1N1 (swine flu) triggered a global pandemic. Fortunately, a safe and effective vaccine was developed and deployed very rapidly, significantly reducing the potential morbidity and mortality resulting from this pandemic. Thus, in a 10-year period of time, two respiratory pathogens caused a worldwide pandemic. Despite this, the world did little to prepare for future pandemics.

L. G. DePaola (✉)
Department of Oncology and Diagnostic Sciences, The University of Maryland School of Dentistry, Baltimore, MD, USA
e-mail: ldepaola@umaryland.edu

R. Windsor · N. Ganesh
Department of Comprehensive Dentistry, The University of Maryland School of Dentistry, Baltimore, MD, USA
e-mail: rwindsor@umaryland.edu; nganesh@umaryland.edu

L. DePaola et al. (eds.), *Infection Control in the Dental Office in the Era of COVID-19*, https://doi.org/10.1007/978-3-031-64611-9_15

15.2 COVID-19: SARS-CoV-2 Virus

On December 31, 2019, a pneumonia of unknown cause was detected in Wuhan, China. The Wuhan Municipal Health Commission China first reported to the WHO [1]. By March 11, 2020, this infection named COVID-19 was declared a pandemic [1]. This disease has the distinction of having had the most dramatic effect on healthcare, inclusive of dentistry, in history. Over 770 million people have been infected and almost seven million have died [2]. SARS-CoV-2 is not ending! It is changing and evolving and mutates very rapidly creating new variants, many of which are more transmissible than previously circulating variants. Therefore, there will be new variants and new COVID-19 infections for the foreseeable future!

15.3 Emergence of Zoonotic Infections

What are zoonotic diseases? They are defined as those diseases and infections naturally transmitted between people and animals. When people and animals interact in close proximity, animal diseases jump species in a process called "spillover"—resulting in human infections. The WHO estimates that, globally, about one billion cases of illness and millions of deaths occur every year from zoonotic infections [3]. Examples of these diseases include HIV, multiple influenza viruses, SARS, Zika, Ebola, West Nile, dengue, and most recently monkeypox, and SARS-CoV-2. Each of these is capable of mutating to a different and/or more transmissible or pathogenic infection. Collectively, this group of pathogens represents a major cause of global morbidity and mortality from infectious diseases. Zoonotic diseases are the most probable source of new global pandemics.

15.4 Will There Be Another Pandemic?

While nothing is absolute, it is almost certain that the world will be confronted by more pandemics. Will it be as bad as COVID-19? Will it be worse? These questions cannot be answered definitively. However, existing conditions favor emergence of another pandemic(s). Ecological changes like "global warming" have disrupted weather patterns and caused displacement of people and animals. International travel allows an infectious agent to circumnavigate the globe in hours rather than days or months. Microorganisms change and adapt creating the potential for new infections. There are demographic and/or behavior changes in populations throughout the world. Global conflicts displace large numbers of people which often cluster in large numbers. Breakdown of public health measures often is associated with this displacement. Clustering creates an ideal environment for the transmission infectious disease(s) [4].

Finally, the re-emergence of vaccine-preventable diseases has opened the door for spread of infections such as measles and polio that were once very uncommon in most of the world. Over the last several years, there has been a significant increase in cases of measles. Thirty-seven countries report outbreaks of measles, which represents a 68% increase from 2021, when 22 countries were reporting large outbreaks. Four regions with the largest outbreaks are in Africa or the Eastern Mediterranean, but many countries worldwide are struggling with increased cases of measles. The global effort to combat vaccine-preventable diseases has struggled to recover in the wake of the COVID-19 pandemic. Using measles as an illustration, just 81% of people worldwide are now estimated to have received the first dose of a measles vaccine, down from 86% in 2019. In low-income countries, vaccination coverage has plummeted from 71% in 2019 to 66% in 2022. Vaccine availability, resistance to be vaccinated, and vaccine safety disinformation, especially in the wake of COVID-19, have all contributed to the resurgence of measles as well as other vaccine-preventable diseases contributing to an increase needless in morbidity and mortality [5].

15.5 How Do Dental Practitioners Deal With This Situation?

The chapters in this publication provide an excellent guide for dental practitioners to follow to establish and maintain a safe environment to practice dentistry. Too often, infection control is not in the forefront of clinician's minds. This must change, and adherence to the principles of infection control as presented in Chaps. 1, 2, 3, 4, 5, 6, 7, 8, 9, 10, 11, 12, 13 and 14 should be of paramount importance in every dental practice. Remember, the next pandemic could be just around the corner.

References

1. World Health Organization. WHO timeline—COVID-19. https://www.who.int/news/item/27-04-2020-who-timeline%2D%2D-covid-19
2. World Health Organization. Coronavirus dashboard. https://covid19.who.int/
3. World Health Organization. Zoonotic disease: emerging public health threats in the region. https://www.emro.who.int/about-who/rc61/zoonotic-diseases.html
4. Morse S. Factors in the emergence of infectious diseases. Emerg Infect Dis. 1995;1(1):7–15. https://doi.org/10.3201/eid0101.950102. https://pubmed.ncbi.nlm.nih.gov/8903148/
5. Centers for Disease Control and Prevention. Progress toward measles elimination—worldwide, 2000–2022. MMWR Morb Mortal Wkly Rep. 2023;72(46):1262–8. https://www.cdc.gov/mmwr/volumes/72/wr/mm7246a3.htm?s_cid=mm7246a3_w

GPSR Compliance

The European Union's (EU) General Product Safety Regulation (GPSR) is a set of rules that requires consumer products to be safe and our obligations to ensure this.

If you have any concerns about our products, you can contact us on ProductSafety@springernature.com

In case Publisher is established outside the EU, the EU authorized representative is:

Springer Nature Customer Service Center GmbH
Europaplatz 3
69115 Heidelberg, Germany

Batch number: 10732044

Printed by Printforce, the Netherlands